Alcoholism
Analysis of a World-Wide Problem

Alcoholism
Analysis of a World-Wide Problem

Edited by
P. Golding
Medical Director, Broadway Lodge
Weston-super-Mare
England

Proceedings of the ALC 82 International
Conference held in Oxford, England,
30 March – 4 April 1982

MTP PRESS LIMITED · LANCASTER · BOSTON · THE HAGUE
International Medical Publishers

Published in the UK and Europe by
MTP Press Limited
Falcon House
Lancaster, England

British Library Cataloguing in Publication Data

Alcoholism.
  1. Alcoholism—Congresses
  I. Golding, P.
  362.2'92   HV5009

  ISBN 0-85200-713-2

Published in the USA by
MTP Press
A division of Kluwer Boston Inc
190 Old Derby Street
Hingham, MA 02043, USA

Library of Congress Cataloging in Publication Data

ALC 82 International Conference (1982 : Oxford,
  Oxfordshire)
  Alcoholism, analysis of a world-wide problem.

  Includes bibliographical references and index.
  1. Alcoholism—Congresses. I. Golding, P.,
1932– . II. Title. [DNLM: 1. Alcoholism—Con-
gresses. 2. Alcoholism—Therapy—Congresses. WM 274
A3544 1982]
RC565.A34 1982   362.2'92   83-14893
ISBN-13: 978-94-009-6609-3   e-ISBN-13: 978-94-009-6607-9
DOI: 10.1007/978-94-009-6607-9
Copyright © 1983 MTP Press Limited
Softcover reprint of the hardcover 1st edition 1983

Typeset by Macmillan India Ltd., Bangalore.

Contents

List of Contributors

S. AHLSTROM
Social Research Institute of Alcohol
  Studies
Kalevankatu 12, 00100 Helsinki 10
Finland

D. ALLEN
Lord Aberdare House
27 Church Road
Whitchurch, Cardiff CF4 2DX, UK

D. ANDERSON
Hazelden Foundation
Box 11,
Center City,
Minnesota 55012, USA

T. ARNGRIM
Aasumvej 337, DK 5240
Odense NØ, Denmark

T. ASUNI
UN Social Def Research Institute
Via Giulia 52, Rome 00186
Italy

H. BAR
Israel Institute of Applied Social Research
Hebrew University
Jerusalem, Israel

R. BAUMAL
Department of Alcoholism Treatment
  Services, 10, Yad Harutzim Street
Talpiot, PO Box 1260
Jerusalem 91000
Israel

C. BLACK
PO Box 8536
Newport Beach
CA 92660, USA

H. BRAMMER
Maschstrasse 18,
2840 Diepholz 1
West Germany

Cdr. G. A. BUNN
Naval Alcohol Rehabilitation Center
Naval Station, Box 80
San Diego, CA 92136, USA

M. CAMERON
District Hospital
Yeovil, Somerset, UK

Rev. K. CAMPBELL
The Parsonage II
3701 E. Monterose #2
Phoenix, Arizona 85018, USA

K. A. CAREY-SMITH
Taranaki Alcohol and Drug Dependence
  Unit, Stratford Hospital
New Zealand

A. B. CECCONI
645 SO Central
Chicago, Ill 60644, USA

J. CLARNO
Parkside Medical Services
1580 N. Northwest Highway
Park Ridge, Illinois 60068, USA

E. COLEMAN
Program in Human Sexuality
2630 University Ave SE
Minneapolis MN 55414, USA

M. CORBIN
333 Colebrook Drive
Rochester, NY 14617, USA

Rev. W. COX
14 Walnut Close
Axbridge, Somerset
BS26 2DT, UK

S. B. CROOS
Alcoholism Information Service
15 Lauries Lane, Colombo 4
Sri Lanka

E. CUTLAND
Broadway Lodge
Oldmixon Road
Weston-super-Mare, Avon
BS24 9NN, UK

M. DAVIES
Centre Revilliod,
5 Route des Acacias
1227 Geneva, Switzerland

M. DIDIER C
Catholic University of Chile
Vicuna Mackenna, 4860 Lo Florida
Santiago, Chile

Rev. J. R. DOLLARD
Belmont Abbey Monastery
Belmont, N Carolina 28012, USA

J. ERWIN
Foothill Family Counseling Center
21297 Foothill Boulevard, Suite #100
Hayward, CA 94541, USA

S. EVANS
2400 Blaisdell Avenue
Minneapolis, MN 55404, USA

J. A. EWING
Center for Alcohol Studies and Depart-
ment of Psychiatry
University of N Carolina
Medical School Building 207H,
Chapel Hill, NC 27514 USA

K. FRUENSGAARD
Department of Psychiatry
Odense University Hospital
5000 Odense C, Denmark

A. GELLER
Smithers Center
474 First Street
Brooklyn 11215 NY, USA

S. GITLOW
1136 5th Avenue
New York, NY 10029, USA

M. GLATT
16 Southbourne Crescent
London NW4 2JY, UK

P. GOLDING
Broadway Lodge, Oldmixon Road
Weston-super-Mare, Avon BS24 9NN,
UK

M. GRANT
Alcohol Education Centre
Maudsley Hospital, 99 Denmark Hill
London SE5 8AZ, UK

J. C. GROVE
Olchfa School, Swansea
South Wales, UK

B. HORE
Withington Hospital
West Didsbury
Manchester M20 8LR, UK

V. HUDOLIN
University Department for Neurology,
Psychiatry, Alcohol and Other
Dependencies,
'Dr M. Stojanović' University Hospital
Vinogradska c.29
41000 Zagreb, Yugoslavia

J. J. HUNTER
Psychology Department
San Francisco State University
San Francisco
California, USA

M. KEEN
Whitchurch Hospital
Cardiff CF4 7XB, UK

Rev. R. LESLIE
Hazelden Foundation, Box 11
Center City MN 55012, USA

V. G. LOKARE
Department of Clinical Psychology
West Park Hospital
Horton Lane, Epsom,
Surrey, KT19 8PB, UK

Sisir K. MAJUMDAR
Elmdene Alcoholic Treatment and Re-
search Unit
Bexley Hospital, Kent DA5 2BW, UK

D. MARJOT
St Bernard's Hospital
Southall, Middlesex, UK

W. MALONEY
The Hazelden Foundation
Box 11, Center City
Minnesota 55012, USA

D. MASI
Department of Health and Human
Services, 412 Watergate E
2510 Virginia Ave NW
Washington DC 20037 USA

T. S. McDADE
Department of Applied Science
College of Technology
College Square East
Belfast, N. Ireland, UK

J. MEDDINGS
Henwood AADAC Box 100
RR1 Edmonton
Alberta, Canada

M. MINIEVIC
Centre for Family Therapy of
Alcoholism, Palmoticeva 37
11000 Beograd, Yugoslavia

P. O'GORMAN
Greenwich District Hospital
London, UK

J. PIPER
Outreach Alcoholism Treatment Center
Scripps Memorial Hospital
9888 Genesee Avenue
Box 28, La Jolla, CA 92038, USA

M. QUINLAN
36 Tirconnell Avenue
Lismore Lawn, Waterford
Ireland

S. RANGANATHAN
TT Ranganathan Clinical Research
Foundation
6 Cathedral Road
Madras 600, 086
India

B. RITSON
University Department of Psychiatry
Royal Edinburgh Hospital
Morningside Park
Edinburgh EH10 5HF
UK

M. de ROUMANIE
Department of Psychiatry
Edinburgh University
Edinburgh, UK

S. SCHAEFER
3238 15th Ave S
Minneapolis 55404, USA

K. SCHMIDT
Yeovil District Hospital
Yeovil, Somerset
UK

R. SCHNEIDER
Institut fur Therapieforschung
Parzivalstrasse 25
D-8000 Munchen 40
West Germany

G. K. SHAW
Elmdene Alcoholic Treatment and Re-
  search Unit
Bexley Hospital
Bexley, Kent, UK

M. STERNE
Chrysalis, a Center for Women
2104 Stevens Ave So
Minneapolis, MN 55404, USA

L. TEEMS
Employee Counselling Services Specialist
US Department of Health and Human
  Services

Allan D. THOMSON
British Journal of Alcohol and
  Alcoholism
140 Harley Street
London W1N 1AH, UK

H.-G. TITTMAR
School of Psychology
Ulster Polytechnic
Newtownabbey
BT37 OQB, UK

Canon L. VIRGO
The Rectory
Skibbs Lane
Chelsfield, Kent, UK

H. VOLLMER
I F T
Parzivalstrasse 25
8000 Munchen 40
West Germany

M. WETHERHORN
1565 South Bragaw
Suite 201
Anchorage
Alaska 99504, USA

W. D. WYSS
Program Director, EAP
University of Minnesota
319 15th Ave SE
Room 307 Minneapolis
Minnesota 55455, USA

H. ZIEGLER
D H S Postbox 1369
Westring 2, 4700 Hamm 1
West Germany

Part 1:
ALCOHOLISM – A WORLD-WIDE PROBLEM

1

Alcoholism treatment in the United Kingdom

B. D. HORE

ACTOR   I've drunk my soul away old one . . .

LUKA   They can cure you of drunkenness now you know, . . .
There's a sort of clinic been built for drunkards, to cure
them you know for free.
They've allowed that a drunk is a human soul, same as
anyone else and they are actually pleased if he
wants to get himself cured . . .

From *The Lower Depths* (Act 2) by Maxim Gorky (first performance 1902).

It is the aim of this review to examine the development of specialized alcoholism treatment services in the United Kingdom in the past 30 years, and to relate this to both governmental and non-governmental influences. Further, it examines inherent problems and suggested responses to the current treatment situation. In descriptive terms, it is perhaps simplest to examine the situation historically.

As in many countries, the first agency of any impact was *Alcoholics Anonymous*, beginning in the late 1940s and steadily growing thereafter, although its geographical spread has been variable. Equivalent self-help groups for the spouse (Alanon) and teenage relatives (Alateen) followed, although the latter have never developed to the same degree as Alcoholics Anonymous. Examination of Alcoholics Anonymous in the United Kingdom has been described by Edwards *et al.*[1] and most comprehensively by Robinson[2]. Alcoholics Anonymous has remained strictly autonomous in the United Kingdom, and links between it and other professions, including the medical profession, do not seem to have been so close as in the United States of America. The role of Alcoholics Anonymous does not seem sufficiently well known to alcoholism professionals, and indeed, rarely features in Summer Schools on Alcoholism.

Following Alcoholics Anonymous in 1951, there was the development of *Alcoholism Treatment Units* (pioneered by Dr Glatt at Warlingham Park Hospital) on a national scale by the government under the National Health Service (private units, until recently, largely did not exist). The original function of such units included being 'a referral sink', provision of specialized treatment techniques (largely unavailable elsewhere) and that of research. Impetus for the development of such units appears to have come from the United States, a prime concept being the benefits likely to result from alcoholics being placed together rather than scattered around mental hospitals. A sample of patients attending Alcoholism Treatment Units was examined by Hore and Smith[3]. Apart from shifts in treatment patterns, e.g. towards more outpatient day care, more emphasis on individual treatment and a reduction of length of intensive programmes, there are fundamental questions being asked regarding the role of such units. They have been criticized for accepting only socially stable cases, reinforcing the disease concept of alcoholism (much under attack by sociologists and psychologists in the United Kingdom) and being irrelevant in terms of numbers of alcoholics requiring treatment. No more units of this type are planned by the government, although (perhaps cause and effect) there has been an increase in private units. It has been suggested that current functions of such units include research, treating patients who are particularly difficult to handle, who could not be dealt with by other agencies, and the education of primary care agencies.

The development of a governmental initiative in 1973, published as *Community Services for Alcoholics*, reinforced the development of two community agencies. These were the *therapeutic rehabilitation hostel* (with abstinence as a treatment goal), and *community based clinics*, working under the aegis of local Councils on Alcoholism. A dilemma of the hostel movement has been the degree to which the hostels are in the 'shelter' business or in the 'change' business. An examination of hostels has come from Otto and Orford[4]. An encouraging report on outcome has come from Edwards[5] who, in an admittedly small sample, found a great improvement in social functioning, and drinking behaviour, several years after entering such hostels.

The majority of such hostels have been provided by voluntary bodies, e.g. Turning Point, 9–12 Long Lane, London, EC1A 9HA, with active notable exceptions, e.g. Manchester, where the Social Services Department of the city provides its own therapeutic hostel and supporting groups (minimum support homes). Such hostels, as described above, have been seen either as a development of aftercare, following treatment e.g. in an Alcoholism Treatment Unit, or, less frequently, a detoxification centre or for patients coming directly from the community. Development of such hostels by voluntary bodies has virtually ceased, due to absence of central government funding and an unwillingness of local government to take on the financial burden. Indeed, there is a danger that some hostels will close.

Councils on Alcoholism developed following examples in the USA and have had, as one of their functions, the development of community-based *low cost* counselling services. Originally, this was largely in terms of information and referral, but more recently such centres have taken on a range of direct counselling services on a walk-in policy. There is evidence (Delahaye[6]) that clients attend here earlier than at other agencies, e.g. Alcoholism Treatment Units and Alcoholics Anonymous. A recent addition has been the use of voluntary counsellors, i.e. lay people (some alcoholic, some not) who in a manner akin to marriage guidance counsellors undertake counselling of the alcoholic or problem drinker after a relatively brief training. The effectiveness of such counselling remains to be established and doubts have been expressed regarding whether adequate professional *support* is always available to such counsellors. It should be realized, however, that such counsellors are often dealing with early cases of alcohol dependence.

Industrial alcoholism programmes (Hore and Plant[7]), with a few notable exceptions, have never gained the popularity of those in the USA. This may reflect a different view of industry in providing treatment for employees under a governmental health service, compared to the situation in the USA. Also, largely absent are special voluntary agencies for women alcoholics, akin to Women for Sobriety.

Detoxification centres have been a very late development in Britain, particularly in relation to the drunken offender (although discussed for over a century). Two such centres have been recently set up, community-based (Leeds) and hospital-based (Manchester) (Hore[8]). The essential aim has been to offer the police an alternative to the 'revolving door' of drunken arrests etc., and to assess patient/client needs and, where appropriate, refer to alcoholism treatment agencies. In Manchester, the centre has recently widened its referral net to include hospital accident/emergency departments and general practitioners' own referrals. From 1977 to 1980 the centre dealt primarily with police referrals.

Redmond[9] examined 235 police referrals in relationship to medical morbidity. Few patients were in need of any emergency medical care at time of admission. Many patients had chronic diseases including bronchitis and ischaemic heart disease. Fifty per cent of patients had liver disease but this was rarely serious. Infestation and T. B. were problems and put staff at risk, as the prevalence of T. B. was significantly higher than in the general population. Very high blood alcohol levels were recorded *without* any concomitant depression of level of consciousness. C. Rossall (personal communication) using the quantitative schedules of Gross et al.[10], found that only 15 % of such patients (primarily a vagrant group of police referrals) had a severe withdrawal syndrome. One factor relating to the degree of severity of the syndrome was length of the immediate pre-withdrawal drinking bout. Makanjoula[11] carried out an intensive follow-up study on the 235 police referrals already mentioned. Patients were randomly divided into an 'intensive' group (given extra support and after-care) and a 'routine' group. Fifty-two per cent of the patients discharged themselves against advice. Of the remaining 48 %, approximately one quarter were referred on to specialized alcoholism agencies. Only 27 % of the patients achieved 3 or more months of voluntary abstinence, and 8.5 % were abstinent for 1 year. However, in terms of social function, there was considerable improvement. Approximately half the patients lived at a settled address, and in general patients' use of general practitioners and casualty departments fell after detoxification dramatically, compared with the pre-detoxification years. A similar fall was seen in hospital admissions. This would suggest the work of the detoxification centre has an important role in reducing the load on general practitioners and casualty and hospital inpatient facilities. Makanjoula found that the intensity of treatment affected outcome, the 'intensive' group showed greater improvement in social and drinking variables.

TREATMENT GOALS

The majority of specialized agencies still recommend abstinence, at least for an initial period, as a treatment goal, particularly in patients physically damaged or suffering from withdrawal symptoms. With less severe cases patterns of controlled drinking may be attempted in both hospital and community clinic.

ROLE OF SPECIALIZED AGENCIES IN THE FUTURE

The Kessel Committee[1 2] recommended that the bulk of treatment had to be carried out by primary care workers − e.g. generic social workers, family physicians − and that services should be locally based. Whether primary care workers have the inclination, *time*, interest and training to deal with such patients remains to be seen. The idea of local multidisciplinary teams (community alcohol teams) to initiate services has been proposed. There thus appears to have been a *devaluation* of specialized services, or at the very least a major change of role. At present however, these radical changes appear to have made little imprint certainly on the demand placed on specialized services already outlined. A more logical approach would seem to be the retention of such specialized services, at least until it can be shown that primary care workers can carry the burden of such cases and, even then, for the more severe case a wide range of specialized services may be required. There is a grave danger that the service provision will fall between the two schools − i.e. a reduction in specialized services not being accompanied by an interest in and take-up of cases by primary care workers. There seems a real danger that alcoholism could become, once again, the forgotten disease.

References

1 Edwards, G., Hensman, C., Hawker, A. and Williamson, V. (1967). Alcoholics Anonymous, anatomy of a self help group. *Soc. Psychiatry*, **1**, 195
2 Robinson, D. (1979). *Talking Out of Alcoholism.* (London: Croom Helm)
3 Hore, B. D. and Smith, E. (1975). Who goes to Alcoholism Treatment Units. *Br. J. Addiction*, **70**, 263

4 Otto, S. and Orford, J. (1978). *Not quite Like Home*. (Chichester: Wiley)
5 Edwards, D. Personal communication. Papers available from Turning Point, 9–12 Long Lane, London, EC1 9HA
6 Delahaye, S. (1977). An analysis of clients using alcoholic agencies within one community service. In Madden, J. S., Walker, R. C. and Kenyon, W. (eds.) *Alcoholism and Drug Dependence – A Multi-Disciplinary Approach*. (London: Plenum Press)
7 Hore, B. D. and Plant, M. A. (1981). *Alcohol Problems in Employment*. (London: Croom Helm)
8 Hore, B. D. (1980). The Manchester Detoxification Centre. *Br. J. Addiction*, **75**, 197
9 Redmond, A. D. (1979). The study of the medical morbidity of chronic drunken offenders at the time of their admission to Britain's first hospital purpose built detoxification centre. *MD Thesis*, Victoria University of Manchester
10 Gross, M., Lewis, E. and Nagaranjan, M. (1973). An improved quantative system for measuring the acute alcoholic psychosis and related states (TSA and SSA). In Gross, M. M. (ed.) *Alcohol Intoxication and Withdrawal – Experimental Studies (Adv. Exp. Med. Biol.,* **35**) (New York: Plenum Press)
11 Makanjoula, J. (1981). A study of police referrals to the Manchester detoxification centre. *PhD Thesis*, Victoria University of Manchester
12 Kessel Committee (1978). *The Pattern and Range of Services for Problem Drinkers*. (London: HMSO)

2
Alcoholism management in New Zealand

K. A. CAREY-SMITH

INTRODUCTION

New Zealand, with 3 million people in an area not much larger than the UK, is now adequately served with a wide variety of organizations and facilities catering for alcoholism, though many are in their infancy[1] (Table 2.1).

The country is well up in the international stakes of high alcohol consumers, with about 9 litres absolute alcohol consumed annually per person (Table 2.2). Heavy beer consumption is customary at social and sports functions, often from early teenage years, and in recent years wine consumption has increased dramatically (seven times in 25 years)[2]. Public bars are still largely drinking barns with standing room only, and with very little of the civilized socializing by both sexes seen in the British pub. There are hundreds of alcohol related road fatalities annually.

Table 2.1 Treatment facilities for alcoholism in New Zealand (total inpatient beds available: approximately 800)

State funded (Hospital based)	State subsidised or voluntary
8 units for inpatients (many having O/P facilities also) = 70 beds	AA: almost 200 groups Alanon & Alateen
5 units for outpatients only	Salvation Army: full range of facilities in 3 main centres = 200 beds
2 long-stay treatment units = 150 beds	Other churches & voluntary agencies (12 hostels) = approx 200 beds
3 psychiatric hospitals with special alcoholism facilities = 100 beds	NSAD: 6 centres (casework etc); 1 hostel = 11 beds.

9

Table 2.2   Estimated consumption of alcohol in New Zealand (litres of absolute alcohol per head of mean population)

Year	Beer	Wine	Spirits	Total
1955	3.96	0.27	1.22	5.45
1965	4.16	0.45	1.22	5.83
1975	5.05	1.23	1.76	8.05
1981	4.87	2.02	1.97	8.86

(Source: NZ Department of Statistics)

A recent report[3] summarizes some of the New Zealander's drinking habits. Information was obtained by interviewing 10 000 people, and some of the findings are as follows:

(1)   9 % of adults were classed as 'heavy' drinkers (over 60 ml absolute alcohol per day). These drink almost two thirds of the total alcohol consumed.

(2)   14 % of males, but only 8 % of women, were 'heavy' drinkers.

(3)   Younger men, and the unskilled/semiskilled, drink larger amounts, but less frequently.

(4)   Managerial/professional people, and well-educated women, have a higher 'drinking intensity', but heavy drinkers are evenly spread through all occupational groups.

(5)   Maori and Pacific Islanders drink more on each occasion, but less frequently, than 'Europeans'; but more Maori/Island women abstain than European women.

(6)   50 % of male 'heavy' drinkers drink mainly beer.

(7)   20 % of male 'heavy' drinkers are unhappy about their intake, and half have wanted to cut down at some stage.

MANAGEMENT OPTIONS IN TARANAKI

Our unit, the Taranaki Alcohol & Drug Dependence Unit, has no shortage of 'customers', especially as our policy is to search out early cases (in the belief that this will reduce our work later), and cover the fields of 'problem' and 'hazardous' drinking, as well as other chemical dependencies.

Our local provincial services are described in order to illustrate current trends in management of alcoholism in New Zealand.

Up to 3 years ago no agencies to help alcoholics existed in Taranaki province (population about 100 000) apart from four or five Alcoholics

Anonymous groups. For a general practitioner in a small country town, there was little help available, even if one *did* detect an alcoholic amongst one's patients. Today the majority can be managed within the province with a variety of facilities.

1. General practice management

I personally consider that a family doctor, even if well informed, is not the ideal person to manage an alcoholic's recovery. Nor am I in favour of home detoxication if inpatient facilities are available locally. General practitioners have little training, even less time, and an inadequate support team. Early and well-motivated 'hazardous drinkers' can, however, often be managed by the GP with strongly worded medical warnings and supportive follow-up, and many of us *have* to cope if local facilities are inadequate. The main function of the GP is in *case-finding*: a good GP with a little tuition and a high index of suspicion should be unearthing between five and ten new cases a year. We keep our GPs informed about how they measure up, comparing referral figures from different areas (Table 2.3) and if the treatment unit is accessible, encouraging, and communicative, the local doctors gradually increase their referral rate. General practice training schemes need a higher input of practical knowledge and experience in the field.

Table 2.3 General practitioner referrals to Taranaki unit*

| | | | | No. of GPs referring | |
Area	No. of GPs	Total patients referred	Nil	1—4 patients	5 or more patients
New Plymouth (city)	21	23	12	8	1
Hawera/Kaponga	7	24	1	4	2
Stratford/Eltham	8	58	0	4	4
Other areas (rural)	12	18	4	8	0

* Approximately, 2½ year period; unit is sited in Stratford

Having uncovered a possible alcoholic, the GP's task is to confront and refer appropriately, and then work with the local team in a supportive role. (AA members known to the doctor can often be very helpful.) If there are no local facilities, the GP should be active in supporting the establishment of a service[4].

The following sections summarize referral options now available.

2. Alcoholics Anonymous

AA (and Alanon) is strong in cities and larger towns, but very patchy in country areas. Our town group had only two or three regular members until the advent of our hospital unit. Now two groups (between eight and 12 members each) provide an essential part of the management plan for most alcoholics we treat.

3. General hospital management

Our local hospital alcoholism unit is typical of several in other provincial centres in New Zealand. Three years ago hospital detoxication units were supported (on paper) by the Health Authorities, but only established with difficulty. The Taranaki Unit was set up in the town of Stratford (population 6000), 30 miles (48 km) from the main centre of population, because of a number of coinciding factors, including local community pressure, support from the medical profession (one of whom volunteered to act as Medical Officer), local political support, available beds and facilities in the local hospital, and encouragement, financial and staffing assistance from the National Society of Alcoholism & Drug Dependence (NSAD — see below). Areas are given a free rein to develop their own provincial service, only limited by finance, thus resulting in much variation and innovation.

Our Unit has six beds (part of the ordinary medical/surgical ward) for initial detoxication and an intensive 1 – 2 week assessment programme (Table 2.4). Staff consists of one full-time director/therapist (who also administers the Unit and manages follow-up, outpatients and educational activities), myself (part-time), a secretary and a 'field officer' stationed in the city 35 miles (56 km) away. The existing hospital staff (nurses, physiotherapist, occupational therapist and others) cover the remainder of the programme. At the end of the assessment period, a future management plan is worked out with the 'patient'.

To summarize, the Unit has these characteristics:

(1)   General-hospital based, with no psychiatric content.

(2)   Small, low budget, utilizing existing facilities and staff.

(3)   Commenced from scratch, and thus able to develop without conflict with other facilities.

(4)   Covering a wide field: 'hazardous' and early problem drinkers, case finding and education, inpatient and outpatient management, follow-up and aftercare, and other 'chemical dependencies'.

(5)   Accepts referrals from a wide variety of sources (Table 2.5).

The Unit has a simple basic management philosophy (discussed later) and reasonable results (Table 2.6). There is much room for improvement, but we feel the approach we use has several advantages, and better results, than the standard UK facility based in a psychiatric hospital. Some areas not already served by a general hospital Unit in New Zealand are planning one, others have a community-based service usually staffed by NSAD workers, with no inpatient beds.

Table 2.4 Taranaki Alcohol and Drug Dependence Unit – assessment programme for inpatients

	Monday	Tuesday	Wednesday	Thursday	Friday	Sat/Sun
8.00	– – – – – – – Breakfast (also Medication) – – – – – – – – –					
8.30	Patient interviews		Staff meeting	Patient interviews		Ward duties
9.30	– – – – – – – – – – Morning tea – – – – – – – – –					
10.00	– – – Physiotherapy (graded exercise programme) – –					Games
10.30	– – – – – Hydrotherapy (hot pool) – – – – – –					Hobbies
11.00	– – – Relaxation therapy (taped) – – – – – – – –					Visit half-way house
11.30	Occup. therapy tutorial	'After-care' Tutorial	Free	Medical tutorial	Free	
12.30	– – – – – – Lunch (also Medication) – – – – –					Hospitality visits
13.00	– – – – – – Occupational therapy – – – – – –					Visitors
15.00	– – – – – – – – Afternoon tea & visitors – – – – – – – –					
15.30– 16.30	Group therapy		'Higher power' group	Group Therapy		Church service (optional)
17.00	– – – – – – – Evening Meal (also Medication) – – – – – – –					
20.00– 21.30	AA (town) (optional)	Group therapy	AA (compulsory)	Free	Free	Free

Table 2.5 Taranaki Alcohol and Drug Dependence Unit – referral sources (approximate)

Self referred	8 %	Prison	15 %
Family/friends	17 %	Probation	4 %
GPs	20 %	AA/Alanon	5 %
Hospitals: base	9 %	Solicitors/clergy	3 %
psychiatric	4 %	Industry	2 %
other	5 %	Other	10 %

Table 2.6 Progress of patients after 1–2 years

	Inpatients	All referrals
Total number	112	251
Abstinent	48 %	36 %
Improved	20 %	16 %
Relapsed	13 %	16 %
Not known	16 %	30 %
Died	3 %	3 %

4. Voluntary organizations

A number of church groups and other organizations help provide services for alcoholics, especially in custodial care and rehabilitation. Several churches in our area responded to a need and established a residential 15-bed 'halfway house' in the country 2 miles (3 km) from our Unit. The House is independent but works closely with the hospital Unit.

5. Long-stay institutions

A number of alcoholics are referred outside the area to several long-stay institutions.

(1)   Queen Mary Hospital: this 117-bed special hospital (state-financed) runs an effective intensive 2–3 month treatment programme in the South Island of New Zealand.

(2)   Salvation Army: in NZ the Salvation Army has 200 beds, and a variety of other services covering all grades of alcoholics.

(3)   Specialized smaller residential hostels (e.g. for young people).

(4)   Psychiatric hospitals: several have special arrangements for alcoholics, who may go either voluntarily or by order under the Alcoholism and Drug Addiction Act (1966). On application by an appropriate person, plus two medical certificates certifying that the proposed subject of the order is an alcoholic as defined by the Act, a magistrate may order detention and treatment in a 'recognized institution' for up to 2 years (normally the alcoholic is released after a few months but remains under supervision). This Act is rarely used, but often acts as a valuable lever if given as one option when confronting a patient.

6. Other organizations involved in alcoholism management

National organizations actively involved in the field of alcoholism are:

(1)   *National Society on Alcoholism & Drug Dependence (NZ) Inc (1956).* This voluntary body, with offices in six centres, takes referrals and provides treatment and information services for chemical dependency. 250–300 new cases are seen monthly, most of whom are referred on to AA or Queen Mary Hospital. NSAD collaborates with any local initiative and encourages the Health Services to take over established treatment facilities.

(2)   *Alcoholic Liquor Advisory Council* (1976). This statutory body is financed from a levy on all alcohol sold. It advises the government, and encourages 'moderation' through financing of educational, research and treatment projects, and programmes in industry. The Council's annual budget is around $NZ 2 million. Projects include TV educational

campaigns, study grants, informative literature, and financing of new treatment projects.

(3) *NZ Medical Society on Alcohol & Alcoholism.* The NZMSAA is open to doctors with an interest in alcoholism, and runs seminars and other educational activities.

MANAGEMENT PHILOSOPHY

Our Unit programme is based on the simple philosophy now to be outlined. Not all NZ treatment units hold similar views, but the majority agree basically with our approach.

(1) Management is based on AA principles, with full sobriety as the main objective. 'Controlled drinking' is not considered a valid option. Abstinence is set as the ideal and goal for 'hazardous' drinkers as well as for the fully dependent alcoholic.

(2) A 'medical model' is favoured, without forgetting psychological, social, spiritual and family factors. Since time and staffing resources are limited, the alcohol problem is attacked first. If major psychological, medical, social or spiritual problems remain after an adequate 'trial of sobriety', these are then dealt with (if necessary by referral).

(3) The approach to counselling is directive, with use of careful but energetic confrontation techniques, bringing all possible ammunition to bear at vulnerable points in the alcoholic's defences (Figure 2.1).

(4) An intensive initial detoxication and management programme is used in about one third of new cases, as previously described.

(5) A concept of 'chemical dependency' results in a policy of withdrawal

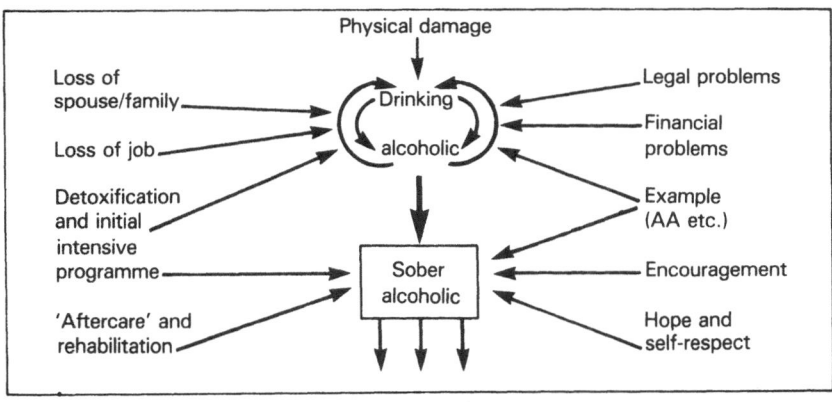

Figure 2.1 'Confronting the alcoholic'

from *all* mind-altering chemicals, apart from a short detoxication regime using chlormethiazole (only in hospital) and occasional use of antidepressants and lithium. No benzodiazapines are used, and a patient in whom alcohol is replaced by a tranquillizer is considered a failure (most are soon drinking again anyway). The use of disulfiram is, however, encouraged.

(6)   Follow-up, aftercare and rehabilitation are carefully planned for and with each alcoholic.

This somewhat rigid and simplistic model is discussed without apology, mainly because it seems to work! No doubt other models also work in the hands of enthusiastic advocates, but each area must adopt an approach to fit in with the staff available to run it. A philosophy that is also held by neighbouring treatment programmes and AA creates much more harmony, with benefit to those we are all trying to help. And I have yet to see hard evidence that the 'model' of alcoholism we use is invalid.

In New Zealand, as in many countries, good alcoholism therapists are rare and therefore their talents are best concentrated first on the patient's alcoholism, rather than floundering around in the bottomless pit of psychosocial factors, personality types and so on. For instance, our Unit, with two therapists, has to manage 250–300 new cases annually (75–100 of these admitted), and still find time for the essential case-finding, public relations and educational work. The approach just described allows all this to be covered, and no one is ever turned away through lack of time.

ALCOHOLISM IN THE MAORI

The Maori's drinking habits have already been briefly mentioned. Maoris have different attitudes to drink, and rarely accept European treatment methods. Problem cases are often heavy 'binge' drinkers ('periodic alcoholics'). 'Professionals' are symbols of 'pakehaism' (the European way of life), communication barriers are significant and many primitive beliefs are still held. The problem will have to be tackled from within the Maori community, and in Taranaki we have made progress because our field officer is a Maori, held in high esteem locally. Support groups for alcoholics and their families have started within the Maori community itself.

CONCLUSION

Although in New Zealand heavy drinking is the 'norm', encouraged by the hotel trade, sports clubs and local tradition, those managing the results are fortunate to have financial support and encouragement from national bodies (ALAC and NSAD), and a reasonably coordinated and growing range of management options, all with similar approaches. The compulsory treatment

Act is sometimes useful (though cumbersome) and there is an increasing awareness in medical and lay circles of the overall chemical dependency problem. The policy of 'separation' from psychiatric institutions I consider to be an additional advantage.

Acknowledgements

The New Zealand Alcoholic Liquor Advisory Council has provided financial assistance and helpful encouragement.

References

1 Alcoholic Liquor Advisory Council (1980). *Directory of Treatment Facilities for Alcoholism in New Zealand.* 2nd Edn. (Wellington: ALAC)
2 *New Zealand Alcohol Related Statistics* (1982). (Wellington: ALAC)
3 Casswell, S. (1980). *Drinking by New Zealanders.* (Wellington: ALAC and Alcohol Research Unit, University of Auckland)
4 Carey-Smith, K. A. (1981). Attacking chemical dependency in a rural general practice. *NZ Family Physician.* **8,** 5

3
Dependencies in the Socialist Republic of Croatia

V. HUDOLIN

INTRODUCTION

Alcoholism, the number one drug dependency in the world, and to some extent other drug dependencies, pose one of the most serious sociomedical problems for contemporary man. It is, therefore, no longer possible today to consider strategies for the control of alcoholism without wide international co-operation. The magnificent plan of the World Health Organization to ensure, by the year 2000, primary health protection for every inhabitant of this planet will not be fulfilled if the problems of dependencies are not attacked through close international co-operation. This meeting should be seen as a major step toward this goal, particularly since in 1982 alcoholism was given priority consideration by the World Health Organization.

BASIC CONCEPTIONS UPON WHICH THE CONTROL OF ALCOHOLISM HAS BEEN ORGANIZED IN SR CROATIA

The subject of this paper is not alcoholism alone, but a review of the extent of this problem and the methods of controlling alcoholism in the Socialist Republic of Croatia, one of the Republics of the Federation of Yugoslavia.

After World War II the medical model approach to alcoholism began to replace the moralistic approach everywhere in the world. In the course of the war, great destruction and devastation had occurred in SR Croatia and all over Yugoslavia. Following the war, health services had to be housed in damaged buildings and the staff was decimated. There was no time to think about alcoholism under these circumstances, especially during the early postwar years. Under the influence of the Russian social school, an expectation prevailed that socialism would automatically solve the majority of social problems, including alcoholism. The private voluntary anti-alcoholic organizations and societies of abstainers which had been active before World War II disappeared in the disaster of war and never recovered completely.

As time passed and the problems of alcoholism seemed to grow worse, and the health service sector was not undertaking any meaningful measures (apart from treating complications – delirium tremens, other psychoses, cirrhosis of the liver), in 1954 the Red Cross Organization took over the programme of combating alcoholism in Yugoslavia, or as it was frequently called at that time the fight against alcoholism. Although the basic function of the Red Cross was prevention, in the beginning dispensaries, consultation and advising stations to help alcoholics and their families were established. Subsequently, the Red Cross passed these institutions on to the health and social service.

The League of the Societies against Alcoholism, a private organization linked with the Socialist League, was established that same year, and served as a social, voluntary organization engaged in the prevention and treatment of alcoholism.

The attention of both these organizations, The Red Cross and the League of the Societies against Alcoholism, was mainly directed at the problem of alcoholism, whereas moderate drinking was accepted as the normal form of behaviour.

This was similar to the way alcoholism and drinking was and still is viewed in all Mediterranean countries.

All these measures, however, did not give serious results either in the prevention of alcoholism or in the treatment and rehabilitation of the alcoholics, since there was no uniform and generally accepted methodology of preventive and therapeutic work.

The Centre for the Study and Prevention of Alcoholism and Other Dependencies was established in Zagreb at that time, i.e. in 1964, and was associated with the Department of Neurology, Psychiatry, Alcoholism and other Dependencies of the Dr M. Stojanović teaching hospital.

A number of investigations, primarily of epidemiological character, were undertaken by the Centre and showed the extent of the problem. Data were thus obtained which came in handy in the elaboration of programmes we deemed necessary to apply in control of alcoholism. The Centre immediately accepted the medical model of approach to alcoholism and was therapeutically oriented at the beginning of its work.

At the very start an inpatient department with 50 beds for the treatment of alcoholics, a day hospital, a partial hospitalization programme, and an outpatient unit each for 50 alcoholics daily were opened.

On 1 January 1965 a Republic Register of Inpatient Alcoholics was established by the Centre in co-operation with the Republic Institute of Public Health. The work of the Register was based on voluntary co-operation with all institutions (mainly those of psychiatric character) engaged in the inpatient treatment of alcoholics in SR Croatia. They sent data about every inpatient alcoholic on to a central office and these data were then computer-processed in the Centre. The medical model was officially accepted throughout the Republic of Croatia in 1964.

Within the scope of the programmes mentioned, some other concepts were accepted from the very beginning. The most important are as follows.

(1) Alcoholism is a disease affecting the entire family and, therefore, the members of the family must be included in the therapeutical process.

(2) An alcoholic can be successfully treated and rehabilitated only if he is motivated to undergo treatment and if he is activated to become the subject in the therapeutical process.

(3) Alcoholism is a disease which must be treated over a long period of time – in our experience – by means of an organized complex approach over a period of at least 5 years. In order to achieve this goal, it is necessary to mobilize paraprofessional workers, and above all the alcoholic himself and his family. We have, therefore, begun with the organization of self-help groups which we named *Clubs of Treated Alcoholics*. The first club was established in 1964.

(4) Alcoholism can be treated only if the alcoholic is instructed to maintain full abstinence.

(5) The alcoholic, the members of his family and the members of the therapeutic team must undergo additional schooling and training.

EPIDEMIOLOGICAL DATA

In addition to data obtained from the Republic Register of Inpatient Alcoholics, a number of epidemiological studies were carried out on samples taken from the general population, samples of youth, representative samples of workers in basic branches of industry etc. A similar model of prevention, treatment and rehabilitation, in addition to epidemiological studies, was adopted in other republics of the Federation of Yugoslavia. However, we shall present here only data from SR Croatia because we started the programme there and conducted the epidemiological investigations. The data which will be presented are for the period of 1965–1978. All investigations were conducted with the aim of obtaining surveys to indicate the extent of the programme and thus offer indispensable elements for the organization of preventing alcoholism and for the treatment and rehabilitation of alcoholics.

SR Croatia is one of the republics comprising the Yugoslav Federation and is bordered by the Adriatic Sea. During the period observed (1965–1978), the population of Croatia numbered approximately 4 500 000.

The period from 1965 to 1978 was chosen because we had at our disposal data obtained by the Republic Register of Alcoholics processed to the end of 1978. From the beginning of 1979 to the present (1982), the same trends were found as for the period reviewed.

Different epidemiological observations made by the Centre had earlier demonstrated that one has to reckon with 15 % alcoholics in the group of the adult male population, and another 15 % of excessive drinkers (problem drinkers). When these data were presented, they caused shock in national and international circles and many did not believe them to be true. Nowadays similar data have been published in many other countries, which until recently refused to admit that alcoholism presented a serious problem (Italy, Great Britain), not to mention the USA, where this problem had been given serious and careful consideration earlier. Different forms of resistance, similar to those in other Mediterranean countries abounding in wine and other natural alcoholic beverages, were encountered in our country. Here, too, the belief in the myth of so-called 'Mediterranean drinking' which allegedly does not result in alcoholism, has been upheld for a long time because Mediterraneans are accustomed to drinking, and in any case 'wine cannot be dangerous since it is a gift of the gods and of nature'.

We were not as successful in investigating in detail and obtaining precise data on drinking and alcoholism among women as we have for men. We do have data on female alcoholics who underwent inpatient treatment for their alcoholism, however.

Attempts have been made to use data on the consumption of alcohol for the purpose of evaluation, but in a country where almost everybody obtains the necessary raw material from his own vineyard or orchard and produces alcoholic beverages at home, and in a country with a relatively highly developed tourist trade, it is difficult to determine precisely the consumption of alcohol among the native population.

Reviewing all the data at our disposal, we found those obtained from the Republic Register of the alcoholics treated on an inpatient basis to be the most accurate. The survey of alcoholism in Croatia is, therefore, based on these data, as being those in accordance with which the continual evaluation and adaptation of our clinical programmes was carried out (Tables 3.1–3.9).

A continuous evaluation of changing trends, indicating the gravity of the problem, was possible on the basis of data supplied by the Republic Register of Treated Alcoholics and from these it was possible to draw some conclusions about alcoholism in Croatia in general, and to revise programmes to control alcoholism according to data obtained.

On the basis of the data reviewed, the following conclusions were drawn:

(1)   Data supplied by the Republican Register of Alcoholics indicated that the number of hospital-treated alcoholics had doubled in the period from 1965 to 1978.

(2)   The increase in the relative number of female alcoholics was more rapid than that in men. A similar trend was observed in women alcoholics in many other countries.

(3)   The number of hospitalization periods for alcoholics was much higher than that of subjects treated, indicating that a number of alcoholics still had relapses after hospital treatment.

Table 3.1 Alcoholics registered for the first time, treated in the inpatient psychiatric institutions of SR Croatia

Year of first hospitalization	Males	Females	Total
1965	2 787	355	3 142
1966	2 660	345	3 005
1967	2 839	385	3 224
1968	3 460	473	3 933
1969	3 646	516	4 162
1970	4 398	668	5 066
1971	4 470	744	5 214
1972	4 323	659	4 982
1973	4 456	660	5 116
1974	4 278	693	4 971
1975	4 663	783	5 446
1976	5 267	852	6 119
1977	5 005	836	5 841
1978	6 138	1 099	7 237
Total	58 390	9 068	67 458

Data: Republic Register of Treated Alcoholics

(4) It became possible to evaluate the programmes applied in the treatment and rehabilitation of alcoholics on the basis of the total number of hospitalizations and partly also to evaluate the programmes for the control, i.e. prevention, of alcoholism in the entire Republic as we were able to follow up alcoholics in individual regions and counties in the Republic.

(5) An increase was also seen in the younger age groups of inpatient male alcoholics at the time of their first treatment.

(6) Usually men in their best years of life suffer from alcoholism.

(7) Alcoholics spent almost half a million days each year in psychiatric institutions of Croatia. According to investigations, the alcoholic loses approximately 10 years of his working life because of the early onset of disablement.

(8) Alcoholics reporting for the first treatment were usually in a serious condition. Specific modifications of treatment and a special programme of post-hospital care outside the institution must be devised for alcoholics with serious complications.

Table 3.2 Number of hospitalizations of alcoholics in the inpatient psychiatric institutions of SR Croatia in regard to sex and the year of treatment

Year of the hospital treatment	Males	Females	Total
1965	3 158	417	3 575
1966	3 562	438	4 000
1967	4 070	522	4 592
1968	5 095	659	5 754
1969	5 631	712	6 343
1970	6 993	949	7 942
1971	7 478	1 091	8 569
1972	7 649	1 012	8 661
1973	8 289	1 051	9 340
1974	8 262	1 197	9 459
1975	9 241	1 330	10 571
1976	10 207	1 435	11 642
1977	9 787	1 437	11 224
1978	12 336	1 866	14 202
Total	101 758	14 116	115 874

Data: Republic Register of Alcoholics

Table 3.3 Age and year of hospitalization of male alcoholics treated for the first time in the inpatient psychiatric institutions of SR Croatia

Year	< 29	30 − 44	45 − 59	60 +	Total
1965	334	1 431	766	256	2 787
1966	344	1 386	706	224	2 660
1967	306	1 484	721	328	2 839
1968	352	1 741	1 006	361	3 460
1969	358	1 858	978	452	3 646
1970	441	2 121	1 293	543	4 398
1971	467	2 231	1 275	497	4 470
1972	504	2 149	1 227	443	4 323
1973	516	2 156	1 266	518	4 456
1974	517	1 985	1 293	483	4 278
1975	630	2 020	1 471	542	4 663
1976	720	2 191	1 709	647	5 267
1977	719	2 024	1 728	534	5 005
1978	721	2 444	2 313	660	6 138
Total	6929	27 221	17 752	6488	58 390

Data: Republic Register of Alcoholics

Table 3.4 Age and year of hospitalization of male alcoholics treated for the first time in the inpatient psychiatric institutions of SR Croatia

Year	<29 %	30−44 %	45−59 %	60+ %	Total %
1965	11.96	51.26	27.52	9.26	100
1966	12.95	52.17	26.52	8.35	100
1967	10.72	52.22	25.57	11.49	100
1968	10.18	50.35	29.06	10.41	100
1969	9.61	50.89	26.97	12.53	100
1970	10.03	48.23	29.40	12.34	100
1971	10.45	49.91	28.53	11.11	100
1972	11.66	49.71	28.39	10.24	100
1973	11.58	48.39	28.41	11.62	100
1974	12.09	46.40	30.22	11.29	100
1975	13.01	43.32	31.55	11.62	100
1976	13.67	41.59	32.46	12.28	100
1977	14.36	40.44	34.53	10.67	100
1978	11.74	39.82	37.68	10.76	100
Total	11.86	46.62	30.40	11.12	100

Data: Republic Register, represented in relative values

Table 3.5 Age and year of hospitalization of female alcoholics treated for the first time in the inpatient psychiatric institutions of SR Croatia

Year	<29	30−44	45−59	60+	Total
1965	43	153	104	55	355
1966	22	159	105	59	345
1967	21	162	139	63	385
1968	44	208	153	68	473
1969	33	196	189	98	516
1970	50	278	238	102	668
1971	66	285	268	125	744
1972	54	250	234	121	659
1973	36	286	231	107	660
1974	54	266	248	125	693
1975	69	286	295	133	783
1976	75	296	325	156	852
1977	66	291	343	136	836
1978	76	341	479	203	1099
Total	709	3457	3351	1551	9068

Data: Republic Register of Alcoholics

Table 3.6 Age and year of hospitalization of female alcoholics treated in the inpatient psychiatric institutions of SR Croatia for the first time

Year	< 29 %	30−44 %	45−59 %	60+ %	Total %
1965	12.64	42.98	29.21	15.17	100
1966	6.34	45.82	30.35	17.29	100
1967	5.40	42.27	35.84	16.49	100
1968	9.24	43.92	32.14	14.70	100
1969	6.13	38.34	36.36	19.17	100
1970	7.48	41.62	35.63	15.27	100
1971	8.87	38.30	36.02	16.81	100
1972	8.19	37.94	35.50	18.37	100
1973	5.45	43.33	35.00	16.22	100
1974	7.79	38.38	35.79	18.04	100
1975	8.81	36.52	37.68	16.99	100
1976	8.80	34.74	38.15	18.31	100
1977	7.89	34.81	41.03	16.27	100
1978	6.91	31.03	43.58	18.48	100
Total	7.81	38.13	36.95	17.11	100

Data: Republic Register of Alcoholics

Table 3.7 Relation between numbers of male and female alcoholics treated as inpatients in psychiatric institutions of SR Croatia from 1965 to 1978

Year	Males	Females
1965	7.85	1
1966	7.71	1
1967	7.37	1
1968	7.31	1
1969	7.06	1
1970	6.58	1
1971	6.01	1
1972	6.56	1
1973	6.75	1
1974	6.17	1
1975	5.95	1
1976	6.18	1
1977	5.98	1
1978	5.58	1
Total	6.44	1

Data: Republic Register of Treated Alcoholics

Table 3.8 Number of days of hospitalization in single years for treating alcoholics in psychiatric institutions of SR Croatia

Year	Males	Females	Total
1965	131 650	19 438	151 088
1966	142 504	23 458	165 962
1967	168 501	28 627	197 128
1968	183 360	27 006	210 366
1969	214 486	34 411	248 897
1970	248 480	37 656	286 136
1971	274 997	48 613	323 610
1972	270 916	48 397	319 313
1973	304 817	54 126	358 943
1974	334 076	56 941	391 017
1975	394 717	73 544	468 261
1976	402 409	63 129	465 538
1977	390 676	58 839	449 515
1978	464 975	64 447	529 422
Total	3 926 564	638 632	4 565 196

Data: Republic Register of Alcoholics

Table 3.9 Number of hospitalizations of alcoholics, treated in psychiatric institutions of SR Croatia, who at moment of admission had diagnosis of alcoholic psychosis

Year	Males	Females	Total
1965	558	54	612
1966	482	71	553
1967	891	126	1 017
1968	1 100	128	1 228
1969	1 559	161	1 720
1970	1 747	205	1 952
1971	1 945	263	2 208
1972	2 173	219	2 392
1973	2 355	259	2 614
1974	2 404	358	2 762
1975	1 894	302	2 196
1976	1 735	249	1 984
1977	1 840	311	2 151
1978	2 349	283	2 632
Total	23 032	2989	26 021

Data: Republic Register of Alcoholics

(9)   A great number of alcoholics was found among the active beneficiaries of health insurance, thus indicating the need for a programme to control alcoholism to be organized within the labour organization.

(10)   Alcoholics die earlier than non-alcoholics.

THE SHORTCOMINGS OF THE MEDICAL MODEL

It was possible to observe clearly during this phase that the complex therapeutic approach which we introduced gave increasingly better results in the treatment and rehabilitation of alcoholics. The impression was gained that the number of alcoholics who undergo inpatient treatment decreased over the past few years in the two largest urban centres of Croatia.

Other parallel investigations, however, showed that the therapeutically oriented medical model was not suitable as the basis of successful prevention of alcohol related problems. In addition, a number of negative factors appeared. I shall mention only a few of them:

(1)   The consumption of alcoholic beverages was slowing but showed still an upward trend.

(2)   There was an increased consumption of alcoholic beverages in young people, especially among children and among women.

(3)   Other alcohol related problems were numerically on the increase (alcohol related road accidents, misdemeanours associated with drinking, etc.)

(4)   At the time of their first inpatient treatment, alcoholics tend to be younger.

(5)   Absenteeism due to drinking and alcoholism showed an upward trend.

All these factors indicated that it was not sufficient to treat and rehabilitate alcoholics, but that all other alcohol related problems must be controlled, too. It became apparent, moreover, that the therapeutically oriented medical model of approach was not sufficient to control all those problems, although a properly conducted medical approach manifoldly improved the results of treatment and rehabilitation.

THE INTRODUCTION OF THE SOCIOMEDICAL MODEL

On the basis of the understanding that the medical model was insufficient for the control of all alcohol related problems, we introduced a somewhat wider approach a few years ago and called it the sociomedical approach. This model required that the activities be enlarged to include all alcohol related problems. The main accent was on preventive action and required that treatment and rehabilitation be carried out as early as possible on an outpatient basis, i.e. in

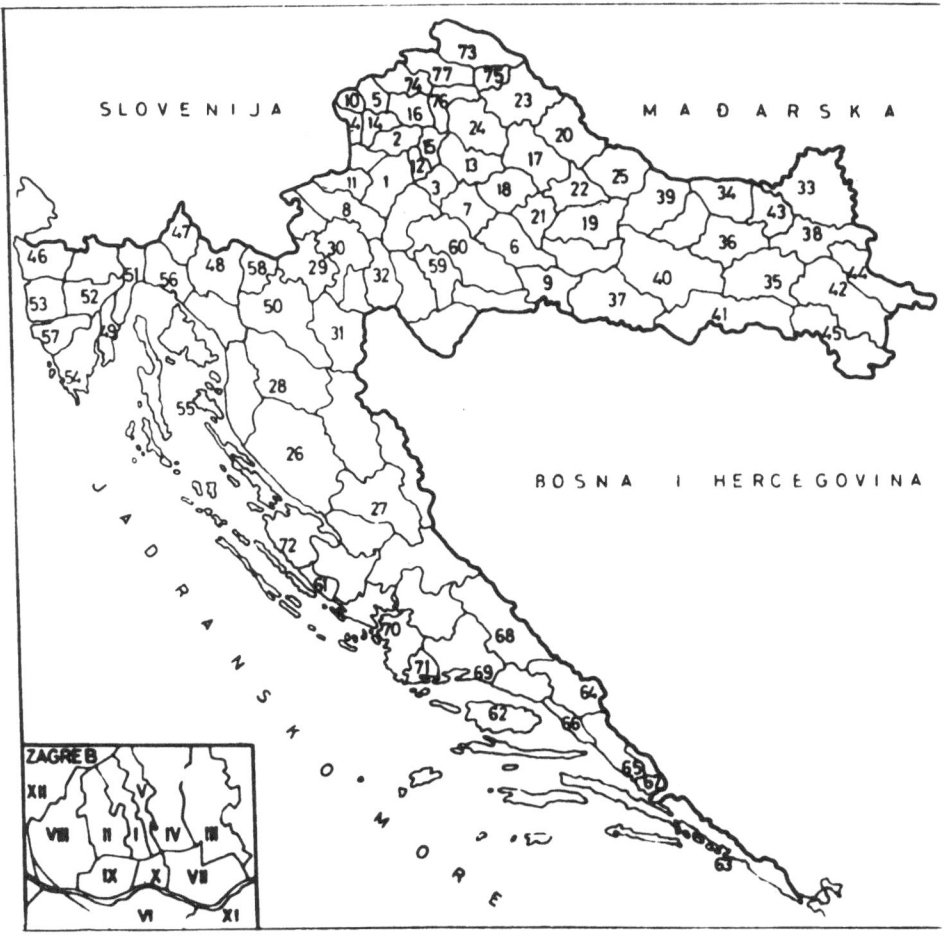

Figure 3.1 Distribution of the clubs of former alcoholics in the Socialist Republic of Croatia. In the bottom left-hand corner (inset), the clubs in the wider metropolitan area of Zagreb are shown. The main map shows the division into counties in the Socialist Republic of Croatia. In every numbered county there are county programmes and clubs of former alcoholics

the local community and within the labour organization. The programmes of the local communities and the labour organizations were to be coordinated with the county programmes. Apart from these, intercommunal and regional programmes were activated and coordinated at Republic level.

The minimum contents of the programme set up by the local community and the labour organization must be health and social education to qualify each individual to apply self-protection and self-help. Paraprofessional workers and all other structures and forces of the local community and the labour organization participate in the implementation of the programme which is conducted by primary health protection (general practitioner). The programme, moreover, takes into account the long term procedure of the alcoholic's rehabilitation and organizes professional teams who work in the Clubs of Treated Alcoholics. Up to now, over 500 Clubs of Treated Alcoholics have been organized in SR Croatia.

The introduction and carrying out of continual training of professional and paraprofessional staff has also been taken into consideration in this programme and for these purposes a special school of social psychiatry, alcohology, and other dependencies has been organized.

PROGRAMMES FOR THE PROTECTION AND PROMOTION OF MENTAL HEALTH

After a certain period of applying the sociomedical approach, it became evident that alcoholism and alcohol related problems could be separated only artificially from other problems involving mental health. It was, therefore, decided that all mental conditions, including alcoholism, should be approached by a common integrated programme of protection and improvement of mental health.

As with the sociomedical approach, the programme was organized on the level of the local community and the labour organization and coordinated on a higher level in the county, on intercommunal, regional and Republic levels. This programme also required intensive education and training of professional and paraprofessional staff. In addition, it was indispensible to introduce health and social education to each member of society and to make them qualified in self-protection and self-help. Protection of mental health and specific programmes of controlling alcohol related problems supplemented each other in this way. Apart from Clubs of Treated Alcoholics, other self-help groups were established (Clubs of Mental Patients, Clubs of Aged People, Clubs of Hypertonics etc.).

The entire programme on the level of the local community and the labour organization depended on the work of the general practitioner, the specialist in labour medicine, the school physician, their professional teams and, above all, the nurse and the social worker.

Special modifications of the programme described were introduced for alcoholics in prisons and for patients with a combination of chronic pulmonary disease, primarily tuberculosis.

EDUCATION

As mentioned, a special School of Social Psychiatry, Alcoholism and Other Dependencies has been established, where professionals and paraprofessionals are trained, starting in the form of short seminars of one week's duration (50 hours) and going on to education extending over the period of 1 year. Suggestions were put forward for specialization in alcoholism and other dependencies to be introduced. Now there exists the possibility of a postgraduate 2-year study course.

Since it is impossible today to control alcoholism and other dependencies without wide international co-operation, in addition to our school, the Mediterranean Organization of Social Psychiatry has organized the Mediterranean School of Social Psychiatry in which experts from all Mediterranean countries act as teachers and the students come from individual Mediterranean regions. So far this school has conducted special educational programmes in Cyprus, Italy, Spain, Greece and Yugoslavia.

RESULTS AND CONCLUSION

Although the programme for the control of alcohol related problems in Croatia has been active for nearly 20 years and although we have studied a great number of cases, the time available is nevertheless too short to enable us to give a review of the general results in controlling alcohol related problems. The results of the treatment and rehabilitation of alcoholics are very good and vary from commune to commune in accordance with the quality of the local programme. The results of treatment and rehabilitation amount to 60 % for the entire territory of Croatia. A good result is considered to be the case of a patient who at the follow-up a year after beginning treatment is still abstinent, has solved his family problems and is working regularly.

According to data collected in two of our largest cities, Zagreb and Rijeka, it became evident that the number of alcoholics was finally beginning to decrease.

The control of other alcohol related problems depends also on society as a whole changing its attitude towards drinking. This, however, is a long term task for which transgeneration studies will have to be devised.

4
Alcoholism in Nigeria

T. ASUNI

INTRODUCTION

Nigeria is a vast country, three times the size of Great Britain and Ireland. It has a population estimated currently to be in the region of 100 million consisting of many ethnic and linguistic groups and different sects. The country is presently divided into 19 states, and there is clamour for more states to be created. Consequently one can hardly make sweeping generalizations about the whole country. Nevertheless, it may be possible to make legitimate statements regarding general trends, and focus attention on the geographical area with which one is familiar. This is precisely what I intend to do in this presentation.

My exposure to the problem of alcoholism is through psychiatry in which I was involved since the beginning of 1957. For many years I was Medical Superintendent of the Neuropsychiatric Hospital, Aro, Abeokuta, which is a complex of a Closed Unit of Landoro Institute, the Open Unit of Aro Hospital, and the adjoining villages in which patients and their relatives were boarded. A fuller account of the hospital has been given elsewhere[1].

Traditionally drinking of alcohol beverages, especially among the Yorubas who occupy the south-western corner of Nigeria, was only on ceremonial occasions – weddings, funerals, festivals, social visits; and it was hardly the practice to drink alcohol beverages as a regular pastime. The popular drink was palm wine or alcohol made out of grain, the alcoholic content of which was quite low until it was left overnight to ferment. A later development was the distillation of these drinks – which initially was an illegal exercise, but has now been legalized.

This traditional pattern is changing rapidly and a clear indicator of this change is the proliferation of modern breweries in the country. There is sometimes more than one brewery in a state. In addition to the breweries, imported distilled alcohol is bottled in the country in the form of spirits. There is now a ban on imported beer. Before this ban, beer to a value of nearly 100

33

million naira was imported in 1 year (the naira is worth between 70 and 80 UK pence).

PROBLEMS OF ALCOHOLISM

The problems which have come to my professional attention have been psychiatric with their attendant social problems. The commonest form of alcoholism is that in which the whole life of the alcoholic revolves around drinking. His performance at work drops, his attendance at work becomes irregular to the extent that he may lose his job or his high position. His family suffers as a result of his inability to carry out his financial responsibility. He gets into debt and loses his social status.

A summary of the findings of a study entitled 'Pattern of alcohol problems as seen in the Neuropsychiatric Hospital, Aro, Abeokuta, 1964–1973'[2] may be appropriate here. One of the major justifications for using this facility for the study was that there was no better place where one could get a collection of people with alcohol problems. The study suggested that the problem was on the increase, but the increasing acceptance of the role of the hospital may also play a part in the apparent increase – in that the hospital was being used more and more.

Of the total number of 60 patients, only 5% were female, 75% were between the ages of 20 and 49; 60% were married, 20% were single, 6.7% were divorced or separated and the status of 12 was not known; 65% of the patients were in non-traditional occupations – they were more westernized, they generally were wage earners.

Sixty-three per cent were Christians, 31% were Moslems – which is understandable. Thirty per cent drank mostly Ogogoro (i.e. distilled local brew), 11.7% drank mainly palm wine, 26.6% drank mainly beer and 31.7% drank different combinations of the above and spirits.

Reasons for admission to the hospital were: dependence and drunkenness 30%, hallucinosis 6.6%, alcoholic psychosis 28.3%, road accidents 1.6%, symptomatic drinking 31.6% and dementia 1.6%.

I am not in a position to talk about the physical problems of alcoholism like cirrhosis of the liver, gastritis, polyneuritis etc., as they would not be brought to the attention of a psychiatrist if the physical problems are the main presenting symptoms, but it will be surprising if there are not many more cases of physical pathology than psychiatric or psychological pathology.

A similar study was that of Odejide[3] which reviewed alcoholics admitted into the 500-bed University College Hospital, Ibadan, with an annual average admission rate of 10 000, 50-odd miles (80 km) from Abeokuta where I was located. Both UCH and the Neuropsychiatric Hospital are located in the same tribal area. It is therefore no surprise that the findings were similar. Of the 42 alcoholics admitted over a period of 10 years (1966–1975), 40 (95%) were males, 36 (86%) were between the ages of 15 to 35. The admissions were into three main units: Emergency Department, 18 cases; Medical Units, 14 cases;

Psychiatric Unit, ten cases. Of the 18 cases admitted via the Emergency Department, eight had delirium tremens, four were involved in road traffic accidents, and six had evidences of liver cirrhosis. Of the ten cases admitted to the Psychiatric Unit, two had social problems, and eight exhibited abnormal behaviour; of the total 42 patients, 30 (71.4 %) were married; six (14.3 %) were single and six (14.3 %) were either separated or divorced. Those with non-traditional occupations totalled 66.7 %; 29 (70 %) were Christians and 12 (29 %) Moslems. No criminal record was noted in any of the cases.

Odejide and Olatawura[4] also did a study of drinking behaviour in a rural community 19 kilometres north-west of Ibadan, the capital of former Western Region, and capital of Oyo State. Of 198 respondents above 15 years of age, 111 were male and 87 female; 68 were abstainers, 29 (26.1 %) male and 39 (45 %) female; 89 were occasional drinkers; 43 (38.8 %) male and 46 (52.7 %) female; 32 were moderate drinkers, 30 (27 %) male and two (2.3 %) female; all nine heavy drinkers were males.

These researchers defined occasional drinkers as those who drink less than twice per month, and on each occasion drink less than a bottle of beer or a shot of spirit, or a pint (about 60 cl) of palm wine or a glass of foreign wine.

Moderate drinkers are those who drink one or two bottles of beer or three glasses of foreign wine or two shots of spirit at a time or 2 pints of undiluted palm wine twice or three times a week.

Heavy drinkers are those who drink more than 3 pints of beer or undiluted palm wine or six shots of spirits or six glasses of foreign wine three or more times a week. Moderate or heavy drinking was uncommon before the age of 35. Of the 32 moderate drinkers 30 (93.8 %) were above 35 years of age, while among the nine heavy drinkers seven (77.8 %) were above 35 years of age.

Most of the respondents (92 %) were Moslems, so were the nine heavy drinkers, six of whom were farmers. This is due to the fact that the villagers are predominantly Moslems.

20.7 % gave health reasons for drinking and these include the assumed value of alcohol as blood tonic, possibly due to the impact of advertising.

These findings, which cannot be reliably generalized to all rural communities, may well be consequences of the nearness to the capital city and its destabilizing effect. This view is supported by the fact that only 63 of the respondents were farmers, and 14 unemployed in any agricultural environment; while the others (118) were engaged in either skilled or unskilled jobs.

In another part of the country, Bendel State, with a different tribal group, Oshodin[5] carried out a study on alcohol abuse among high school students in the state capital, Benin City, and another[6] in a secondary school in a rural area of Benin District. He found that 87 % of the students in Benin City and 71 % of the students in the rural area used alcohol; 18 % of the students in the rural area could be classified as alcohol abusers. They used alcohol more for social than psychological reasons in contrast to the situation observed in the urban area (Benin City) where psychological reasons predominated.

Ebie and Pela[7] also found that 66 % of their series of high school students in Benin City admitted the use of alcohol.

ATTITUDE TO ALCOHOLISM

Except in situations where a close friend or member of one's family is alcoholic the public does not seem to be very acutely aware of the individual and social problems of alcoholism. Even in situations where personal involvement brings the problem into focus, people are not aware of the services to use. Of course the traditional healer is consulted as the problem is often considered to be caused by evil machination of others, or violation of taboos, curse etc.

The attitude to alcoholism appears to be rather tolerant but not condoned and advice and admonition are lavishly given by relatives and friends who are not drinking colleagues. It is only when it becomes an overt problem by frequent disturbing behaviour socially, domestically and occupationally that efforts are made to seek outside help — usually from traditional healers, and religious healing sects, in the first instance.

TRADITIONAL TREATMENT

It is not known how effective traditional intervention is in the problem of alcoholism. One situation which was brought to my attention was that of an important chief who was unsuccessfully treated by traditional methods. By virtue of his position, he had access to the most renowned and powerful traditional healers.

One method used by traditional healers is making superficial incisions under the lower lip and rubbing some powdered herbs into the incision like an inoculation. The efficacy of this method needs to be assessed.

PSYCHIATRIC TREATMENT

Rarely does a person with drinking problems come by himself for treatment. Even when he does, treatment is not initiated without the involvement of his relatives and friends directly or indirectly. This is the tradition of the hospital where I worked, where in the treatment of all psychiatric cases the active collaboration of relatives is part of the regime. We are indeed reluctant to initiate treatment without this active collaboration.

Secondly, it is considered futile to attempt treatment on an outpatient basis except when the relatives can guarantee to follow rigidly the instructions given, which is very rare. This procedure of inpatient treatment was confirmed by a patient who had once been treated on an outpatient basis in another psychiatric facility in the country — he said that they wasted their time on him as he continued drinking during the treatment.

The first approach is to rely on the patient's willingness to have treatment, even though this may be spurious or half-hearted. He is treated in an open ward with strict instructions to obey the rules, the most important of which is that he does not drink. If he violates the rule by going out to drink, he is deprived of his clothing − thanks to the weather − and his liberty is increasingly curtailed.

It has been known that a patient not properly clothed has gone out of the hospital to drink. In this case, he was transferred to a closed unit from where he could not readily get out. Even in this situation, he was able to get out by wearing another patient's clothes and he had to be put under tighter surveillance − not to be out of sight of members of the staff in the hospital compound. He was not kept in a room by himself so that he could still interact with other patients.

This was a patient who had been brought by his mother, having lost his job, lost his wife, and his behaviour had been disgraceful to say the least. The patient admitted that he had brought shame and opprobrium to himself and his family and he was the black sheep of the family. He claimed that he wanted to be rid of his drinking problem.

Treatment is considered to be a continuum from 'drying out' to weaning to rehabilitation. There is no demarcation between stages of treatment but considerable overlapping. The problem of sobering up hardly arises because patients are not brought to hospital initially in the state of intoxication. Rather, it is during the course of treatment in the hospital that they go out to drink and return to the hospital inebriated. The reaction to this behaviour is to regard it as a break in the treatment chain and we have to start again as if the patient is being introduced to treatment for the first time.

The agreement reached with the patient and his relatives during the initial interview is that the patient has to remain dry continuously for at least 3 months before we can consider his discharge. If at any time in that period he breaks the chain and drinks, the whole programme is cancelled and he has to start again. So the more he breaks the chain, the longer he stays in the hospital.

Another agreement reached before the beginning of treatment is that if the patient breaks his word repeatedly regarding his co-operation, the hospital is entitled to take whatever step considered to be in his best interest, and acceptable to his relatives. The extreme step is transfer from an open unit to a closed unit where his freedom of movement is considerably curtailed.

The patient is exposed to the necessary treatment modalities. He participates in the group therapy with other patients with mostly dissimilar problems. He has individual psychotherapy to explore problem areas in his life with the aim of modifying these. A change of job may be necessary if this exposes him to the temptation of alcohol. A change of friends and associates from those who are drinking companions is necessary since the patient's lifestyle and social support must be modified. The foundation for these changes is developed while the patient is still in the hospital, with the understanding and collaboration of his relatives.

The physical conditions associated with alcoholism are treated, and these include malnutrition, vitamin deficiencies and any medical complications or illnesses associated with excessive drinking. Clordiazepozide (Librium) or similar anxiolytic or major tranquillizers are used to lower his anxiety and avert withdrawal symptoms. Chlorpromazine is also used.

Conditioned therapy has not been used, but it has occasionally been considered. Disulfiram (Antabuse) was seriously considered in a particular case, but was not used because the patient asked for it out of desperation when he was suicidal.

Unfortunately, we are not in a position to say much about the success rate of this regime, as follow-up was not aggressively pursued, and very few patients continue on an outpatient basis as advised. Some of the failures we hear about. There was one patient who died in an unusual circumstance, and we suspected suicide.

None of the alcoholics that we have dealt with had any criminal charge, and we have never been called to testify in court in either civil or criminal cases involving the use of alcohol. Even though some of our patients had been violent and physically aggressive and must have violated the law, the total situations indicated medical rather than judicial intervention. It is also noteworthy that among the vagrants collected in Lagos in 1958 and the vagrant psychotics collected, studied and treated in Abeokuta in 1966[8], there was no alcoholic.

There is no voluntary organization like Alcoholics Anonymous operating in Nigeria yet.

CRIMINAL OFFENCES

Criminal offences associated with drunkenness must be many but they are not recorded in Nigeria in such a way as to focus on drunkenness. The most serious of these offences is driving under the influence of alcohol leading to road accidents, involving loss of limb or life. Of course when the drivers involved also die in the accident, there is no one to prosecute. It may call the attention of the authorities to the seriousness of the problem of alcohol if the involvement of alcohol in such serious criminal offences is appropriately recorded.

Of course, there is the problem of the scarcity of the technology and manpower to measure alcohol blood levels. Apart from the big cities with fairly well equipped hospitals and laboratories, it is not possible to carry out blood examinations. If the question of alcoholic intoxication ever arises in a police case, and the accused is taken to hospital, the doctor, limited by lack of facilities, can only rely on his clinical examination of speech, motor coordination and smell of alcohol in the accused's breath.

How many drunken pedestrians and cyclists are killed on the roads is not known. Vehicle drivers involved in such fatal accidents, especially on isolated roads, do not usually stop.

In summary, the problem of alcohol appears to be increasing in Nigeria,

with higher earnings, ready availability of alcohol enhanced by the proliferation of breweries, urbanization, loosening of traditional social control of
extended family and neighbourliness. Public attitude to the problem appears
to be tolerant until it gets to be very disruptive and shameful.

It does not appear to be appreciated by many that this is an area in which
psychiatry can be helpful, and even when it is so appreciated there is reluctance
to use psychiatry because of the stigma associated in some quarters with
psychiatric hospitals. The effectiveness of traditional healers' intervention is
not known. The long term effect of modern psychiatric intervention cannot
be reliably ascertained because of failure of patients to come for follow-up, but
cases of relapses are known.

Treatment regime is a continuum from drying-up to rehabilitation; it relies
on collaboration of relatives and friends and it consists of different modalities.

The problem of the right of the alcoholic regarding treatment has never
arisen, as the patient is brought by his relatives and it is assumed and confirmed
that he is willing to have treatment, even though the willingness may be
spurious at first. We do not recall any situation where an alcoholic has been
forced to come to hospital except perhaps in case of frank alcoholic psychosis
when the patient has lost touch with reality. In any case, we are emboldened to
enforce initial treatment with the consent of relatives where treatment is
indicated and the patient is unwilling or unable to give the consent. After this
initial treatment, the situation is discussed with the patient to get his consent
and co-operation.

We have never been challenged in court for violation of the human rights
of our patients — certainly not by alcoholics.

References

1 Asuni, T. (1967). Aro Hospital in perspective. *Am. J. Psychiatry*, **124**
2 Asuni, T. (1975). Pattern of alcohol problems as seen in the Neuropsychiatric Hospital, Aro,
Abeokuta 1964–1973. In *Proceedings of the 1974 Workshop of the Association of Psychiatrists in
Africa — Alcohol and Drug Dependence*. (Lausanne: International Council on Alcohol and
Addictions.)
3 Odejide, A. O. (1978). Alcoholism: a major health hazard in Nigeria. *Nig. Med. J.*, **8**, (3)
4 Odejide, A. O. and Olatawura, M. O. (1977). Alcohol use in a Nigerian rural community.
Afr. J. Psychiatry, **1**, (2), 69
5 Oshodin, O. G. (1981). Alcohol abuse among high school students in Benin City. *Drug Alc.
Dependence*, **7**, 141
6 Oshodin, O. G. (1981). Alcohol abuse; a case study of secondary school students in a rural
area of Benin District, Nigeria. *Drug Alc. Dependence*, **8**, 175
7 Ebie, J. C. and Pela, O. A. (1981). Some aspects of drug use among students in Benin City,
Nigeria. *Drug Alc. Dependence*, **8**, 265
8 Asuni, T. (1980). Vagrant psychotics in Abeokuta. *Afr. J. Psychiatry*, **6**, (III & IV)

5
Alcoholism in Sri Lanka – a general survey

S. B. CROOS

Sri Lanka (Ceylon) is a pear-shaped island at the southern end of the Indian subcontinent, between 5 ° 55′ and 9 ° 51′ of north latitude and 79 ° 41 ′ and 81 ° 53 ′ east longitude, separated from India by a narrow strip of shallow water − the Palk Strait, approximately 22 miles (35 km) wide. The island has an area of approximately 25 300 square miles (65 000 km²). The island's greatest length − north to south − and breadth − west to east − are 270 miles (440 km) and 140 miles (229 km) respectively. Due to its strategic position in the Indian Ocean, Sri Lanka has been subject to varied international influences throughout history.

Tables 5.1−5.5 show the classified distribution of population.

Drinking alcoholic beverages in this multiracial, multilingual and multidenominational island is an accepted social custom among the majority of the people. Most people drink occasionally, and even regularly, and for the majority, alcohol appears to present no real difficulty. The fact remains, however, that a very significant number of people do have a very real and often unidentified problem caused by drink. Since most of those involved spend their time concealing their failing from themselves and from others, it is not surprising that drinking problems seem much rarer than they in fact are. Everybody is aware of the effects and dangers of drink, but in general, the majority manage to enjoy the pleasures and avoid the complications. The paradox of drink is that it appears to be a boon to many and a scourge to a few.

Although there are many alcohols, the kind in alcoholic beverages is known as 'ethyl alcohol' or 'ethanol' with the chemical formula C_2H_5OH. As a food, alcohol provides only 'naked' calories, thus lacking in the essential amino acids and vitamins, and its prolonged consumption therefore causes malnutrition and other complicated anaemic conditions.

However, alcohol is also classified as a drug due to its dramatic effects on the central nervous system, and is one of the few substances which needs no

Table 5.1 Population (thousands)

Year	Males	Females	Total
1971	6 489	6 119	12 690
1972	6 619	6 242	12 861
1973	6 738	6 353	13 091
1974	6 837	6 447	13 284
1975	6 950	6 546	13 496
1976	7 060	6 657	13 717
1977	7 176	6 766	13 942
1978	7 296	6 894	14 190
1979	7 441	7 030	14 471
1980	7 578	7 100	14 738
1981	7 539	7 311	14 850

Source: Statistical Pocket Yearbook, Department of Census and Statistics and Ministry of Plan Implementation

Table 5.2 Population by race (thousands)

	1946	1953	1963	1971	1977	1978
All races	6 657	8 098	10 582	12 690	13 940	14 190
Low country Sinhalese	2 903	3 470	4 470	5 426 }	10 204	10 402
Kandyan Sinhalese	1 718	2 147	3 043	3 705 }		
Ceylon Tamils	734	885	1 163	1 424 }	2 644	2 669
Indian Tamils	781	974	1 123	1 175 }		
Ceylon Moors	374	464	627	828	954	978
Indian Moors	36	48	55	27	29	29
Europeans	5	7	—	—	—	—
Burghers and Eurasians	42	46	46	45	48	48
Malays	23	25	33	43	48	48
Veddahs	2	1	1	—	—	—
Other	41	32	20	16	13	15

Source: Statistical Pocket Yearbook, Department of Census and Statistics and Ministry of Plan Implementation, 1979

Table 5.3 Population by religion

Religion	1963	1971	%age distribution 1963	1971
Buddhists	7 003 300	8 567 600	66.18	67.40
Hindus	1 958 400	2 239 300	18.51	17.62
Christians	884 900	986 700	8.36	7.76
Muslims	724 000	909 900	6.84	7.16
Other	11 400	7 600	0.11	0.06

Source: Statistical Pocket Yearbook, Department of Census and Statistics and Ministry of Plan Implementation, 1979

Table 5.4 Population by age and sex (thousands)

Age Group	1972 M	1972 F	1973 M	1973 F	1974 M	1974 F	1975 M	1975 F	1976 M	1976 F	1977 M	1977 F	1978 M	1978 F	1979 M	1979 F
15—19	698	680	711	692	721	703	733	713	744	726	757	737	769	751	784	766
20—24	648	640	660	651	669	661	681	671	692	682	703	693	714	707	729	721
25—29	485	482	494	490	501	497	510	505	518	514	526	522	535	532	545	542
30—34	383	357	390	363	395	369	402	374	408	380	415	387	422	394	430	402
35—39	372	363	378	370	384	375	390	381	397	387	403	394	410	402	418	410
40—44	318	276	324	281	329	285	335	290	340	294	345	299	351	304	358	310
45—49	293	259	299	263	305	265	308	271	313	276	318	280	323	286	330	292
50—54	230	194	234	197	238	200	242	203	245	206	249	210	254	214	259	218
55—59	195	159	198	162	201	165	204	167	208	170	211	173	215	176	219	180
60—64	153	119	155	121	158	123	160	125	163	127	165	129	169	132	172	134

M = male; F = female

Table 5.5   Marital status by age and sex (census of population, 1971)

Age group	Sex	Total	Married
15–19	Male	688.7	3.9
	Female	671.2	69.8
20–24	Male	639.5	84.9
	Female	631.1	289.4
25–29	Male	478.9	221.2
	Female	475.1	348.8
30–34	Male	377.7	277.3
	Female	352.0	302.1
35–39	Male	366.8	311.9
	Female	358.6	318.9
40–44	Male	314.3	278.7
	Female	271.8	236.1
45–49	Male	289.6	258.0
	Female	255.1	213.0
50–54	Male	227.0	200.2
	Female	190.9	145.4
55–59	Male	192.1	167.0
	Female	157.3	109.6

Source: Statistical Pocket Yearbook, Department of Census and Statistics and Ministry of Plan Implementation, 1979

digestion, but is rapidly absorbed by the body tissues. Due to its affinity to water, within minutes of ingestion the alcohol rushes to all parts of the body.

The vast majority of physical problems caused by drink are those affecting the central nervous system and the digestive system, the common conditions being

intoxication (mild to moderate)
alcoholic stupor
alcoholic coma
alcoholic tremulousness
alcoholic hallucinosis
alcoholic convulsive seizures
alcoholic polyneuropathy
delirium tremens
gastritis
cirrhosis
impotence
pancreatitis

However, besides the direct changes in the physical and psychological conditions of a human being, it is invariably to the economic and social disturbances associated with alcohol use and abuse and alcoholism that very great importance is attached. It is very important, therefore, to find an answer to the question as to why man, confronted with the many disadvantages of alcohol consumption, including its abuse which is its consequence in many cases, nevertheless firmly adheres to it. This question has been answered in different ways, and it has also been said that the economy would suffer if alcohol production and consumption ceased to be a market factor.

Whatever the answers, the fact is that in our society today, the pressures towards drinking are fast increasing, and since alcohol is easily and readily obtainable, drinking is freely and regularly indulged in at all levels, unmindful of its disastrous consequences. A further frightening development in recent times is the increasing numbers of teenagers and women taking to drink.

A noticeable feature in teenage drinking in Sri Lanka is the fact that most young people start drinking carelessly and recklessly whilst at college, often due to peer pressure. This type of drinking is seen especially at the various 'big' school cricket encounters, often resulting in antisocial behaviour. A further factor encouraging this type of drinking is the fact that the alumni of these schools celebrate these occasions annually in reminiscing about their younger days, and also joining in the fun and frolic with excessive drinking, and often paying scant respect to social norms. The students therefore unwittingly imitate their elders and end up in much trouble in fights and with the law.

In the universities too, this pattern is observable, especially at the annual Conventions, Convocations and 'Colours Nights.' Although often this pattern of drinking appears to be a passing phase in normal growth, there are a significant number, like the author, who ultimately 'progress' into alcoholism.

A new feature that has further encouraged increased drinking is the ever-expanding and profitable tourist industry. To cater to the enormous influx of tourists, the hotel trade too has expanded considerably, thereby opening up more outlets for drinking (Tables 5.6, 5.7).

Although a large number of these tourists usually come to Sri Lanka on short holidays, there are a significant number, including the 'hippies', who stay over for very long periods and some have even made Sri Lanka their

Table 5.6 Tourists arrivals in Sri Lanka (by purpose of visit)

	Number of tourists		
Purpose of visit	1977	1978	1979
Holiday	144 148	177 824	227 218
Business (official and private)	6 221	11 651	18 131
Other	3 296	3 117	4 815

Source: Ceylon Tourist Board

Table 5.7   Employment in tourist industry

Category of establishment	Number of establishments		Total employees	
	1978	1979	1978	1979
Hotels and restaurants	194	203	10 066	11 834
Travel agents etc	118	140	2 267	2 831
Airlines	14	16	982	1 147
Agencies providing recreational facilities	11	13	84	84
Tourists shops	125	172	1 661	2 195
National Tourist Organization	1	1	344	381

Source: Ceylon Tourist Board

permanent residence. The majority of these persons have adapted themselves to the local style of living and to drinking local liquor including the illicit brews.

The problem worries physicians, psychiatrists, social workers, business and industry, trade unions, the clergy, counsellors, the legal profession, the lay public and the government, and continues to assume alarming proportions.

The enormous scale in which alcohol is consumed is revealed by the figures for profit on the sale of arrack (the popular cheaper licensed distilled spirit) alone annually from 1966/67 to 1973, shown in Table 5.8.

Table 5.8   Profit on sale of arrack (Rs. Mn.)

1966/67	107
1967/68	110
1968/69	110
1969/70	124
1970/71	149
1971/72 (15 months)	305
1973	220

Source: Estimates of Revenue and Expenditure of the Government.

Further details of production, sales and prices of liquor, and Government revenue from this source, are given in Tables 5.9–5.16.

In Sri Lanka today, a large number of people are wholly or partly dependent on the manufacture and sale of alcoholic beverages for their livelihood (Table 5.17).

However, the demand far outstrips the supply of legally-distilled alcohol especially for arrack and toddy which are the cheaper and more popular licensed liquors, and this has encouraged a flourishing and lucrative industry in

Table 5.9 Sugar industry – alcohol sales

Sales – by-products	Unit	1970	1971	1972	1973	1974	1975	1976	1977
	Bn. Gls.*								
Dry gin		8 031	4 968	10 994	16 650	4 595	5 062	2 971	440
Lemon gin		899	567	1 620	4 093	1 470	826	537	499
Orange gin		450	290	1 193	1 574	510	840	277	419
Brandy (STD)		13 002	8 048	10 342	13 178	5 475	7 864	7 255	6 459
Whiskey		1 033	118	481	995	2 184	1 286	1 105	762
Rum (white)		691	437	818	1 290	2 507	726	305	100
Finest blend arrack		8 109	8 650	23 475	32 465	77 117	90 856	57 879	39 319
Special white arrack								4 486	9 319
Cane arrack								10 766	64 938
Orange Liquor								230	25
Brandy (very special)								200	260
Rum (red)								2 206	1 831
Methylated spirits	Bottles			272 379	249 357	558 228	487 158	854 077	641 592

* 1 000 000 000 gallons = 45 460 000 hectolitres

Table 5.10 Sri Lanka Sugar Corporation – annual output of alcohol

	Unit	1975	1976	1977	1978	1979
Kantalai Factory						
Spirits	kilolitres	1 145	2 594	3 274	2 645	3 466
Gal Oya Factory						
Spirits	kilolitres	1 362	3 998	2 440	3 270	3 211
Dry gin	litres	20 962	17 484	17 281	32 026	38 575
Lemon gin	litres	3 510	1 005	3 214	4 981	10 492
Orange gin	litres	1 082	–	1 282	940	1 298
Beehive Brandy	litres	35 596	31 236	30 115	88 917	44 384
Gregson's Whiskey	litres	3 578	4 010	3 578	10 639	10 971
Rum	litres	10 401	723	8 192	30 592	33 415
Arrack	litres	428 551	324 407	265 426	357 130	538 946

Source: Statistical Pocket Book, Department of Census and Statistics and Ministry of Plan Implementation, 1980

Table 5.11 Sri Lanka Sugar Corporation – spirits production and sales (in thousand gallons)

	1976	1977	1978	1979
Kantalai				
Production	571	720	581	178
Sales	621	678	571	192
Gal Oya				
Production	879	548	705	758
Sales	902	524	706	772

Source: Review of the Economy, 1979 – Central Bank of Ceylon

Table 5.12 State Distilleries Corporation – production and sales (proof gallons) of arrack (seeduwa)

	1975	1976	1977	1978	1979
Production	306 089	456 609	41 703	514 727	1 442 522
Sales	306 089	456 609	41 703	514 727	1 204 505

Source: Review of the Economy, 1979 – Central Bank of Ceylon

the manufacture and sale of cheap, potent illicit brews. These are:

(1) Pot arrack (or 'Kasippu' as it is popularly termed) – so called because an earthenware vessel resembling a pot was used in its manufacture. It was a cottage industry in the very early days. The process of manufacture was by condensing of steam emanating from a pot of boiling toddy (or more recently 'sugar cane juice') into another vessel.

(2) Tea Cider – brewed with tea leaves and fermented with yeast. This constitutes a very potent drink.

(3) Other brews: plantain skins, orange peel, pineapple shavings, dates, potatoes and other assorted substances are used, the products carrying identifiable names. In recent times, unscrupulous manufacturers use substances such as cement, battery acids, methylated spirits and barbed wire, and these are highly poisonous.

Most of these brews, carrying popular brand names, are made surreptitiously, and often in the jungles or scrub land, not easily accessible to the law, under very crude and unhygienic conditions, so that they are highly contaminated with various potent substances seriously injurious to the drinker's health, thereby also posing an increasingly grave national health hazard.

Table 5.13   Government revenue from liquor taxes (in rupees)

	1971/72	1973	1974	1975	1976	1977	1978	1979
Arrack tavern rents	21 098 054	19 332 862	21 758 101	26 340 558	24 381 429	19 043 426	21 486 126	31 252 253
Toddy tavern rents	9 389 279	8 336 156	8 861 734	8 523 261	8 335 045	7 889 086	5 117 280	5 299 383
Tapping licence fee	184 132	92 862	114 112	343 645	278 181	178 880	126 178	113 292
Country liquor licence fee	1 073 140	1 155 560	983 701	673 402	1 425 493	885 221	1 032 588	1 177 116
Foreign liquor tavern rents	127 647	11 468	222 935	486 416	116 401	216 964	1 029 898	1 075 813
Foreign liquor licence fee	750 266	156 290	228 063	12 459	481 739	245 546	314 418	694 899

Source: Estimates of Revenue and Expenditure of the Government of Ceylon

Table 5.14 Sale price of arrack as at 21.2.1980* (in rupees and cents)

Quality	By the glass		Per 750 ml	As sealed bottles	
	Per 100 ml	Per 50 ml		Per 375 ml	Per 185 ml
	Rs cts	Rs cts	Rs cts	Rs cts	Rs cts
1. Special arrack	3 40	1 70	25 50	12 75	6 40
2. Coconut arrack	3 90	1 95	29 25	14 65	7 35

* In Foreign Liquor Licensed premises licensed for the sale of liquor to be consumed on the premises

Table 5.15 Sale price of liquor by bottle as at 21.2.1980* (in rupees and cents)

Quality	Alcohol content %	750 ml Rs cts	375 ml Rs cts	185 ml Rs cts
1. Ten-year-old coconut arrack	27—29	50 80		
2. 'Old Seeduwa' (double distilled) arrack	27—29	42 80		
3. Double distilled arrack	27—29	38 80		
4. Very Old Special Arrack	34—36	36 60		
5. Coconut arrack	40—42	27 80	13 90	6 95
6. Special arrack	40—42	24 20	12 10	6 05
7. Seven-year-old arrack	34—36	37 00		
8. Palmyrah arrack		29 80		

* In Foreign Liquor Retail (Off) Licensed premises licensed for the sale of liquor by bottle only

Table 5.16 Government revenue from liquor (in rupees)

Year	Duty on country-made liquor*	Duty on other country liquor
1971/72	27 380 659	1 785 477
1973	24 481 906	2 551 057
1974	19 523 212	196 416 259
1975	17 774 788	188 361 806
1976	23 062 177	167 220 955
1977	32 103 602	208 879 740
1978	36 001 824	518 627 011
1979	49 895 912	448 158 044

* Includes revenue from beer, gin, rum and rectified spirits
Source: Estimates of Revenue and Expenditure of the Government of Ceylon

Table 5.17 Employment in liquor-related industry

	1975	1976	1977	1978	1979
Sri Lanka Sugar Corporation	3068	3705	4023	5162	
State Distilleries Corporation	149	n.a.	160	1410	1449

At present there are in Sri Lanka over 350 hotels, 400 retail sales points and 100 taverns where licensed liquor is available at restricted hours for sale and/or consumption. The illicit consumption which, therefore, is apt greatly to exceed the amount of licensed liquor consumed, is also associated on the one hand with traditional production for home consumption and, on the other, with the circumstances that curtail the establishment of increased retail sales points, restricted times of sales together with recent rapid price increases. Further, the illicit trade (including unlicensed social clubs, boutiques, gaming joints etc.) has now mushroomed in every part of the country to meet the escalating demand of the ever-increasing clientele who appear to have been forced by necessity to switch over to a cheaper drink.

Although stern legal measures are enforced to combat the manufacture, transportation and sales of these illicit brews, the turnover in terms of money income far exceeds the comparatively negligible costs of being prosecuted and fines imposed by the courts.

Drinking alcoholic liquor has now become an inescapable part of public and private life, an invariable accompaniment of births, marriages, deaths, business deals, conferences and similar occasions, and is so interwoven into the social life of the community that rarely does one meet a person who does not drink. It was also no uncommon thing in the past for prominent members to come into parliament intoxicated. Presently, however, a healthy trend has been established by Government in ensuring that a code of ethics is observed by public officers and other public figures both at public and other functions.

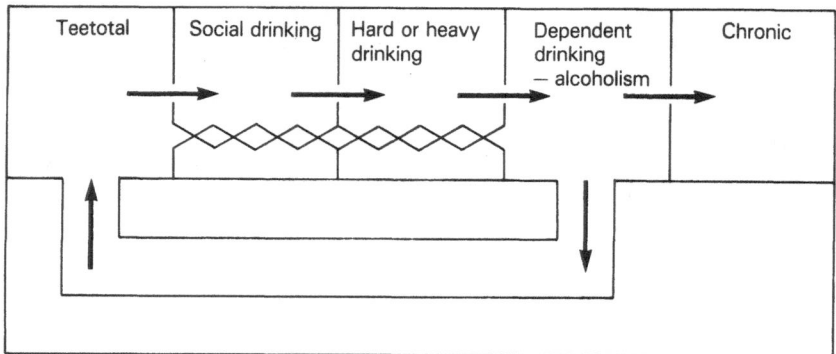

Figure 5.1

For an appreciation of the alcohol problem, it is well to recognize the different types of drinkers. The following classification gives a rough estimation regarding the individual's attitude toward alcohol:

(1)   Moderate drinkers (acceptable in many but not all human groups)

(2)   Excessive drinkers
    (a) occasional intemperate
    (b) habitual heavy
    (c) alcohol addicts − compulsive or dependent − alcoholics
    (d) symptomatic
    (e) chronic

The factors that encourage alcoholism in Sri Lanka appear to be:

(1)   weakened social patterns and kinship ties due to deculturation by Western influences (see Appendix),
(2)   drinking being synonymous with hospitality and social functioning,
(3)   difficult living conditions,
(4)   increased production of licensed liquors,
(5)   proliferation of illicit liquor distilleries,
(6)   non-disapproval of drunkenness and drunken-aggressive behaviour,
(7)   breakdown of the family unit,
(8)   disintegration of spiritual values,
(9)   lack of educational programmes,
(10) sudden influx of wealth to a fair section of the people.

When I describe alcoholism or alcohol dependency, I am referring to a pattern of drinking behaviour which differs from what I regard as normal drinking behaviour. In fact, not only are many people remarkable for their intemperate use of intoxicating liquors, but intemperance appears to have already entered into and formed part of our new national culture.

Although no island-wide survey on alcoholism has so far been done, the Department of Psychiatry of the University of Sri Lanka had carried out a community survey of alcoholism at Etul Kotte, an urban area on the outskirts of the City of Colombo, in 1974. The survey revealed a prevalence rate of 6.5 per 1000, and as there were no female alcoholics, this figure is reported to be equivalent to 13.1 per 1000 of the male population.

It is interesting to mention here that the Sunday newspaper *Weekend*, in its issue of 18 February 1979, revealed the following findings of its 'Insight' team:

'While in many government departments drunkenness has become rampant, the incidence of alcohol being the cause for family strife has risen and so has the incidence of lawlessness due to consumption of liquor. . . .

'In Germany, a country reputed for the drinking habit, only 8 %, or half of Sri Lanka's percentage, are under the influence of liquor while at work. This 15 % is exclusive of those who "spend the day" at the bar. . . .

'There are more than 20 bars within a radius of 2 square miles [5 km²] in the Fort and Pettah, where the greater majority of workers − both State and otherwise, are supposedly working. In Jaffna alone, there are 250 toddy taverns, according to the Excise Commissioner. . . .

'In Colombo, an estimated 5000 gallons of arrack is consumed each day. The volume is only from the six city taverns and not counting the hordes of clubs, bars and retail outlets.'

Regarding the manufacture and sale of illicit brews, this same team reported thus:

'While the government has ensured the closure of arrack taverns between Avissawella and Embilipitiya-Deraniyagala, the 'Insight' team found out how villages from a hamlet in the vicinity of the confluence of the Kelani Ganga and Sitawaka tributary are in the thick of manufacturing Kasippu − "at home". . . . Their business . . . has now become established as a regular means of supplying "spirits" under the various brand names to an estimated 75 000 persons today.'

Besides the general hospitals (State run) which also treat alcoholics for their medical complications, there are two mental hospitals in the out-stations − one at Mulleriyawa, and the other at Angoda − which treat alcoholics as indoor patients too. The psychiatric ward in the general hospital in Colombo treats about 50 alcoholic indoor patients annually. There is also a permanent waiting list of about 25 patients suffering from alcoholism seeking admission as only about two or three beds are allocated for alcoholic patients.

Apart from the effect of alcoholism on the individual, the most immediate and disruptive effect is on the family. Alcoholism is rightly termed a 'family illness' and many families are unable to cope with or withstand the overwhelming crises that arise, and finally disruption of the family unit is inevitable.

In Sri Lanka today, alcoholism appears to be a major cause for many divorces and separations in the family, and the Family Courts which were set up recently to adjudicate matters of family disputes have found that alcohol is a major contributory factor in the majority of cases.

Alcoholism in Sri Lanka continues to take its toll not only on the alcoholic and his family, but also indirectly in other ways, by its contribution to fatal road accidents, crime rates, absenteeism in the workplace and unemployment.

Its effects in the employment field are seen in the below-standard work, the wastage of material and time, the disturbance of morale, damage to equipment and material, increase in labour grievances, and increase in hospital/medical/surgical claims. Its effects in social costs include the costs of hospitals, courts, jails, police, welfare and relief measures.

Table 5.18 shows the factual employment Leave Record of the author during his 'pre-alcoholic', 'alcoholic' and 'recovery' stages, and still in the same employment.

Table 5.18

Year	Casual leave	Vacation leave	Sick leave	No-Pay leave	Duty leave
Pre-alcoholic					
1958	7	29	–	–	$4\frac{1}{2}$
1959	14	$16\frac{1}{2}$	18	1 (strike)	2
1960	14	$16\frac{1}{2}$	6	–	6
1961	14	$9\frac{1}{2}$	–	–	$2\frac{1}{2}$
Alcoholic					
1962	14	13	24	5	–
1963	14	13	24	153*	–
1964	14	$34\frac{1}{2}$	24	17	2
1965	14	22	24	$\begin{cases}30\frac{1}{2}\\63†\end{cases}$	–
1966	14	24	24	$71\frac{1}{2}$	–
1967	14	24	24	29	–
1968	14	24	18	20	–
1969	14	24	24	71	–
1970	14	24	24	19	–
1971	14	24	24	34	–
Recovery					
1972	14	24	18	–	–
1973	14	24	19	–	–
1974	14	24	22	–	–
1975	14	$13\frac{1}{2}$	8	–	–
1976	14	32	18	–	–
1977	14	$20\frac{1}{2}$	$21\frac{1}{2}$	2 (strike)	–
1978	14	30	24	$\frac{1}{2}$	–
1979	14	24	24	$12\frac{1}{2}$	–
1980	14	24	24	4	–

* Extended 'half-pay' leave on account of motor accident necessitating long term hospitalization

† Additional 'half-pay' leave on account of hospitalization

Note: No 'No-pay' leave post-1972 on account of alcoholism i.e. after 'recovery' from alcoholism

Because of the enormous diversity of ethnic and religious backgrounds in this 'melting pot' nation, not to mention the regional and social-class variations, it becomes impossible to generalize about the use and abuse of alcohol in Sri Lanka as a whole. To confound the matter further, people who are interested in the subject tend traditionally to approach it in a partisan spirit, turning deaf ears to scientific findings. This much can be agreed upon, however – the earlier stereotype of the alcoholic as a marginal and hopeless derelict has been considerably revised. Nevertheless, the havoc caused by alcoholism is colossal. The steadily increasing incidence of the disease is threatening to reach epidemic proportions. Yet it appears that the magnitude and seriousness of the disease of alcoholism are insufficiently appreciated. Alcoholism as a particularly complicated disease goes far beyond the sphere of medicine. It creates numerous difficulties not only medical, but also psychological, social, economic, legal and spiritual.

The causes of alcoholism are so many and appear in such differing constellations from person to person, that one cannot consider treating alcoholism as if it were a simple illness with an identifiable and specific aetiology, a known course and a proven response to a particular drug or treatment modality. Alcoholism is a result of complex and interacting forces, and the only characteristic shared by most alcoholics appears to be the repeated abuse that acts as a form of 'self-treatment' for the sufferer.

CHALLENGES TO BE MET

There are thus clearly urgent challenges for

(1) early diagnosis,
(2) effective treatment,
(3) rehabilitation,
(4) education and
(5) prevention.

Diagnosis

The early diagnosis of alcoholism is however, not made any easier by the secretive attitude of the alcoholic, and often the relatives and friends who mistakingly shield him and in industry cover up for him. Very often alcoholics seek treatment for complications arising out of alcoholism, vehemently 'denying' their excessive consumption of liquor, thus misleading the physician as to the actual condition.

The definition and recognition of typical traits of personality can however, be very helpful for correct diagnosis.

Treatment

Unfortunately, in Sri Lanka there are no specific detoxification centres. At present, affluent alcoholics generally seek either inpatient or outpatient medical treatment in private hospitals or nursing homes, not necessarily for alcoholism, which they 'deny' (denial syndrome), but mostly for the various physical complications arising out of their excessive consumption of alcoholic beverages.

Many of the less fortunate also seek either inpatient or outpatient treatment in the medical wards of the State hospitals, also mainly for the physical complications arising out of their excessive and prolonged consumption of alcoholic beverages − 'denying' their 'dependence' on alcohol.

However, many do seek inpatient treatment for alcoholism in the State mental hospitals and the psychiatric clinics in the State hospitals.

The disadvantage here is that the 'ordinary' addicts are also mixed up with the 'psychopathic' alcoholics, so that the specialized treatment so necessary for alcoholics cannot be afforded. Further, there is also the disadvantage that not all patients are alcoholics, and alcoholics are accommodated and treated along with both drug addicts and other psychiatric patients, and whose conditions and behaviour may alternate from mild to severe or violent.

Even where alcoholics seek outpatient treatment at the psychiatric clinics of the State hospitals, the present shortage of staff and lack of the necessary facilities and time act as deterrents to the special attention and treatment needed.

It should be mentioned here that besides the normal scientific medical treatment available, many persons, especially in the villages, resort to treatment from 'Kattadiyas' (a type of witch doctor) who perform complicated, tedious, psychologically exacting and costly ceremonies − 'devil dancing' or 'thovil' ceremonies − which include the use of fire, the loud beating of drums and various other rituals including the loud chanting of various stanzas ('charms') and the dancing of the 'Kattadiya' around the patient.

These 'Kattadiyas' attempt to invoke the assistance of the various deities to drive away the 'evil spirits' supposedly haunting the patient − the patient being said to be 'possessed' of the 'evil spirit.'

At the end of the ceremonies, which may last from about 2 or 3 days to a week, a yellow 'charmed' thread is usually tied round the arm of the patient by the 'Kattadiya'. This thread is supposed to ward off any maleficent influences.

The following types of the more scientific treatment are however, generally used:

(1)   conditioned reflex aversion,
(2)   psychotherapy,
(3)   acupuncture,
(4)   disulfiram (Antabuse),
(5)   chemotherapy,
(6)   Alcoholics Anonymous.

The first three modalities are generally centred in a hospital environment.

Rehabilitation

In the case of rehabilitation, very unfortunately, in Sri Lanka we have no 'half-way' houses, rehabilitation centres or the like. Therefore alcoholics, treated in a hospital environment, on returning home are faced with the former domestic, job and environmental problems which they have not learned to cope with or withstand, and thus many do relapse into drinking.

However, groups of Alcoholics Anonymous for the alcoholic, and the Al-Anon family groups for the family and friends of the alcoholic are spread around the City of Colombo, Kandy and in Wennappuwa, and are the mainstay of the many alcoholics in their 'sobriety.'

Alcoholics Anonymous and Al-Anon family groups have also been formed at the psychiatric ward of the General Hospital in Colombo, and an Al-Ano club has been established in Wennappuwa. This Club, besides affording space for the meetings of the AA and Al-Anon groups, also provides recreational and other facilities for alcoholics. Alcoholics Anonymous groups claim a successful recovery rate of around 50%.

Besides the above facilities, the author has also kept 'open-house' at his home where alcoholics and their families can meet regularly to enable them to integrate more closely in a 'homely' environment — a neglected but essential element in rehabilitation.

Education

A vital factor in the treatment and rehabilitation of the alcoholic is the education not only of the alcoholic but also the alcoholic's family and those close to him. Further, on the primary preventive side, it is essential that public education programmes aimed not only at the adult public, but also young people, especially at school level, be organized with special stress not so much on alcoholism education but especially on alcohol education.

Unfortunately in Sri Lanka there are no Alcoholism Information Centres or the like to assist in this vital aspect. The 'National Council on Alcoholism' which started somewhere in 1972 wound up somewhere in 1973; the 'Ceylon Association for the Rehabilitation of Alcoholics' which also started about the same time, ceased prematurely.

Efforts are continuing to be made by organizations like the National Temperance Movement and the National Temperance Association of the Seventh Day Adventists, both strong advocates of total abstinence and prohibition. Total abstinence from alcohol, drugs, tobacco and beef is also being strongly advocated by temple organizations and the temperance societies formed in a number of government departments and Buddhist schools, especially in these schools where the young people are organized to take an oath to refrain from using alcohol, drugs, tobacco and beef for the rest of their lives. But it appears that in a changing religious atmosphere, their former influence has waned. However, they remain an essential link in the chain of action against the products concerned.

Interest in this field has also been shown by the Department of Social Services, the School of Social Studies, the Sri Lanka Sumithrayo (a branch of Befrienders International), the Sarvodaya, the Family Services Institute, the Family Counselling Centre of the National Council of Churches and other social service organizations.

On the other hand, Alcoholics Anonymous, a fellowship of recovering alcoholics, and Al-Anon, a fellowship of spouses, relatives and friends of alcoholics are working quietly and with considerable effect, being interested only in people with drinking problems and their families.

AA does not preach temperance, but through open public meetings aided by extensive newspaper reports it has proved that alcoholism is a disease that can be 'arrested.'

Starting from a single group with a handful of members conversing only in English in 1962, AA has now six groups in the City of Colombo, one group in Kandy (72 miles (115 km) from Colombo city) and one group in Wennappuwa (36 miles (57 km) from Colombo city). The Wennappuwa group is necessarily a Sinhala-speaking group.

There are also Al-Anon groups functioning in these three centres.

Notwithstanding the above developments which can hardly scratch the surface, it was the firm conviction of the author, that there still was a gaping void in this field. Motivated by the fact that he was a 'recovered' alcoholic, and accepting the 'challenge' to open more avenues to tackle this problem, the 'Alcoholism Information Service' was started privately, in the belief that health education directed toward increasing public awareness of the use and abuse of alcohol can help as a deterrent to the emergence of problem drinking and alcoholism.

Literature in English, Sinhala and Tamil was published and issued free of charge.

It was also possible to organize for the first time in December 1974 a 'Seminar on Alcoholism' under the distinguished patronage of the then Deputy Minister of Defence and Foreign Affairs, Mr Lakshman Jayakoddy, MP and Chairman, Sri Lanka Narcotics Bureau, where the various disciplines of clergy, both Buddhist and Christian, legal, medical, counselling and AA were represented.

Up to date the author, as Director/Counselor of the Alcoholism Information Service, has been involved in making the subject of alcoholism better understood and has been commended by Mr Yvelin Gardner of the National Council on Alcoholism in the United States as a 'One-Man National Council'.

However, this Service has its limitations especially financially as it is run on the author's personal finances.

For the first time in the history of the trade union movement in Sri Lanka, the Central Bank Employees' Independent Trade Union was able to venture into the field of alcoholism with special reference to the labour force due to the singular efforts of the author who was its Honorary Secretary, Occupational Health (Alcoholism), and has thus far conducted a number of seminars.

Due to his involvement in the trades union field, the author was able to establish, for the first time in Sri Lanka, the 'Sri Lanka National Trades Unions Council on Alcoholism' representing a number of the major trade unions at the first 'Sri Lanka National Trades Unions' Seminar on Alcoholism' held under the patronage of the Hon. the Deputy Minister of Trade and Shipping, Mr M. S. Amarasiri MP on 9 and 10 June 1979.

The Honourable Minister among other things said that 'the liquor menace had retarded the Government's development work. . . . Despite the fact that we have a number of world religions that denounce consumption of liquor, the spirits have made us more "spiritual" in this field. . . . I view this Seminar on Alcoholism as an important event and therefore, I am hopeful that the outcome of this Seminar would bring about some solutions to the question of Alcoholism. . . .'

As President of this Council, the author has delivered talks at a number of education seminars organized by the various trade unions in Sri Lanka. An encouraging feature is that the government-sponsored trade union – the Jathika Sevaka Sangamaya – too has included the subject of alcoholism in its trade union education seminars where the author is involved.

It should be mentioned that the Trades Unions Council on Alcoholism was established owing to a generous financial grant given by the International Federation of Commercial, Clerical and Technical Employees (FIET) in Geneva, through its Secretary for Regional Activities, Mr Hans J. Schwass. Further, FIET and its affiliates together with the generous assistance of Dr Eva Tongue, Assistant Director of the International Council on Alcohol and Addictions, had also helped the author to attend both the 24th and 25th International Institutes on the Prevention and Treatment of Alcoholism held in Zurich in 1978 (where he read a paper) and in Tours (France) in 1979.

Special mention must also be made of Mr Gary R. Nebeker, Assistant Director, Department of International Affairs of the United Food and Commercial Workers' International Union in Washington, DC for all the encouragement and special assistance afforded to the author in this field.

Prior to the formation of the Sri Lanka National Trades Unions Council on Alcoholism the author had already felt an urgent need to subscribe positively to the multidisciplinary approach to this problem of alcoholism, and steps were therefore taken to form a national association. The inaugural meeting comprising a select group of prominent interested persons was held on 5 March 1979, at the Holiday Inn in Colombo – the new association being called the Sri Lanka National Association on Alcohol and Drug Dependence.

The official inauguration of the Association and induction of office-bearers took place at a seminar at the Galle Face Hotel in Colombo on 22 March 1980.

The Honourable Minister of Health, Mr Gamini Jayasuriya MP, who was inducted Patron of the Association, declared that '. . . . the formation of this Association was very significant as the problem of alcoholism and drug dependence were assuming formidable proportions.' He said that he was appreciative of the keenness displayed by the Association and emphasized the importance of a citizens' organization like it to tackle the problem.

Following this seminar, a 'Resource Persons Educational Seminar on Alcoholism and Drug Dependence', in collaboration with the Drug Advisory Programme of the Colombo Plan through the good offices of Attorney Pio A. Abarro, Drug Adviser, Colombo Plan countries, and sponsored by Hotel Lanka Oberoi, was held on 20 September 1980, under the distinguished patronage of the Hon. the Deputy Minister of Defence and Chairman, Narcotics Control Board of Sri Lanka, Mr T. B. Werapitiya, MP.

Among other things the Minister said: 'I must also very specially thank the Sri Lanka National Association on Alcohol and Drug Dependence for taking the initiative in organizing this very valuable Seminar in collaboration with the Colombo Plan Bureau. The Sri Lanka National Association on Alcohol and Drug Dependence which was formed recently, has to its credit, during the last few months of its existence several very worthwhile programmes conducted by them. In fact, I have had very good reports of their activities in the twin fields of prevention of alcoholism and drug dependence. . . . the Government alone cannot tackle this problem. It needs the support of international organizations and non-governmental bodies to train such personnel. . . . There is a dearth of trained personnel in this country. I think this Seminar fills a long-felt gap in this field.'

The Association is now, among its other activities, carrying out an intensive education programme, especially in the schools island-wide.

To enable more disciplines to be involved in this field, which is vitally necessary, the author set about organizing a clergy council inviting the various clergy especially from the Christian denominations, and on 12 January 1981, with the assistance of the Sri Lanka National Association on Alcohol and Drug Dependence and the Colombo Young Men's Christian Association, the first 'Sri Lanka National Christian Clergy Seminar on Alcoholism' was held under the patronage of the Right Reverend Oswald Gomis, Bishop of Colombo.

The Bishop among other things remarked: 'One reason for the fact that the clergy here are not involved as they should be in helping alcoholics is because they need more knowledge of alcoholism to do something really effective. . . . This will then form the spring-board for definite action to overcome the problems of alcohol.'

Subsequent to this seminar, the first Sri Lanka National Christian Clergy Council on Alcoholism was established in June 1981. One of the aims of the Clergy Council is to 'educate the clergy on alcoholism, and to foster and promote educational, counselling, spiritual and pastoral care of alcoholics and their families'.

The official inauguration of the Council and induction of the office-bearers was held at a seminar sponsored by De Rance Inc., of Wisconsin in the United States of America, on 24 October 1981.

The author is at present the Council's *pro-tem* Honorary Secretary. He is also the Honorary Secretary/Treasurer of the Sri Lanka National Association on Alcohol and Drug Dependence. Professionally, he is a Staff Assistant attached to the Central Bank of Ceylon.

As an initial step in its educational programmes at parish level, a seminar on alcoholism under the aegis of the Cottage Group of St Mary's Church, Dehiwela, was held on 30 June 1981. Similar programmes will also be organized in the various parishes throughout the island.

It is also the author's plan now to invite (1) business and industry, (2) drug manufacturers and (3) banks (both State and private) to form similar associations.

It is therefore the author's fervent prayer that the more affluent organizations in the developed countries would give their fullest support especially financially, not only for the expansion of the present organizations but also for the opening up of more avenues in this much neglected public health field.

APPENDIX

'The onset of the disintegration of Ceylon found expression in different facets of national life; apart from . . . there came the gradual inflow of Western social customs until their adoption became the fashion . . . the ancient religion and way of life were on the eve of displacement and dissolution. . . .

'But the scandal had grown that legislation was introduced to diminish the sale of liquor; among the addicts were women and children.

'There is one subject which I cannot be silent and that is the extension of drunkenness throughout the island. English rule has given to Ceylon . . . but we have at the same time extended a curse throughout the island, which weighs heavily on the other scale namely, drunkenness. . . .

'Drunkenness is gradually extending itself to the villages, where it was unheard of before, and even women are accustoming themselves to intoxicating drink.

'To wear Western dress, to eat Western food, to drink liquor of Western brew became a hall-mark of distinction.'

(N. E. Weerasooriya (1971). *Ceylon and Her People*. Vol. III, pp. 225–228. (Ceylon: Colombo Printers).)

6
Alcohol-drinking habits of the Israeli public

H. BAR and R. BAUMAL

1. INTRODUCTION

The consumption of alcoholic beverages, and especially wine, has been a widespread phenomenon ever since the early days of humanity. Apart from its nutritional and medical value, alcohol was – and still is – used in religious worship and rituals. In addition to its social function, abuse of alcoholic beverages is also widespread, and hence a source of concern, reference to which may be found both in our own sources (e.g. the story of Noah and his daughters) as well as in other cultures such as the Greek mythology.

The excessive and problematic use of alcoholic drinks, whether in private or on cultural and social occasions, has always been a difficult health and social problem which requires intervention. Alcoholism, which is a consequential phenomenon of exaggerated use of alcoholic drinks, and common to all social strata, constitutes today one of the most serious medical and social problems both in Western society and in Eastern (Communist) society. In the USA, for instance, this problem comes next to heart disease, cancer and mental illness.

Alcoholism is not only the problem of the user himself, but also that of his environment and especially his family, and hence the number of people harmed by alcoholism, directly or indirectly, is much greater than that of the actual abusers.

A matter which greatly adds to the severity of the problem is the inclination of abusers to deny and/or ignore their condition, and thus delay applying for help for many years. (Indeed, according to a survey conducted by the Unit for the Prevention of Alcoholism, it appears that an average of 19 years elapses between the starting of heavy drinking and applying for help.)

In Israel, alcoholism is not as widespread as in other Western countries, and up to recently there has been a tendency to ignore the problem, on account of the myth that alcoholism does not exist among Jews.

About 10 years ago, the Ministry of Labor and Welfare (then the Ministry of Social Welfare) set up a unit for the prevention of alcoholism, which presently operates ten anti-alcoholism centres throughout the country, and which has to date treated 1800 alcoholics and their families.

The present study was conducted at the request of the Unit for the Prevention of Alcoholism at the Ministry of Labor and Welfare, and was prompted by the lack of sufficient and reliable information regarding drinking habits (attitudes and behaviours) of the Israeli public. Though this unit has some information on those who apply for treatment, it is not sufficient for throwing light on the drinking habits of the general public − which is the objective of this study.

An additional and very important aspect of the present study is to examine the scope, nature and extent of the problem related to use of alcoholic beverages in the general public (versus the help-seeking population) in order to locate the population at risk, throw light on its specific characteristics and help in assessing the extent of the problem in Israel.

To the best of our knowledge, this is the first time findings have been published in Israel regarding the Israeli adult Jewish population (excluding kibbutzim) − hence the importance of this preliminary comprehensive survey which, incidentally, will serve as a point of departure for further studies on this topic.

The research objectives

These are

(1)   To study assessments and perceptions of the public regarding drinking of alcoholic beverages − with respect to customs, motives and consequences.

(2)   To study the scope, nature and extent of the problematics related to use of alcoholic beverages among the Israeli public.

(3)   To attempt to specify the characteristics of populations at risk, and not only from the aspect of actual alcohol abuse.

(4)   To attempt to assess the problem of alcoholism in Israel in order to assist the responsible bodies and the treatment agencies in their planning of operations.

The sample, and data collection

The findings reported in this study are based on the Continuing Survey* of the Israel Institute of Applied Social Research, conducted from 14 February to 22 March 1982. In this framework 1033 respondents were interviewed in 34

* The Continuing Survey of the Israel Institute of Applied Social Research is conducted jointly with the Hebrew University Communications Institute

The mapping sentence

Respondent(s) assesses the extent of $\begin{Bmatrix} A \\ \text{actual} \\ \text{potential} \end{Bmatrix}$ $\begin{Bmatrix} B \\ \text{use} \\ \text{knowledge} \\ \text{positive attitude} \\ \text{readiness} \\ \text{recognition} \end{Bmatrix}$

of $\begin{Bmatrix} C \\ \text{self} \\ \text{spouse} \\ \text{family member} \\ \text{youth in general} \\ \text{others} \\ \text{treating agencies} \\ \text{in general} \end{Bmatrix}$ regarding the $\begin{Bmatrix} D \\ \text{harm} \\ \text{benefit} \\ \text{in general} \end{Bmatrix}$ of $\begin{Bmatrix} E \\ \text{situation} \\ \text{treatment} \\ \text{in general} \end{Bmatrix}$

of $\begin{Bmatrix} F \\ \text{self} \\ \text{family members} \\ \text{others} \\ \text{'drinkers'} \\ \text{society} \\ \text{in general} \end{Bmatrix}$ with respect to $\begin{Bmatrix} G \\ \text{drinking} \\ \text{cessation of drinking} \end{Bmatrix}$ of $\begin{Bmatrix} H \\ \text{one} \\ \text{more than one} \end{Bmatrix}$

$\begin{Bmatrix} I \\ \text{small glass} \\ \text{bottle} \end{Bmatrix}$ of $\begin{Bmatrix} J \\ \text{wine} \\ \text{beer} \\ \text{alcoholic drinks} \end{Bmatrix}$ at frequency of $\begin{Bmatrix} K \\ \text{regular — daily} \\ \text{weekly} \\ \text{monthly} \\ \text{occasional} \end{Bmatrix}$

$\begin{Bmatrix} L \\ \text{alone} \\ \text{in company} \end{Bmatrix}$ for motive of $\begin{Bmatrix} M \\ \text{personal — ease tention} \\ \text{relaxation} \\ \text{improving mood} \\ \text{pleasure} \\ \text{familial} \\ \text{social — social affiliation} \\ \text{ease loneliness} \\ \text{personal-physical — ease pain} \\ \text{blood circulation} \\ \text{treatment of cold} \end{Bmatrix}$

$\begin{Bmatrix} N \\ \text{routine} \\ \text{festive occasion} \\ \text{religious ritual} \\ \text{mourning} \\ \text{driving} \\ \text{unspecified} \end{Bmatrix}$ $\begin{Bmatrix} O \\ \text{at home} \\ \text{in coffee house} \\ \text{in restaurant} \\ \text{community anti-alcoholic centre} \\ \text{general hospital} \\ \text{mental hospital} \\ \text{mental health centre} \\ \text{social welfare bureau} \end{Bmatrix}$

$\longrightarrow \begin{Bmatrix} \text{positive} \\ \text{to} \\ \text{negative} \end{Bmatrix}$ assessment, with respect to drinking of alcoholic drinks.

settlements throughout the country, which constitutes a representative sample of the Jewish adult (20 +) population.*

During each interview, which took place in the respondent's home, the questions were posed to the respondent and his answers recorded on the spot by a team of trained interviewers. The work of the interviewers, which was performed under direct supervision of local fieldwork supervisors, was checked and verified for reliability at several stages of the fieldwork.

The content universe of the study

The main study variables were based on a theoretical basis which encompassed the topic of alcoholic drinking and the study objectives. The content universe of the aspects related to this comprehensive topic is formulated by means of a mapping sentence, as follows.

Upon analysing the findings and re-examining the universe of the investigated contents, changes were introduced in the mapping sentence, then revised for reading as follows.

$$
\text{Respondent(s) expresses}
\begin{Bmatrix} A \\ \text{instrumental} \\ \text{cognitive} \\ \text{affective} \end{Bmatrix}
\begin{Bmatrix} B \\ \text{attitude} \\ \text{involvement} \end{Bmatrix}
\text{of}
\begin{Bmatrix} C \\ \text{self} \\ \text{others} \end{Bmatrix}
\text{regarding}
$$

$$
\text{situation of}
\begin{Bmatrix} D \\ \text{self} \\ \text{others} \\ \text{in general} \end{Bmatrix}
\text{with respect to}
\begin{Bmatrix} E \\ \text{always problematic} \\ \text{sometimes problematic} \\ \text{non-problematic} \end{Bmatrix}
$$

$$
\text{drinking of alcoholic drinks at frequency of}
\begin{Bmatrix} F \\ \text{regular} - \text{daily} \\ \text{weekly} \\ \text{monthly} \\ \text{occasional} \end{Bmatrix}
$$

$$
\begin{Bmatrix} G \\ \text{alone} \\ \text{in company} \\ \text{in general} \end{Bmatrix}
\text{for motive of}
\begin{Bmatrix} H \\ \text{personal-physical} - \text{general health} \\ \text{ease pain} \\ \text{psychological} - \text{ease tension} \\ \text{relaxation} \\ \text{improve mood} \\ \text{pleasure} \\ \text{social} - \text{social affiliation} \\ \text{ease loneliness} \end{Bmatrix}
$$

$$
\text{in framework of}
\begin{Bmatrix} I \\ \text{festive occasion} \\ \text{religious ritual} \\ \text{mourning} \\ \text{driving} \\ \text{unspecified} \end{Bmatrix}
\longrightarrow
\begin{Bmatrix} \text{high} \\ \text{to} \\ \text{low} \end{Bmatrix}
\text{assessment}
$$

with respect to drinking of alcoholic drinks.

* Excluding the kibbutz population — 4%

The report structure

Following Section 1, which presents the background and the content universe of the study, are five sections presenting the research findings.

Section 2 deals with the drinking behaviour of the general public, and presents the scope of non-problematic drinking of alcoholic beverages.

Section 3 presents cognitive attitudes of the public regarding the consequences of drinking.

Section 4 deals with the scope of and acquaintance with problematic drinking of alcoholic drinks.

Section 5 presents the relationships between worry with regard to drinking on the one hand, and each of the study variables, on the other.

Section 6 presents the intercorrelations and the structure of interrelationships among the respondents' attitudes on the topic.

Finally, Section 7 is designed to classify population subgroups — those which are more and those which are less liable to drinking — by background characteristics as well as by extent of exposure to alcoholic beverages.

2. DRINKING HABITS

Five per cent of the respondents report consuming alcoholic drinks at least every 2 or 3 days, apart from any drinking on religious occasions. An additional 10% drink approximately once a week. One third of the respondents report no drinking at all (apart from any on religious occasions) and an additional 25% drink only very rarely.

On occasions of social gatherings, about one fourth (24%) of the respondents usually or always serve alcoholic drinks to guests, while at a festive dinner the proportion that usually or always serves alcoholic drinks rises to about one third (33%). Yet a large proportion of the respondents report that they serve alcoholic drinks only very seldom or not at all (62% in social gatherings, and 54% at festive dinners).

Sixteen per cent of the respondents report that they drink alcoholic drinks, at least often, in the framework of rituals related to mourning after the dead.

Drinking on occasions of mourning was found to be related to religious observance: the greater the observance, the higher the extent of drinking on occasions of mourning. Likewise, it was found that such drinking (in mourning) is more prevalent among respondents born in Asia–Africa (24%) than among Israeli-born (13%) or European–American-born (12%) respondents.

Drunkenness is also reported. Fifteen per cent of all respondents, which constitutes 24% of the 'drinking' respondents, report that they themselves have got drunk, even if rarely. Three per cent of the 'drinkers' get drunk at least once a month.

In this study we also attempted to investigate respondents' motives for drinking alcoholic drinks, even if drinking occurs only seldom.

The most frequent motive for drinking was for pleasure, to feel good, and to improve one's good mood (39 % of all respondents, which constitutes 57 % of the 'drinking' respondents).

The second most frequent motive was in order to be accepted in society and not to be exceptional (13 % of all respondents, which constitutes 19 % of the 'drinking' respondents).

15 % of the respondents (22 % of the 'drinkers') report a motive that may be considered a risk, since frequent consumption of alcoholic drinks may result in dependence and even addiction. (It is evident that part of these respondents are already in some such stage.) These motives include:

to improve bad mood, depression	4 %
to relax, to ease tension	3 %
to ease pain	3 %
to escape from worries and forget troubles	2 %
to sleep better at night	2 %
to overcome a feeling of hopelessness or helplessness with regard to the future	1 %

3. THE IMPLICATIONS OF DRINKING

Forty-six per cent of the respondents believe that alcoholic drinks help, a person, at least to a certain extent, to improve his bad mood (63 % of this group think that the help in this sense is small). Only about one fourth of the respondents believe that drinking alcoholic drinks prevents improving a bad mood.

The assessment that alcoholic drinks help a person forget worries and troubles is reported by 38 % of the respondents (over two thirds of this group think that the help in this sense is small). About one fourth of the respondents think that drinking is an impediment to forgetting worries and troubles.

Only 19 % think that drinking an alcoholic beverage helps a person, at least to some extent (the majority of them think the help is small), to be acceptable in society. On the other hand, 45 % think it an impediment.

In the opinion of the Israeli public, drinking is more effective for the purpose of improving a person's mood than for any other purpose. Yet the public believes that drinking, more than anything else, prevents a person from being acceptable in society.

Sixty-one per cent of the population think that drinking has a harmful effect on health, while a great majority (80 %) think that a dose of three small glasses of an alcoholic beverage has a harmful, or even very harmful, effect on the ability to drive a car. Only a very slight proportion think that drinking has a beneficial effect on health and driving, while 25 % think that drinking has no special effect on health and 10 % think it does not affect the ability to drive.

Are there any differences in the assessment of the consequences of drinking among respondents of different sex, age, education, income etc.?

Respondents with little education (0–8 years of schooling), more than those in all the other education brackets, express the opinion that drinking alcoholic drinks hampers a person greatly in forgetting his worries or improving his bad mood, and it is especially harmful to being accepted in society. They also think it is very deleterious to health. However, there are no meaningful differences by education on the assessment of the effect of three small glasses of an alcoholic drink on the ability to drive.

Thus it seems that respondents with little education are more extreme in their negative attitudes toward drinking than respondents of higher education groups, and indeed they abstain from drinking on social occasions — but they get drunk more than the others. In other words, the gap between their attitudes and their personal behaviour is more pronounced than in the other education groups.

Respondents in the youngest age group (20 – 24) more than the middle groups, and much more than the oldest (55 +) age group, think that drinking may help a person forget and escape from his troubles, improve his bad mood and also be acceptable in society.

Respondents in the oldest age group express the most extreme attitudes both regarding the opinion that drinking hampers fulfilling these needs, as well as with regard to its harmful effect on the ability to drive. And indeed, this age group drinks less. In other words they behave in great accord with their extreme attitudes.

There is no disagreement among the various age groups regarding the deleterious effect of drinking on health.

Respondents with high income also behave in accordance with their attitudes. They do not express extreme opinions that drinking hampers fulfilling the various needs, and they believe less than others that drinking is very deleterious to health. But there are no differences between them and the other income groups in their assessments regarding the effect of three small glasses on the ability to drive.

Religious respondents, more than the secular, but also somewhat more than the traditional respondents, think that drinking is harmful to health and to the ability to drive; in their opinion it is also very harmful to being accepted in society, to improving bad mood and also to escaping from worries.

Men, slightly more than women, think that drinking can help, even though to a small extent, in improving bad mood and in making one acceptable in society (but there are no differences between men and women regarding forgetting and escaping from troubles). Furthermore, fewer men than women think that drinking is deleterious, or very deleterious, to health and harmful with respect to the ability to drive.

Respondents of Asian–African origin have more extreme attitudes regarding the effect of drinking on the fulfilment of each of the needs mentioned. However, no meaningful differences were found in the assessments of respondents from different ethnic origin with regard to the influence of drinking on health. Respondents of European–American origin, somewhat more than the others, consider that drinking three small glasses has a very harmful effect on the ability to drive.

As expected, respondents who do not drink often think, more than the others, that drinking is harmful, or very harmful, to being acceptable in society, but also hampers the forgetting of troubles and improvement of bad mood. Likewise they believe, more than the others, that drinking is very harmful to health and to the ability to drive.

It is of interest to note — and difficult to know whether it could have been predicted — that those who drink often think, more than the others, that drinking can even be helpful, mainly in improving bad mood and forgetting troubles, but also in being acceptable in society. Those who drink think, more than the others, that drinking has no special influence on health or on the ability to drive (though the latter to a lesser extent).

Acquaintance with people who drink is also related to the assessment of drinking as a factor in fulfilling needs (except for being acceptable in society, which was found not to be related to acquaintance with people who drink).

A finding which may be surprising is that respondents who know people who drink think (and the more they are acquainted with such people the more they think so) that drinking can help a person improve his bad mood and forget his troubles. They also think less that drinking three small glasses is harmful to driving. In other words, acquaintance with people who drink is a moderating factor in this sense.

As for the effects of drinking on health, there are no meaningful differences by acquaintance with people who drink.

For the relationships between concern and the cognitive attitudes of respondents, see Section 5.

4. DRINKING AS A PROBLEM

When can drinking be perceived as a problem? An answer to this question is not provided here; this study only expresses the Israeli public's attitudes on this topic.

Forty-six per cent of the respondents are certain that a person who drinks alcoholic drinks every day has a drinking problem, and the same is true with regard to a person who drinks by himself in order to relieve tension; only 8 % are certain this is not so (31 % think — as distinct from being certain — that there is a problem, while 15 % think there is not).

Drinking of alcoholic beverages every day is considered by the majority of the respondents to be a problem; however, this fact, which does not take into consideration the quantity and its behavioural implications, cannot serve as an indication of posing a problem. Findings show that 2 % of the Israeli public drink alcoholic beverages every day, and 61 % of the respondents think that regular drinking (at least three times a week) has a bad or very bad effect on health, and this explains the public's attitude to regular drinking.

One of the definitions of the target population of the Unit for the Prevention of Alcoholism of the Ministry of Labor and Welfare is: 'All persons who suffer from their own or from a family member's consumption of alcoholic drinks'. This definition implies that every person who is directly or indirectly involved in the problem related to drinking is entitled to receive aid from the Unit.

Despite the fact that only 2 % of the public drink regularly every day and 5 % drink at least every 2–3 days, 14 % of the public are very worried, or very worried indeed, at the fact that they themselves or one of their family (spouse, parents or children) drink alcoholic drinks – and this finding in itself ought to be a warning against future development of the problem.

The following findings may also be considered as indications of drinking problems in Israel.

(1) 3 % of the respondents report getting drunk about once a month

(2) 29 % of the respondents report acquaintance with at least two people who drink regularly every day

(3) 15 % of the respondents report knowing at least two alcoholics (defined as 'a person who cannot function properly without taking an alcoholic drink every day')

(4) 17 % of the respondents report that they themselves drink (even if only occasionally) for motives which may cause addiction

From the above findings it seems that the assessment made by the Unit for the Prevention of Alcoholism that there are about 7200 alcoholics in Israel is a rather careful assessment; apparently it does not encompass the entire problem in Israel. The findings of this study may hint at an intensification of the problem in the future.

5. WORRY AND ATTITUDES ON THE TOPIC OF DRINKING

This section is designed to provide an answer to the question 'What is the relationship between affective involvement – which is manifested by an expression of worry regarding own or family member's drinking – and attitudes on the topic?'

Involvement in this topic may be of various types. Often, the involvement is cognitive, e.g. giving thought to, research or interest in the topic. Another type is instrumental involvement, e.g. being actively involved, or discussing the problem; still another type (the one to be dealt with here) is affective involvement, e.g. feelings of excitement and happiness, or, in the negative sense, worry.

What then, is the relationship between involvement and attitudes on the topic? There is no reason to assume a monotonic relationship; there is no basis for assuming that increased involvement must be more strongly correlated with positive attitudes than with negative attitudes, or vice versa. The theory of components of scalable attitudes[1–3] proves that one can predict involvement from attitude – but not vice versa – and by politonic relationship[4].

Interrelationships between worry and drinking habits

Abstaining from serving alcoholic drinks among those who seldom or very seldom serve at social gatherings and festive dinners is characteristic similarly of those who are very much worried and those who are not at all worried about the topic.

*Serves alcoholic drinks at every social gathering − very seldom or never:

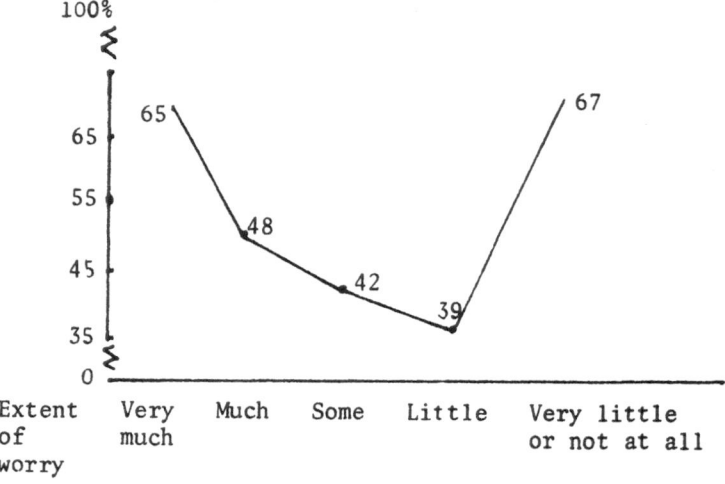

* The following diagrams present graphically one column of percentages from a crosstabulation. For example:

Worried by own or family member's drinking	Serves alcoholic drinks			
	Always or usually	Often	Seldom or never	Total
Very worried	21	14	65	100
Worried to a great extent	27	25	48	100
Worried to a certain extent	29	29	42	100
Worried to a little extent	44	17	39	100
Worried to a very little extent or not at all	21	12	67	100

These percentages are not cumulative and hence do not amount to 100%; therefore, in the graph the connecting line between the percentages is not a summation curve but is intended to help the reader grasp instantly the differences between the groups, and especially to demonstrate the pattern that was found, namely, that the most involved and the least involved are more similar to each other than to the rest of the groups

Serves alcoholic drinks at every festive dinner — very seldom or never:

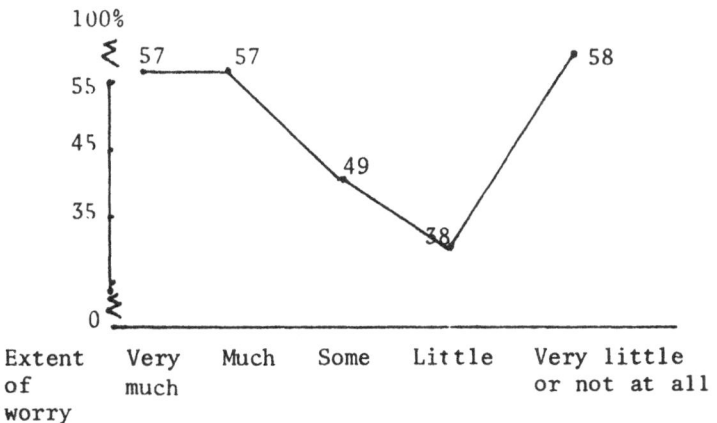

The less the worry (except for the least-worried group, which behaves exactly like the most worried group) the more the inclination to serve alcoholic drinks always or usually at social gatherings.

Serves alcoholic drinks at every social gathering — always or usually:

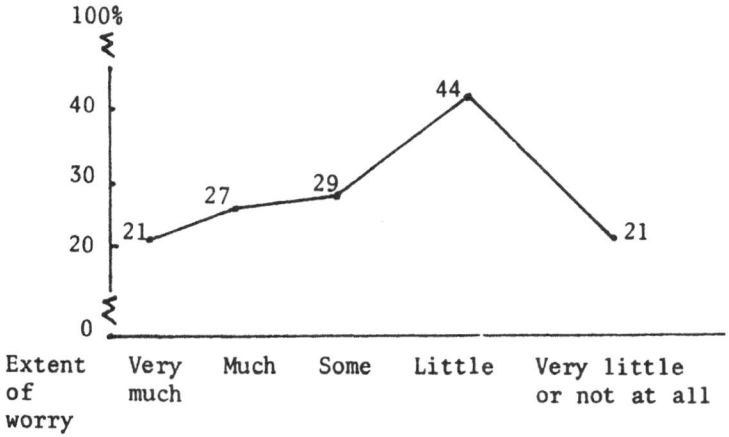

The least and the most worried tend less than the others to serve alcoholic drinks as part of mourning ritual.

Tends to drink alcoholic drinks as part of mourning ritual — seldom or never:

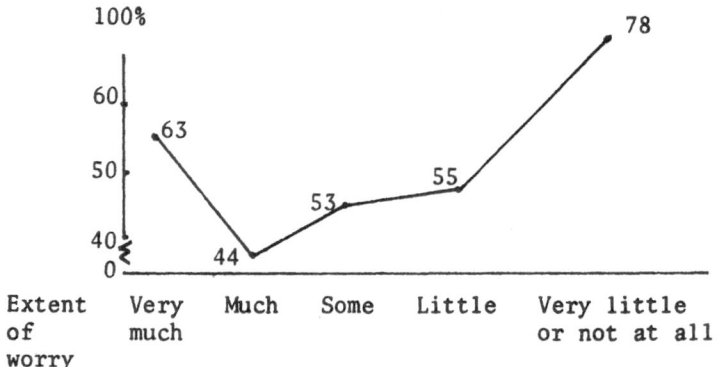

The most worried of own or family member's drinking report more on own abstinence from drinking. (The less one is worried the less one reports on abstinence, except for the least worried group).

Does not drink at all:

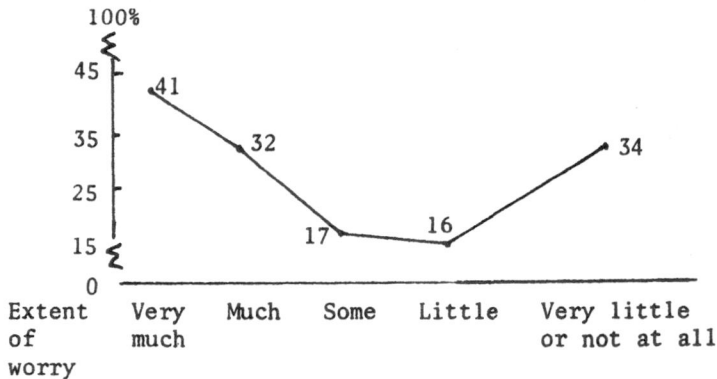

Frequent drinking is more characteristic of the medium groups (*vis-à-vis* worry), and less so of the extremely worried groups.

Drinks at least once a week:

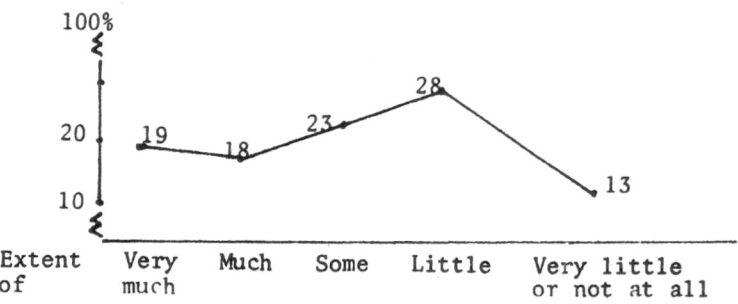

Also with regard to the motives for drinking, the similarity between the extreme groups is strong. The most worried and the least worried respondents drink more than the others in order to feel good; and they drink less than the others for motives which may induce addiction such as improve bad mood, depression, escape from worries, and in order to overcome a feeling of hopelessness and despair.

Drinks for pleasure or to feel good, have good mood:

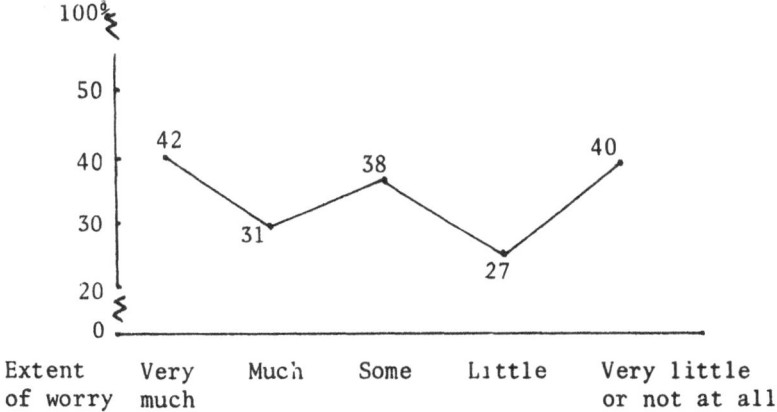

Support of this finding, which refers to all respondents whether they drink or not, is found with respect to drinking motives among respondents who reported drinking.

Drinks for motives which may induce addiction (only among 'drinkers'):

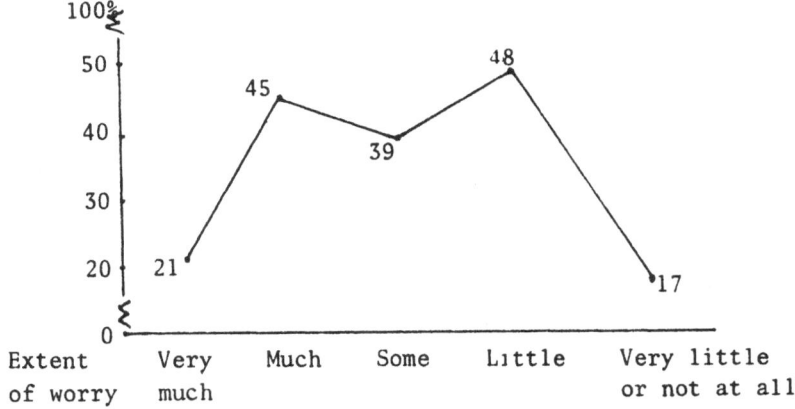

As for the relationship between worry and drunkenness among the 'drinkers', it was found that the least worried, followed by the most worried, reported more than the others never having got drunk.

Got drunk (even if only once) during past year (only among 'drinkers'):

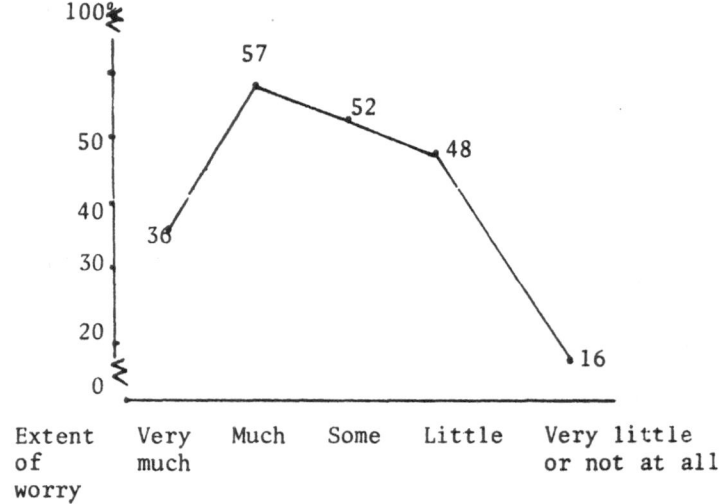

Relationship between worry and assessment of consequences of drinking

Respondents who are most worried with the topic of drinking think more than others — at least twice as much — that drinking is a great impediment to being accepted in society (40 % versus 12–20 % in the other groups), while the least worried believe it helps achieving this goal.

Drinking is a great impediment to being accepted in society.

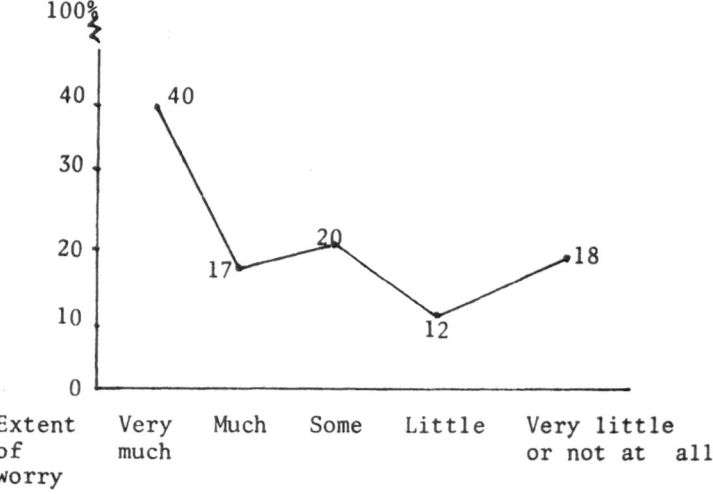

The same trend is apparent with regard to the influence of drinking of alcoholic drinks on improvement of bad mood.

Drinking of alcoholic drinks is a great impediment to improving bad mood:

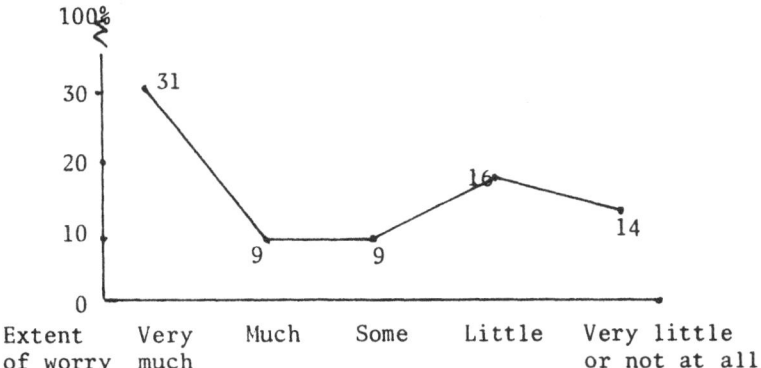

A similar trend — though not as strong — is also apparent regarding the assessment that alcoholic drinks help forget one's troubles and escape from worries.

Drinking of alcoholic drinks is a great impediment to forgetting troubles and escaping from worry.

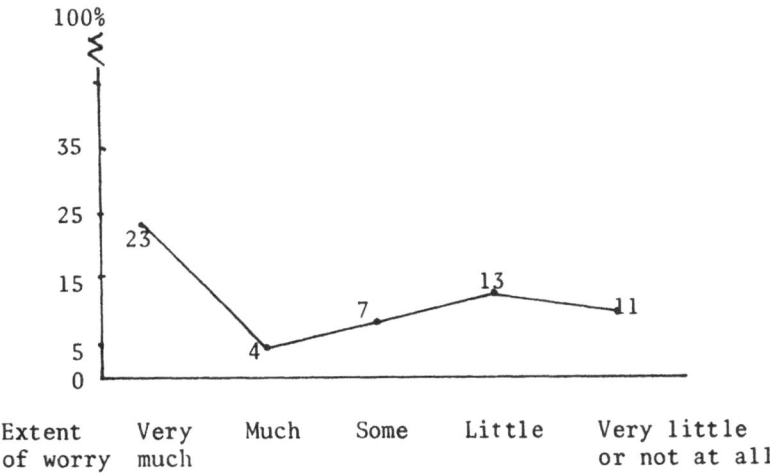

The most worried and the least worried express similar assessments that regular drinking — of at least three times a week — affects badly and very badly one's health.

Regular drinking of at least three times a week has bad and very bad influence on health:

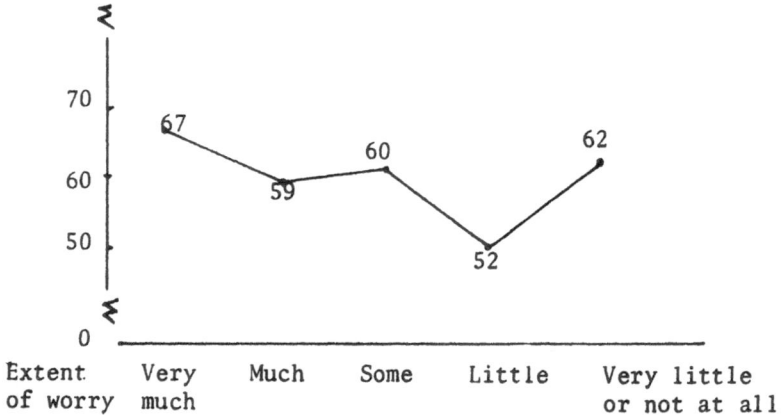

The most worried, followed by the least worried, think more than the others that drinking three small glasses of an alcoholic drink affects very badly the ability to drive.

Drinking three small glasses of an alcoholic drink affects very badly the ability to drive:

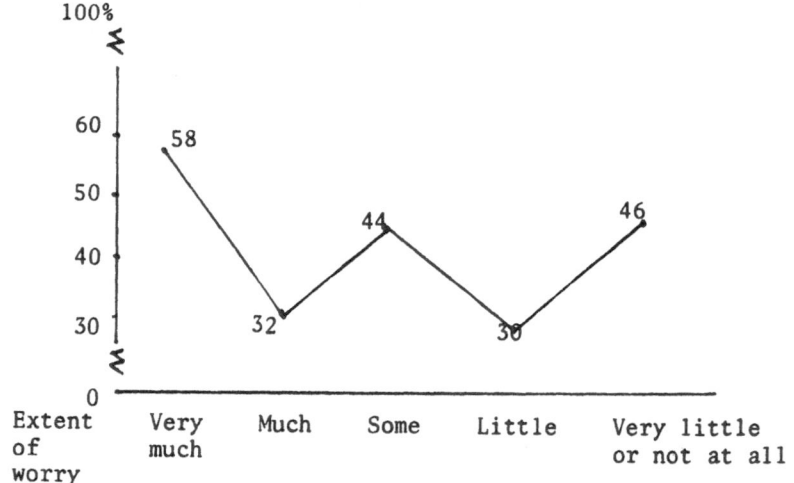

Relationships between worry and attitudes toward problematic drinking

In this area too a similar tendency exists, namely, that the most worried, followed by the least worried, more than the other groups define a person who drinks regularly every day, and a person who drinks by himself in order to relieve tension, as a person with a drinking problem.

Definitely thinks that person who drinks daily has a drinking problem:

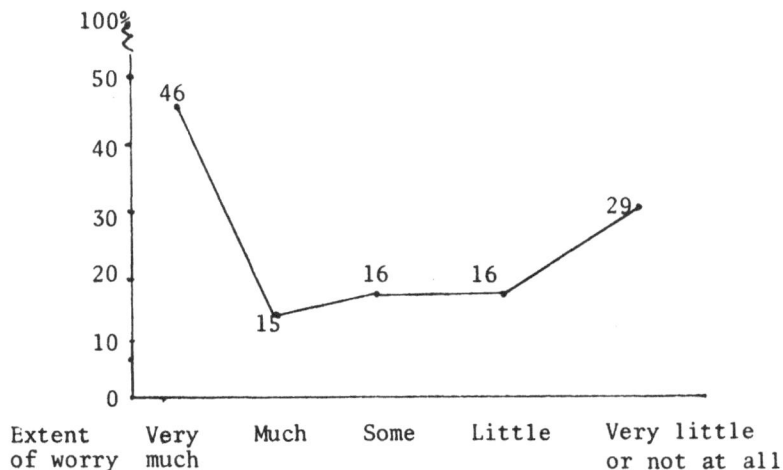

Definitely thinks that person who drinks alone in order to relieve tension has a drinking problem:

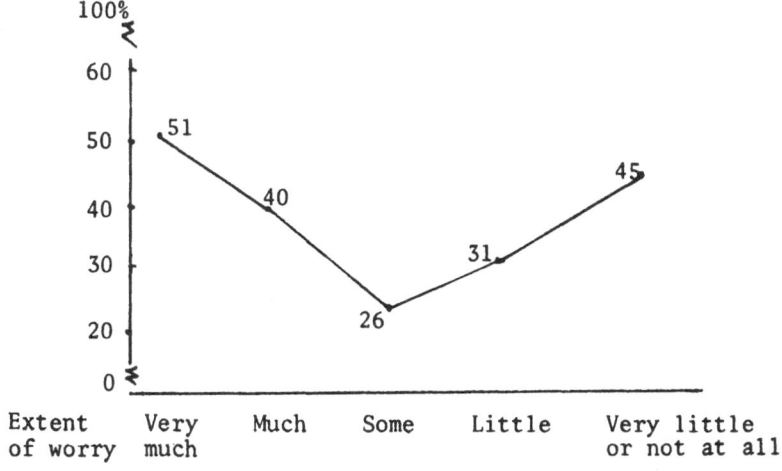

The least worried, followed by the most worried, report, more than the others, that they don't know anyone who drinks daily, nor anyone who may be defined as a problematic drinker.

Doesn't know anyone who daily drinks an alcoholic drink:

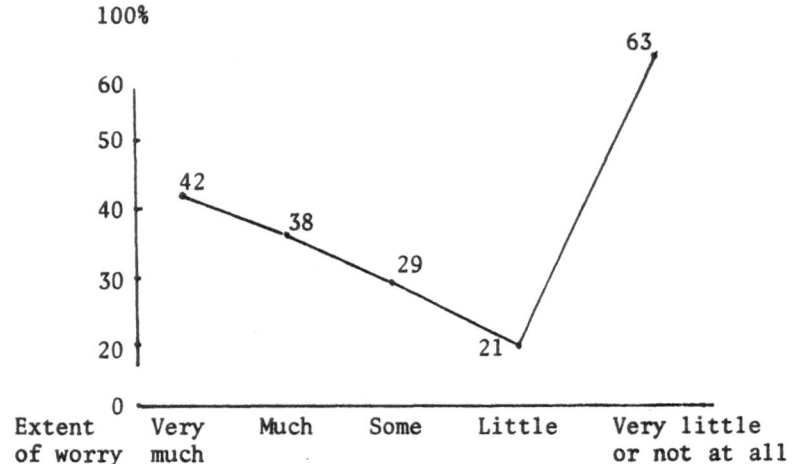

Doesn't know anyone who could be defined as a problematic drinker:

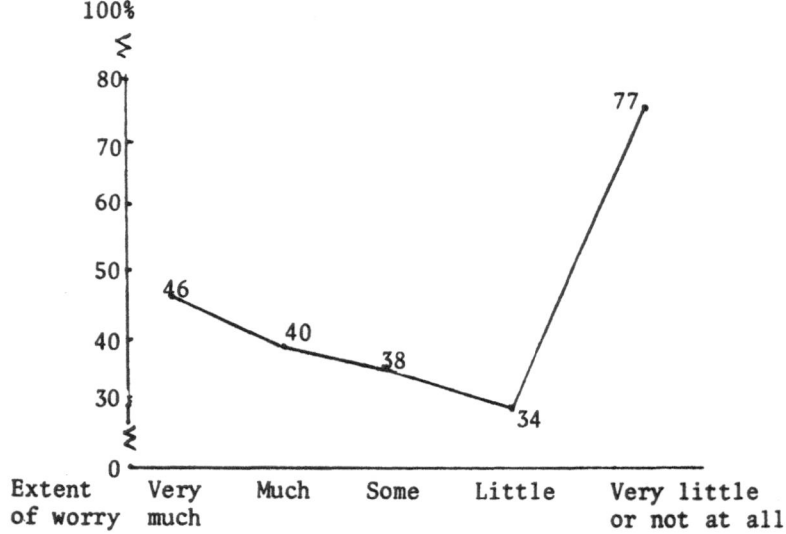

Yet, the more one is worried about one's own or a family member's drinking, the more one knows people who drink daily, as well as people who can be defined as problematic drinkers.

Knows at least six people who drink daily:

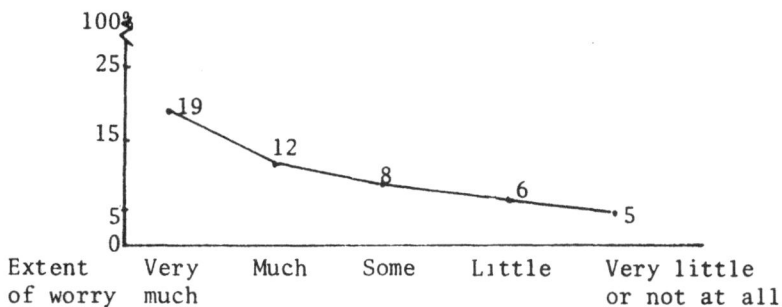

Knows at least two people who may be defined as alcoholics:

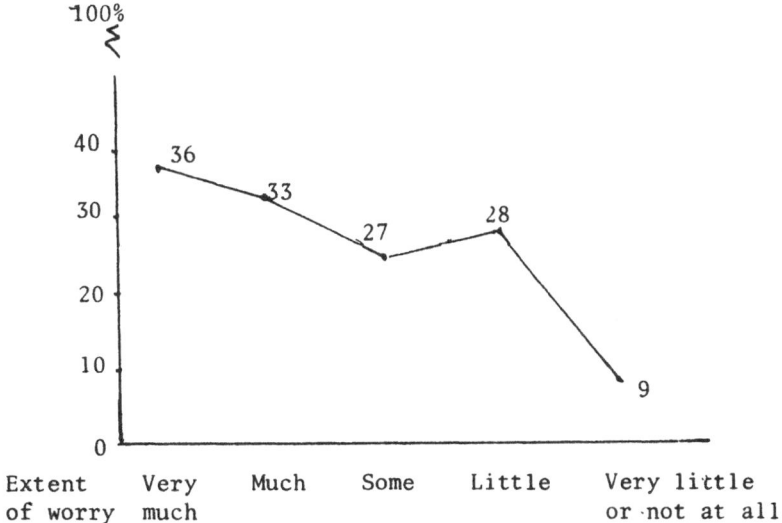

To sum up, in general it may be said that respondents who are most affectively involved in the topic of alcoholic drinking, and respondents who are least involved, are more similar to each other than to other groups in their extreme attitudes both with respect to drinking behaviours and consequences of drinking, as well as in expressing extreme attitudes toward the topic of problematic drinking. Only with regard to one aspect is there a monotonic relationship with worry, namely, acquaintance with people who drink daily and with alcoholics.

6. STRUCTURE AND INTENSITY OF INTERRELATIONSHIPS AMONG THE VARIABLES

In the previous sections we discussed the various aspects of consumption of alcoholic drinks, and the attitudes toward consumption. We shall now deal with the *structure of the interrelationships* among the various attitudes. Is drinking related to acquaintance with people who drink daily? Is the assessment of the consequences of drinking on health related to the assessment of the consequences on driving? An attempt will be made here to answer these and other questions.

First, let us examine the interrelationships among the universe of our variables. These relationships are expressed by means of (weak) correlation coefficients* which were calculated for each pair of attitude variables. The variables were classified in accordance with the common range of the mapping sentence, given in section 1. Although each variable had its own range of categories, all variables were classified by the common range, from high positive attitude to low positive attitude toward drinking.

The main findings from the interrelationship analysis are as follows:

(1)   The absolute majority of the coefficients are positive. The few negative coefficients that were found were low (ranging between −0.02 and −0.10). In other words, in general there were no contradictions between attitudes of one type and attitudes of another type

(2)   The positive relationships range between 0.01 and 0.86, which means that some attitudes are strongly correlated and some are weakly correlated with each other

The variables that are most strongly correlated with other variables are:

(1)   Frequency of drinking of alcoholic drinks. (The lowest correlation values of this variable with other variables are the highest among all lowest correlation values of other pairs of variables, 0.19 and 0.32)

(2)   Frequency of drunkenness in the past year

These variables express instrumental attitudes, and two of them deal with actual consumption of alcoholic drinks.

In order to facilitate perception of the structure of interrelationships among variables, we shall present a graphic presentation of a smallest space analysis

---

* The correlation coefficient expresses the extent to which responses to one question are more positive inasmuch as the responses to the other question are more positive; there is no assumption of linearity. This coefficient ranges between −1 and +1, +1 expressing a full monotone relationship. −1 also expresses a full monotone relationship but in the opposite direction, i.e. when one variable rises the other declines. A zero coefficient points to a lack of a monotone relationship

Table 6.1 Intercorrelations* of variables related to drinking of alcoholic drinks (u_2)

	0	1	2	3	4	5	6	7	8	11	13	14	12	9	10
Serves alcoholic drink at social gathering	1	—														
Serves alcoholic drink at festive dinner	2	84	—													
Drinks on occasion of mourning	3	62	44	—												
Drinking helps being accepted in society	4	56	48	39	—											
Drinking helps improve bad mood	5	50	38	46	66	—										
Drinking helps forget worries and troubles	6	39	33	27	50	81	—									
Influence of regular drinking on health	7	40	33	22	57	51	50	—								
Influence of drinking 3 glasses on driving	8	30	25	32	41	36	29	53	—							
Frequency of drinking	11	65	57	46	55	50	35	46	34	—						
Acquaintance with people who drink daily	13	36	33	39	17	24	24	21	32	42	—					
Acquaintance with problematic drinkers	14	21	19	42	−05	01	07	08	23	30	86	—				
Frequency of drunkenness in past year	12	43	28	40	31	30	28	19	31	79	43	46	—			
Daily drinkers have drinking problem	9	14	−02	04	23	01	−09	21	18	32	10	−10	31	—		
A person who drinks in order to ease tension has a drinking problem	10	08	−04	05	06	−02	−06	11	06	19	07	06	27	81	—	

* Decimal points omitted

(SSA)*, wherein each variable is represented by a point in the space. The closer two points are on the space, the higher the correlation between the variables represented by these points, and conversely, the farther away two points are on the map, the lower the correlation between the variables represented by them.

The smallest space analysis of the data showed that the matrix of interrelationships presented in Table 6.1 can be graphically presented by a three-dimensional space, the regions in the space corresponding to the facet elements of the mapping sentence.

Basically, the structure of the interrelationships among the variables is a three-dimensional one, but a four-dimensional SSA was required in this case in order to demonstrate this structure. Two dimensions describe the scattering of the variables along a cylindrical axis†, and two additional dimensions describe the circular arrangement of the base of the cylinder.

The scattering of the points may be observed as if in a cylinder. A schematic description of the interrelationships among variables related to alcoholic drinking is presented in Figure 6.1.

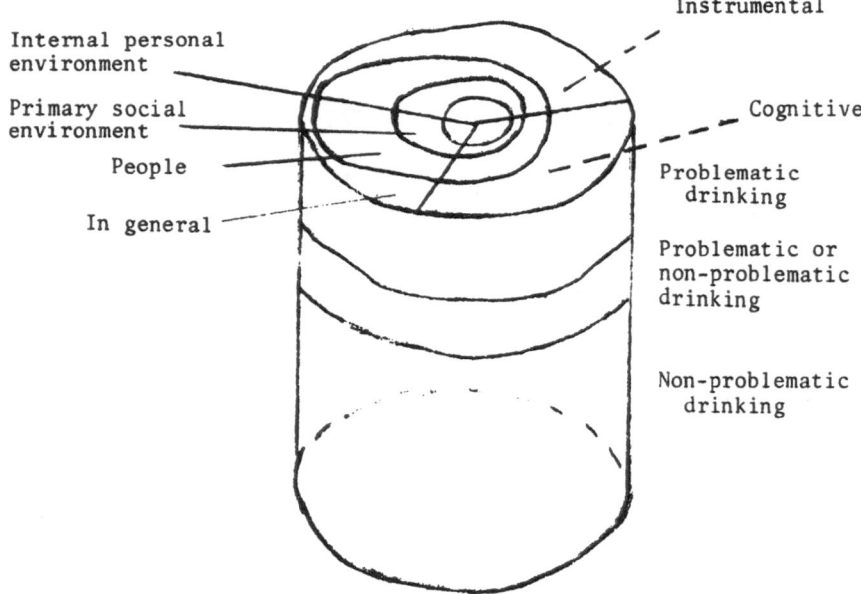

Figure 6.1 Schematic description of the interrelationships among variables referring to drinking of alcoholic drinks

* Smallest Space Analysis is one of the non-metric multivariate data analysis methods developed by Professor Louis Guttman, see references 5 – 7

† One dimension determines the length of the axis, and the other stems from 'noise'

The vertical (cylindrical) axis corresponds to Facet E. The variables referring to problematic drinking are located at the lower part of the cylinder, while those referring to non-problematic drinking are located at the upper part of the cylinder, with variables which sometimes refer to problematic and sometimes to non-problematic drinking appearing between these two extremities.

In each cross-section of the cylinder there is an additional partitioning by two facets, D and A, as described in Figure 6.2.

The inner circle contains all variables relating to internal-personal environment. The second circle refers to the social primary environment. Next is the circle referring to people in society, and the external circle contains variables which refer to drinking in general, without specification of the reference framework. Therefore, the reference framework facet is a modulating facet.

A modulating facet is a facet that is ordered in a certain sense (but not every ordered facet has a modulating role).

As aforesaid, the circular order of the variables may be additionally partitioned by cognitive attitudes on the lower right hand side of the space, and instrumental attitudes throughout the rest.

7. EXPOSURE TO DRINKING

By background variables

It is important to examine which groups are more and which are less exposed to alcoholic drinks, since there is a positive relationship between exposure to and problematic use of alcoholic drinks. In societies in which the exposure to alcoholic drinks is small, that is, where drinking of alcohol is unusual (e.g. Islamic countries), the problem of alcoholism is rare, while in societies where exposure is great, the problem is more frequent.

Identifying the groups that are more exposed to alcohol will therefore assist in locating populations that are at greater risk than others, and may assist those who engage in the prevention of alcoholism in Israel in their work.

Sex

In general it may be said that there are significant differences between men and women in the extent of use and exposure to alcoholic drinks. Frequency of drinking was found to be clearly related with sex. Women avoid drinking more than men (40% avoidance among women versus 24% among men), and frequency of drinking is greater among men.

Twenty per cent of the men drink at least once a week, as compared to 11% among women (7% of the men drink at least every 2–3 days, versus 3% among women).

The research findings reveal that although women of Asian–African origin avoid alcoholic drinks somewhat more than women of European–American

- 29 -

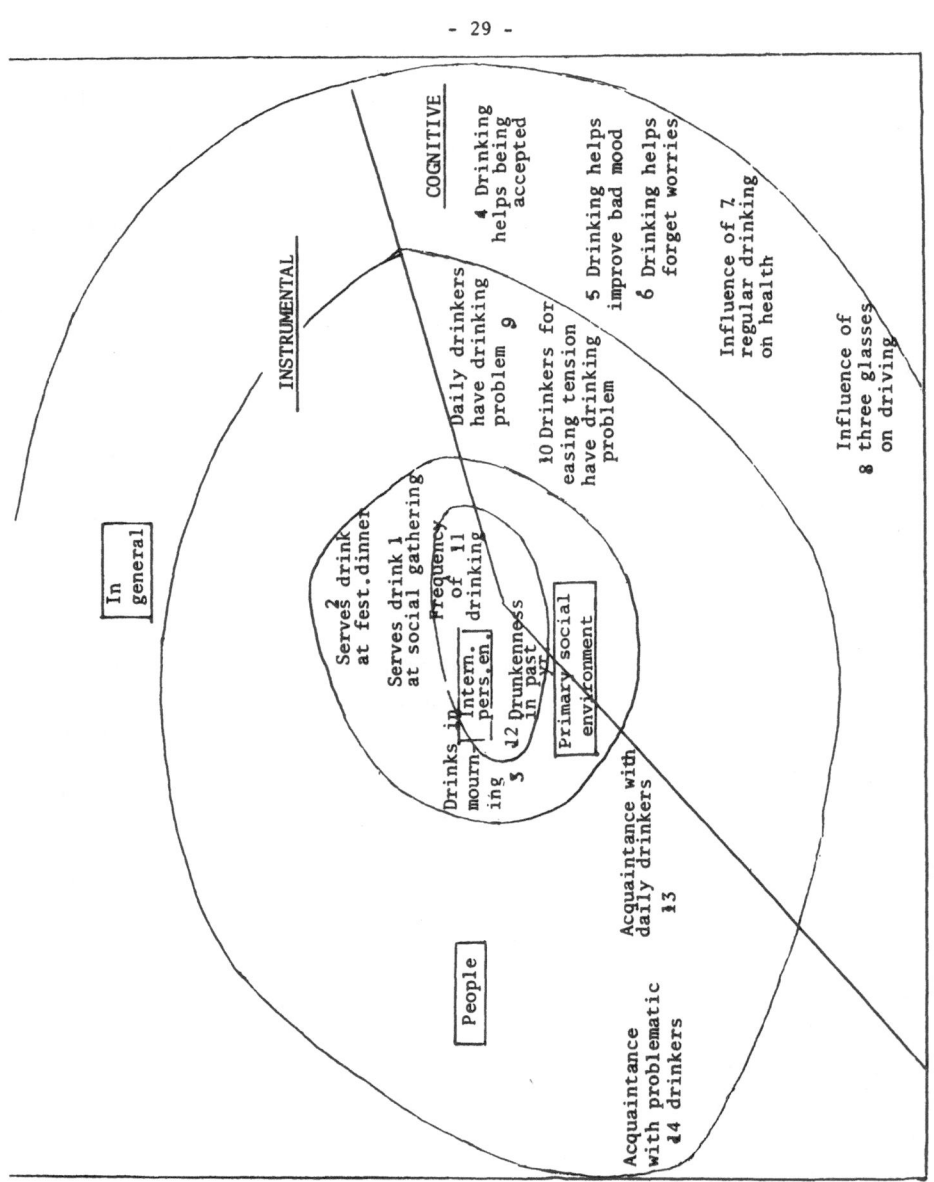

Figure 6.2 Circular partitioning of the SSA space: a two-dimensional projection of the four-dimensional space

origin, the former drink more frequently; this is particularly true with regard to the category 'once a week' (23 % versus 14 %).

No differences by country of origin were found among men with regard to actual drinking and frequency.

With regard to drunkenness (among those who use alcoholic drinks) the difference between men and women is smaller, yet men still get drunk more often than women (29 % of the men versus 23 % of the women).

With regard to serving alcoholic beverages at social gatherings or festive dinners, or at mourning rituals, there are no significant differences between men and women, though here too men use alcoholic drinks somewhat more than women.

Men, somewhat more than women, are acquainted with alcoholics, and with a greater number of them (37 % of the men know an alcoholic versus 30 % of the women, and 17 % of the men know at least two alcoholics versus 14 % of the women).

As for the motive for drinking among those who drink, even if rarely, women somewhat more than men (27 % versus 21 %) report a motive that could be considered as risky and could bring about addiction. Among women who drink alcoholic drinks, those of European–American origin drink more than those of Asian–African origin for social motives, i.e. 'in order to be accepted by society and not be different' (28 % versus 23 %).

Among men no differences were found by country of origin with respect to motive.

Age

In general, no significant differences were found by age, with respect to exposure to alcohol.

Among the various age groups (20–24, 25–34, 35–54 and 55+) there are no meaningful differences with regard to actual drinking or frequency, but among those who drink alcoholic drinks, drunkenness was indeed found to be related to age.

In the younger age group (20–24) 14 % report drunkenness, even if only once in several months, versus the oldest age group (55+) of which only 5 % report so (the 25–34 age group reports 9 % and the 35–54 age group 12 %). Furthermore, drinking without getting drunk is reported by 59 % of the youngest age group, versus 86 % of the oldest age group, and 75 % in the intermediate groups (76 % in the 25–34 and 74 % in the 35–54 age groups). Thus, in the three main age groups – young, old and intermediate – it appears that among those who drink alcoholic drinks there is an inverse relationship between age and drunkenness: the higher the age, the lower the frequency of drunkenness.

Serving alcoholic drinks at each social gathering and each festive dinner is more common in the youngest age group (20–24) (11 %) than in the others, while among the oldest age group (55+) it is least common (4 % at social gatherings and 7 % at festive dinners). Moreover, the latter group, more than the other age groups, serves alcoholic drinks at social gatherings and festive dinners 'very rarely or not at all' (45 % at social gatherings and 40 % at festive dinners).

Regular or frequent drinking of alcohol at mourning rituals is less common among the older age group than among the other age groups (5 % versus an average of 11 % in the other groups among which there is no significant difference), and the oldest group is also more entirely abstaining than the others (80 % versus an average of 70 % of the other groups among which there is no significant difference). Although the youngest age group (20—24) report drinking 'always' at mourning rituals less than the intermediate groups, this group also reports drinking on such occasions 'rarely or never' somewhat less than the other age groups — a finding that may suggest use of alcoholic drinks by this group as a rule, regardless of its non-acceptance of the ritual as such.

No meaningful and consistent differences were found between the age groups with regard to acquaintance with an alcoholic or the motive for drinking.

Education

By respondents' reports, alcoholic drinking, and bearing no relation-ship to frequency, rises with the rise in education. Among respondents with 8 years of schooling, use of alcohol (or non-abstention) is 57 %, in 9—11 years of schooling it is 66 %; 12 years of schooling it is 68 % and in 13 + years of schooling it is 73 %.

When we consider the entire sample of respondents, there are almost no differences by education in the percentage of those who drink at least once a week. But when we consider the population of alcoholic drinkers, then those with the lowest education (0—8 years of schooling) drink a little more frequently (28 % versus 21 % in the three other education groups).

Despite the fact that drinking rises with the rise in education, drunkenness (among those who use alcoholic drinks) and its frequency is inversely related to education: the lower the education, the more common the phenomenon, and the more frequent its occurrence. Among the lower educated (0—8 years of schooling) 14 % get drunk at least every few months and 65 % drink without getting drunk, while among the higher educated (13 + years) 7 % get drunk at least every few months and 79 % drink without getting drunk.

As for serving alcoholic drinks at social gatherings and festive dinners, there are no meaningful differences between the education groups.

Actual drinking — even though rarely — as part of a mourning ritual does not differ greatly among the various education groups; yet those with 11 or less years of schooling drink on such occasions more often than those with 12 or more years of schooling.

Acquaintance with an alcoholic, and with a larger number of alcoholics, rises as education declines, and among those who drink, the lower the education the more potentially addictive the motive.

Origin

Up to recent years there was an ongoing myth that alcoholism is not widespread among Jews. Pnina Eldar and Reuven Bauml[8] claim that this myth stems from an erroneous generalization about Jews in studies concerning European Jewry. According to them, Jewish communities in Europe have adopted limited drinking habits in order to avoid conflict with their non-Jewish environment where alcoholism prevailed. The European Jews are compared with the Jewish communities of Asia and North Africa who adopted more liberal drinking habits, since their Moslem environment abstained from drinking and thus did not have an alcoholism problem which could serve as a pretext for conflict with the Jewish community.

In general, it may be said that the assumption of Eldar and Bauml regarding different drinking habits of European and Asian/African Jews finds support in the present study, and our findings point to different drinking habits in accordance with origin.

By country of birth or father's country of birth (for Israeli-born), it was found that there are no significant differences in actual use of alcoholic drinks, but frequency of drinking was found to be a little higher among those of Asian–African origin (18% drinking at least once a week among them, versus 13% among European–American respondents). This finding regarding the differences between respondents of Asian–African and European–American origin persists when we consider only the country of birth, but the Israeli-born respondents behave with respect to drinking in much the same way as non-Israeli-born respondents of corresponding countries of origin.

Furthermore, and even more distinctly, drunkenness (among the 'drinkers') is more prevalent and more frequent among those of Asian–African origin than among their European–American counterparts (14% drunkenness at least every few months among Asian–African respondents, versus 5% among European–American respondents).

Also with regard to drunkenness the Israeli-born behave like non-Israeli-born of corresponding origin (Israeli-born of Asian–African origin: 15% drunkenness at least every few months, versus 8% among Israeli-born of European–American origin).

Serving alcoholic drinks at social gatherings and dinners, as well as at mourning rituals, is also more prevalent among Asian–African respondents, and here too Israeli-born respondents behave in similar fashion to non-Israeli-born respondents of the same origin.

As for acquaintance with alcoholics, here too there are differences by ethnic origin. More Asian–African respondents know an alcoholic, and also a greater number of alcoholics, than their European–American counterparts. Twenty per cent of Asian–African-born respondents know at least two alcoholics, versus 10% of European–American-born respondents. The extent of acquaintance of Israeli-born respondents of European–American origin with alcoholics is similar to that of their non-Israeli-born counterparts, but that of Israeli-born of Asian–African origin is lower than that of their non-

Israeli-born counterparts, but still higher than their European–American counterparts.

As for motives for drinking (among the 'drinkers'), the differences by origin are not as great as for use of alcoholic drinks and acquaintance with alcoholics, though here too, a similar trend exists. Asian–African respondents drink somewhat more than European–American respondents for motives that may induce addiction (27 % versus 22 %). But this difference disappears when we consider country of birth (25 % in both groups), when 29 % of Israeli-born of Asian–African origin drink for motives that might induce drunkenness, compared to only 17 % of the Israeli-born of European–American origin. This finding may be useful in the guidance of personnel engaged in the prevention of alcoholism.

Status

As an indicator for socioeconomic status, a combination of two variables was used, namely education and income. A respondent was graded as low on status if his education was 8 or less years of schooling and his gross income (including all family members') was 7 000 shekels or less per month. A respondent whose education was 13 years or more, and with gross income of 12 000 or more shekels per month, was graded high. The remaining respondents were classified as intermediate. Accordingly, 77 respondents (9 %) were graded low, 668 (77 %) intermediate, and 125 (15 %) high.

On the basis of this classification, there are indeed considerable differences in the extent of exposure to and use of alcoholic drinks. Drinking of alcoholic drinks — extent and frequency — was found to be clearly related to status. Abstention from drinking declines as status rises (51 % among the low, 31 % among the intermediate, and 24 % among the high status), and frequency of drinking rises with the rise in status (at least every week: 10 %, 15 % and 20 % among low, intermediate and high status respectively).

To summarize, the higher the socioeconomic status, the more respondents drink, and also they drink more often.

Despite the fact that respondents of higher status report more drinking, findings show that among respondents who reported drinking 'sometimes', the lower the status the more frequent the occurrence of drunkenness (36 %, 26 % and 20 % respectively among the low, medium and high status respondents).

In general, then, it may be said that people of low status drink less but, when they do drink, it more often involves drunkenness.

As a general rule, serving of alcoholic drinks at social gatherings and dinners is more prevalent as status rises, but as for serving 'always' or 'generally', the pattern is not uniform. At social gatherings, the higher the status the less they serve 'always' or 'generally', but at dinners the higher the status the more they serve 'always' or 'generally'.

Although drinking alcoholic drinks in connection with mourning rituals is apparently prevalent in all strata of the population, our findings show that the lower the status the higher the use, and the less respondents report drinking 'seldom' or 'never'.

With regard to acquaintance with alcoholics, it is clear that the higher the status the less the acquaintance, and, moreover, the lower the status the higher the number of alcoholics one knows.

As for the motives among the 'drinkers', the lower the status, the more respondents report drinking (even if seldom) for motives that may induce drunkenness. Among 'drinkers' 14% of higher-status respondents report drinking for such motives, as compared to 23% and 33% of the intermediate and low status, respectively. Also with respect to motive, the findings clearly show that respondents of low status drink very little, as compared to intermediate and high status respondents, for the motive 'to be acceptable in society, not to be different' (15% of low status versus 21% and 24% of intermediate and high status respectively).

Religious observance

Use of alcohol prevails less among religious and traditional respondents as compared to the secular respondents (60%, 58% and 83% respectively), but among the 'drinkers' there are no significant differences in the frequency of drinking.

As for drunkenness (among the 'drinkers'), the religious more than the traditional and secular report drunkenness at least every few months (13% versus 9% and 8% respectively) and also somewhat more drinking without getting drunk (69%, 77% and 75% respectively).

In general, secular respondents drink more than the traditional or religious, but among the 'drinkers' the religious tend more to get drunk than the others. Serving alcoholic drinks at social gatherings and dinners is more customary and gets more frequent among the secular than among the traditional and the religious, but as for mourning rituals, differences are not as distinct, though still there is a slight tendency for more drinking on such occasions as religiosity rises.

Acquaintance with alcoholics was found to be related to religiosity. The higher the religiosity the more the acquaintance. Although use of alcohol in general is more prevalent among the secular, among the 'drinkers' the religious, more than the traditional and secular, drink more for motives that may induce drunkenness (30% among religious versus 21% and 19% among the traditional and secular, respectively).

By profile of direct contact with drinking

Up to now this section has dealt with a comprehensive description of the background characteristics of respondents in relation to drinking in general and problematic drinking in particular. We shall now deal with the profile of contact with drinking of each respondent, as produced by the POSAC programme[9-11]. This programme presents a two-dimensional partial order scalogram for profiles comprising, in our case, four variables: frequency of drinking, frequency of drunkenness, acquaintance with people who drink every day, and worry with respect to drinking. These variables are ordered from low to high, in accordance with a common contextual range, namely, the extent of contact with alcoholic drinking.

As aforesaid, all variables were so ordered as to enable comparison with respect to extent of contact, starting with no contact at all (simultaneous consideration of all the aspects examined) on the one hand, and ending with much, close and frequent contact, on the other.

Table 6.2 shows in detail the profiles of contact with alcoholic drinking by the four variables that were examined, and the number of respondents represented by each profile.

Figure 6.3 is a schematic representation by POSA of Table 6.2.

As can be seen in Figure 6.3, the POSA has a 'joint' (vertical) axis, which represents the extent of contact with alcoholic drinking. Respondents with much contact, i.e. who themselves drink very frequently, get drunk, know people who drink daily, and who are greatly worried by the topic of drinking, are located at the bottom and constitute 1 % of the respondents included in this partial order.

At the top are located 26 % of all respondents, and these are respondents with the least contact.

The POSA also has a lateral axis (horizontal) which represents the mode of the contact. On the right hand side, the contact is affective, i.e. respondents are worried whether they themselves drink or not. On the left hand side the contact is instrumental, i.e. direct and personal. This division was obtained because both drinking and worry are basic variables which explain, respectively, the x and y axes of the profiles map.

It should be noted that the position of the variable 'acquaintance with daily drinkers' in the partial order is interesting. High values of this variable are in profiles which are located in the centre of the rhombus. Variables with high values located on the lateral axis have a moderating role. The division of categories by this variable is presented by means of a broken line in Figure 6.4, which is a schematic presentation indicating the position of this variable. (The variable is the third from the left in each case and its values are either 1 or 2, and appear in the diagram as 1/2.)

This variable distinguishes between respondents who are worried by the topic but don't drink themselves, on the one hand, and on the other respondents who drink but are not worried; two additional subgroups are those whose level of contact in these two aspects is low. In other words, acquaintance with people who drink moderates the extremeness of both attitude and involvement. When respondents do not know people who drink they become more extreme. This may be explained by 'prejudice' towards something unfamiliar, while familiarity (in our case, exposure to drinking) is a moderating factor.

Table 6.2 Contact with drinking of alcoholic drinks (in absolute numbers)

Extent of worry	Acquaintance with people who drink every day*	Frequency of drunkenness*	Frequency of drinking	Profile	N
very little/not worried at all	don't know any such people	don't drink	don't drink	4433	249
very little/not worried at all	don't know any such people	don't drink	very seldom	3433	189
very little/not worried at all	don't know any such people	don't drink	at least once a week	2433	261
very little/not worried at all	don't know any such people	don't drink	at least every 2–3 days	1433	26
Worried to some or little extent	don't know any such people	don't drink	don't drink	4432	22
worried to some or little extent	don't know any such people	drink but don't get drunk	very seldom	3332	21
worried to some or little extent	don't know any such people	get drunk rarely	at least once a week	2232	67
worried to some or little extent	know one person	drink but don't get drunk	at least every 2–3 days	1322	9
worried/very worried	know at least 2 people	don't drink	don't drink	4411	52
worried/very worried	know at least 2 people	get drunk at least every few months	seldom	3111	30
worried/very worried	know at least 2 people	get drunk at least every few months	at least once a week	2111	32
worried/worried	know at least 2 people	get drunk at least every few months	at least every 2–3 days	1111	11
			Total number of respondents		969

* This table and Figure 6.3 present 'pure' profiles of only the two basic variables, i.e. drinking and worry. The other two variables were not taken into consideration here

The table represents respondents having a profile of contact with alcoholic drinking; they comprise 94 % of the total number of respondents in this study

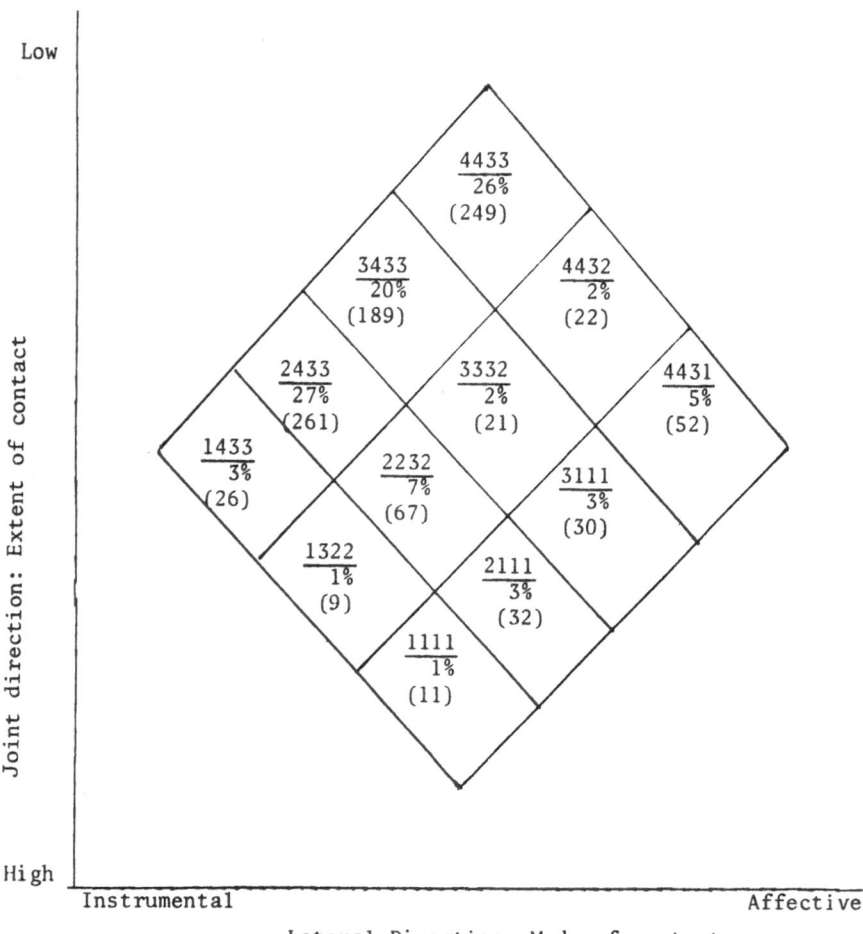

Figure 6.3 A Partial Order Scalogram Analysis of contact with drinking of alcoholic drinks ($n = 969$)

8. SUMMARY

The purpose of this study was to investigate the occurrence of use of alcoholic drinks among the Israeli public, and the aspects related to problematic use of such drinks.

The research findings show that in Israel today, both the behaviour and the attitudes towards use of alcoholic drinks are still different from those of other Eastern and Western countries, though a tendency for change in this respect is apparent.

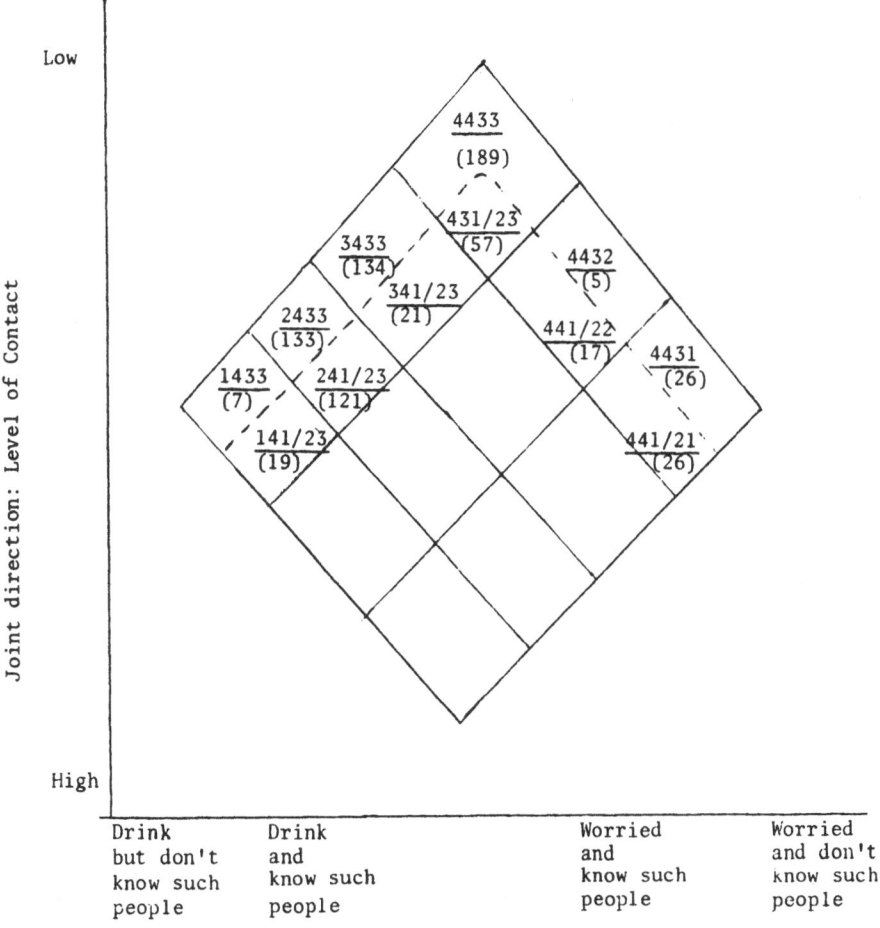

Figure 6.4   Partial Order Scalogram Analysis of contact with drinking of alcoholic drinks which includes the variable 'Acquaintance with people who drink every day'

Findings regarding behaviour and attitudes towards drinking

The main findings that express the situation in the Israeli public today with regard to drinking are:

(1)   58 % of the Israeli public drink very seldom or not at all (33 % don't drink), except for on religious occasions,

(2)   33 % of the Israeli public do not serve or seldom serve alcoholic drinks at every social gathering,

(3)   29 % of the Israeli public do not serve or seldom serve alcoholic drinks at every festive dinner,

(4)   Of those who use alcoholic drinks, 74 % have never got drunk,

(5)   72 % of the Israeli public are 'very little' or 'not at all' worried by their own or a family member's (spouse, parents, children) drinking,

(6)   55 % of the Israeli public are not acquainted with even one person who drinks daily alcoholic drinks (67 % do not know any alcoholics).

However, these patterns of behaviour are accompanied by the following attitudes.

(1)   61 % of the Israeli public believe that regular drinking − at least three times a week − has a bad or very bad effect on health.

(2)   46 % of the Israeli public are certain that a person who daily takes an alcoholic drink has a drinking problem.

(3)   In general, 26 % of the Israeli public express a very low level of contact with alcohol drinking − they neither drink at all and have never got drunk, nor do they know people who drink daily; they are also not at all worried by their own or a family member's drinking.

Reference to the various subgroups in the Israeli public shows that:

(1)   Use of alcohol is more prevalent, and at greater frequency, among men − whatever their origin. Differences are not so distinct between men and women with regard to drunkenness. Of the women who consume alcoholic drinks, more are of Asian−African origin.

(2)   The younger respondents (aged 20−24) report more than the others on drunkenness, and more than the others serve alcoholic drinks at social gatherings and festive dinners.

(3)   With the rise in education, use of alcohol rises, but drunkenness declines.

(4)   With the decline in education, acquaintance with alcoholics increases, as do motives for drinking that induce addiction.

(5)   The extent of use of alcoholic drinks is similar among respondents of different origin, but greater frequency of drinking, drunkenness and serving of drinks at social gatherings and festive dinners and at mourning is reported more among respondents of Asian−African origin, as compared to European−American respondents. It is important to note that in all aspects related to use of alcoholic drinks, there is a strong similarity between Israeli-born respondents and non-Israeli-born respondents of corresponding origin.

(6)   Use of alcoholic drinks is more prevalent among secular respondents than among the traditional and religious, but drunkenness, acquaintance with alcoholics and drinking for motives that may induce addiction are reported more by the former.

(7)   The higher the social status (based on education and income and related to origin and religious observance), the more the extent of drinking, its frequency, and serving alcoholic drinks at social gatherings and festive

dinners, and the less the extent of drunkenness, acquaintance with alcoholics and drinking for motives that induce addiction.

Findings regarding existence of actual or potential problem

The above findings present a picture showing the existing situation in Israeli society. We shall now present findings that may hint at the possibility of the existence of a problem, whether actual or potential.

(1) 2 % of the public drink alcohol every day (apart from drinking on religious occasions) (15 % drink at least once a week). Daily drinking is not necessarily problematic drinking, but it may be assumed that in this group of 'drinkers', more than in the other groups, there may be problematic users of alcohol who may need help, whether they are aware of it or not.

   The researchers are aware of the fact that to confess before an interviewer to daily drinking is harder than to respond to the other questions. Presumably, a number of respondents found it hard to confess to daily drinking or to drunkenness, and 'boasting' of drinking is probably unlikely; hence, 2 % of daily drinking may be considered as the minimum likelihood.

(2) 5 % of the Israeli public get drunk at least every few months (1 % at least once a week).

   The researcher's comment on the previous item (1) applies here too.

(3) 13 % of the Israeli public are worried or very worried about the fact that they themselves or someone in their family (spouse, parents, children) drink alcoholic drinks. In other words, reports on such direct personal worry may be interpreted as either indirect reporting of actual personal problematic use or an expression of fear regarding a family member.

   The topic of worry is a rather complex and interesting one. In general, the most worried and the least worried are similar in their extreme attitude towards the topic, both with regard to drinking behaviour and its impact, as well as problematic drinking.

   This research does not answer the question whether respondents are worried because of their own drinking or that of a family member; it also does not answer the question to what extent the Israeli public is worried about the use of alcohol in general.

   Nevertheless, taking into consideration the target population as defined by the Unit for the Prevention of Alcoholism, this finding most emphasizes the need for a service that could provide answers to needs which stem from either direct or indirect problematic use of alcohol.

(4) 15 % of the Israeli public drink (even if rarely) for motives that may induce addiction. It is possible that this population uses alcoholic drinks for these motives without being aware of the danger of addiction, and preventive programmes should take this into consideration.

(5)   29% of the Israeli public know at least two people who daily take alcoholic drinks; this finding, again, may hint that daily drinking is perhaps more prevalent than actually reported on direct questioning of the respondents.

(6)   The finding that most testifies to the existence of a problem related with drinking is that 1.1% of the Israeli public are at the highest level of contact with alcoholic drinking. (Respondents in this group drink at least every 2−3 days, get drunk at least every few months, know at least two people who drink daily, and also are worried or very worried by their own or a family member's daily drinking.)

It is obvious that this group requires help (even if only for its worry): yet it need not be assumed that respondents of the other contact levels do not need professional help.

(7)   From the structure of interrelationships among the various research variables, it appears that frequency of drinking is the variable that is most related to all the other variables. Furthermore, the relationship is so strong that the lowest coefficients of this variable with all the other variables are the highest among the low coefficients of other inter-relationships. (The second strongest relationship is that of drunkenness.)

This finding may point to the fact that a change in drinking habits will bring about a change in all the other variables, and the change apparently is in both directions.

Main conclusions

The main conclusions of this research are as follows:

(1)   Although Israel differs, with respect to use of alcohol, from Western and Eastern Societies, a changing tendency in this respect is apparent, and Israeli society should expect this.

(2)   The assessment of the Unit for the Prevention of Alcoholism regarding the existence of about 7200 alcoholics in Israel is a very cautious assessment and probably does not encompass the entire problem in Israel.

(3)   It is worth while to look again and more deeply into the higher inclination of young people, as compared to the other age groups, to serve alcoholic drinks at social gatherings and festive dinners, their inclination to attribute to alcoholic drinks effects on the psychological and social functioning and their greater tendency to get drunk. Such an examination is necessary since the younger age group has not yet reached its full potential with regard to the use of alcoholic drinks, and the process that leads to alcoholism is a lengthy one.

(4)   The question of worry with respect to drinking, in all its complexity, requires further study; likewise, a special research effort should focus on the populations at high risk (rather than the entire public) in order to

answer the question regarding the proper structure and scope of activities necessary for meeting the specific needs related to problematic use of alcoholic drinks in Israeli society.

(5) Finally, the false belief that alcoholism does not exist among Jews in general, and among Israelis in particular, should be uprooted and eliminated.

References

1 Guttman, L. (1954). The principal components of scalable attitudes. In Lazarsfeld, P. F. (ed.) *Mathematical Thinking in the Social Sciences*, pp. 216–257. (New York: Free Press)

2 Levy, S. (1978). Involvement as a component of attitude: theory and political examples. In Shye, S. (ed.) *Theory Construction and Data Analysis in the Behavioral Sciences*. (San Francisco: Jossey-Bass)

3 Adler, I. and Guttman, L. (1975). *Prediction of the Extent of Viewing of Broadcasting of the Olympic Games in Montreal in 1976*. (Jerusalem: Israel Institute of Applied Social Research)

4 Levy, S. and Guttman, L. (1976). *Values and Attitudes of Israeli High School Youth. Second Study*. (Jerusalem: Israel Institute of Applied Social Research)

5 Guttman, L. (1968). A general nonmetric technique for finding the smallest coordinate space for a configuration of points. *Psychometrika*, **33**, 469

6 Lingoes, J. C. (1973). *The Guttman–Lingoes Nonmetric Program Series*. (Ann Arbor: Mathesis Press)

7 Lingoes, J. C. (1979). *Geometric Representations of Relational Data*. 2nd Edn. (Ann Arbor: Mathesis Press)

8 Eldar, P. and Bauml, R. (1981). *Alcoholism in Israel*.

9 Shye, S. and Elizur, D. (1976). Worries about deprivation of job rewards following computerization: a partial order scalogram analysis. *Hum. Relations*, **29** (1)

10 Shye, S. (1978). Partial order scalogram analysis. In Shye, S. (ed.) *Theory Construction and Data Analysis in the Behavioral Sciences*. (San Francisco: Jossey-Bass)

11 Shye, S. (1981). *An Integrated Method for Scaling Subjects and Structuring their Multivariate Attributes: Description and Illustration of Partial Order Scalograms and Lattice Analysis*. (Jerusalem: Israel Institute of Applied Social Research)

Part 2:
ALCOHOLISM – TREATMENT

7

A continuum of care: treatment, training, prevention

Cdr. G. A. BUNN

Dedicated to my beautiful and supportive wife, Nan, and our expanded family –
James, Kathleen, Kelly, Tane, David, and Danny.

INTRODUCTION: A CONTINUUM OF CARE

The US Navy's Alcohol Program has long been considered one of the finest
treatment programmes in the world. Through the combined leadership and
guidance of Capt J. J. Zuska, MC, USN (Ret.) and recovering alcoholic, Cdr
R. Jewell, USN (Ret.), the Navy's programme began its effort at the Naval
Regional Medical Center (NRMC) Long Beach, California in 1965. From
this modest but highly successful 'grass roots' beginning, the treatment effort
has grown to encompass over 30 inpatient facilities with a yearly throughput
of more than 5000 patients.

However, just as the alcohol problem can be viewed on the basis of a
continuum from abstinence to acute alcoholism, the Navy's Program is one of
a continuum of care. The Naval Alcohol Rehabilitation Center (ARC) San
Diego, California has the largest treatment and training facility dealing with
alcohol in the world, and is the focal point for this effort. It is staffed both in
San Diego and at its satellite offices with full time and part time employees
numbering over 800 and with a yearly operating budget of approximately $6
million.

The ARC was established in 1973 to meet the needs of the military
community for the treatment and rehabilitation of the alcoholic, and to
provide training and education for Navy Alcoholism Counselors assigned to
treatment facilities and Collateral Duty Alcoholism Advisors (CODAA)
assigned to commands stationed throughout the world. The ARC also
became, in 1976, the headquarters for the administration and management of

the world-wide Navy Alcohol Safety Action Program (NASAP), the Navy's prevention effort.

As the efforts of the ARC began to impact the military community, a need to emphasize an eclectic approach to treatment became apparent. Ongoing research showed a gradual shift in patient population from the older, more easily identified chronic alcoholic to the younger, more difficult to diagnose and treat alcohol misuser or poly-drug client.

Methodologies that are effective for the alcoholic do not always achieve the same results with the misuser, namely the change from negative behaviours to positive behaviours. For the alcoholic, treatment focusses on changing *behaviour* with a resultant change in *attitudes*; however, experience, especially from the efforts of NASAP and other research, has demonstrated that the reverse approach (changing attitude, with subsequent change in behaviour) was most effective with the alcohol misuser. We are striving to encourage the use of NASAP for this latter population, thus freeing treatment facilities from the burden imposed by these inappropriate referrals and allowing treatment personnel to deal more specifically with the alcoholic. Data also suggested the need for a training programme designed to provide knowledge in specific areas and to develop skills and characteristics determined to be more responsible to both patient and fleet needs. This development is being accomplished through the Institute in Alcoholism Studies (IAS) Course which relies heavily upon supportive interaction between the Treatment and Training Departments.

The author, in his eighth year with the Navy's Alcohol Program and currently the Commanding Officer of the Alcohol Rehabilitation and Training Center, San Diego will discuss the various elements within this continuum of care, specifically the following.

(1) *Treatment.* ARC San Diego treats within its 6 week residential programme 650 patients per year, including all active military, retired and dependents. Special focus in treatment is on the family.

(2) *Training.* Three principal courses of skill creative training will be discussed detailing curricula. These courses are:

    (a) Alcoholism Administration, Training and Advisor (ATA) Course taught 15 times (2 weeks in length) per year around the world. The 4000 graduates include those from all branches of US service, other federal agencies and several foreign military. Its graduates serve within every Navy command as advisors and resource managers.

    (b) Institute in Alcoholism Studies (IAS), taught four times per year, 10 weeks per cycle in San Diego, develops the second stage product for service in inpatient facilities throughout the world. The 400 graduates include all US military and military from Canada, Australia, New Zealand and Britain. These graduates first become Navy Alcoholism Treatment *Interns* (ATI); once they serve a year's internship and pass a certification exam, they then become Alcoholism Treatment *Specialists* (ATS).

(c) Awareness workshops – tailored training to meet the needs of the various levels of supervisory responsibility from flag rank to petty officers.

(3) *Prevention.*

(a) Navy Alcohol Safety Action Program (NASAP) – this is the Navy's secondary prevention effort designed to deal with alcohol problems prior to the addictive or seriously destructive stage. After 7 years of operation it has reached over 100 000 students. The thrust and success of this effort will be discussed.

(b) Navy Drug Safety Action Program (NDSAP) – based on the experiences of the NASAP effort, this Program has just completed its first pilot year and the recently completed evaluation of the effort will be discussed.

All of the effort described above is tied together with one of the most extensive audiovisual (A/V) and media programmes in the field, encompassing everything from videotape recorder (VTR) coverage of all patient and student group dynamics to production of training tapes for world-wide distribution (Figure 7.1).

TREATMENT

The Treatment Department at the ARC is composed of three divisions, Counseling, Medical and Professional Support. The Department is directly responsible for the 24 hour, 7 days per week care of the patients in coordination with the Administrative Department and the Chief Master-at-Arms.

Counseling Division

The Counseling Division, under the management of the Senior Military Counselor has direct military responsibility for all the patients and their primary counselors. In this capacity the Senior Military Counselor reports directly to the Commanding Officer for *all* patient disposition. The ARC's current patient capacity is 82 (ten female beds) with expansion plans for an additional 50 beds by October 1983. These beds remain continually in full use with an ongoing waiting list of 6–8 weeks. The patients are randomly assigned to one of seven groups with a primary counselor as their manager. In addition to the seven primary counselors, there is an indoctrination/orientation counselor who processes and re-evaluates each newly-reporting patient. The staff, like the patient population, has representation from the Navy, Marine Corps and Coast Guard as well as civilian personnel.

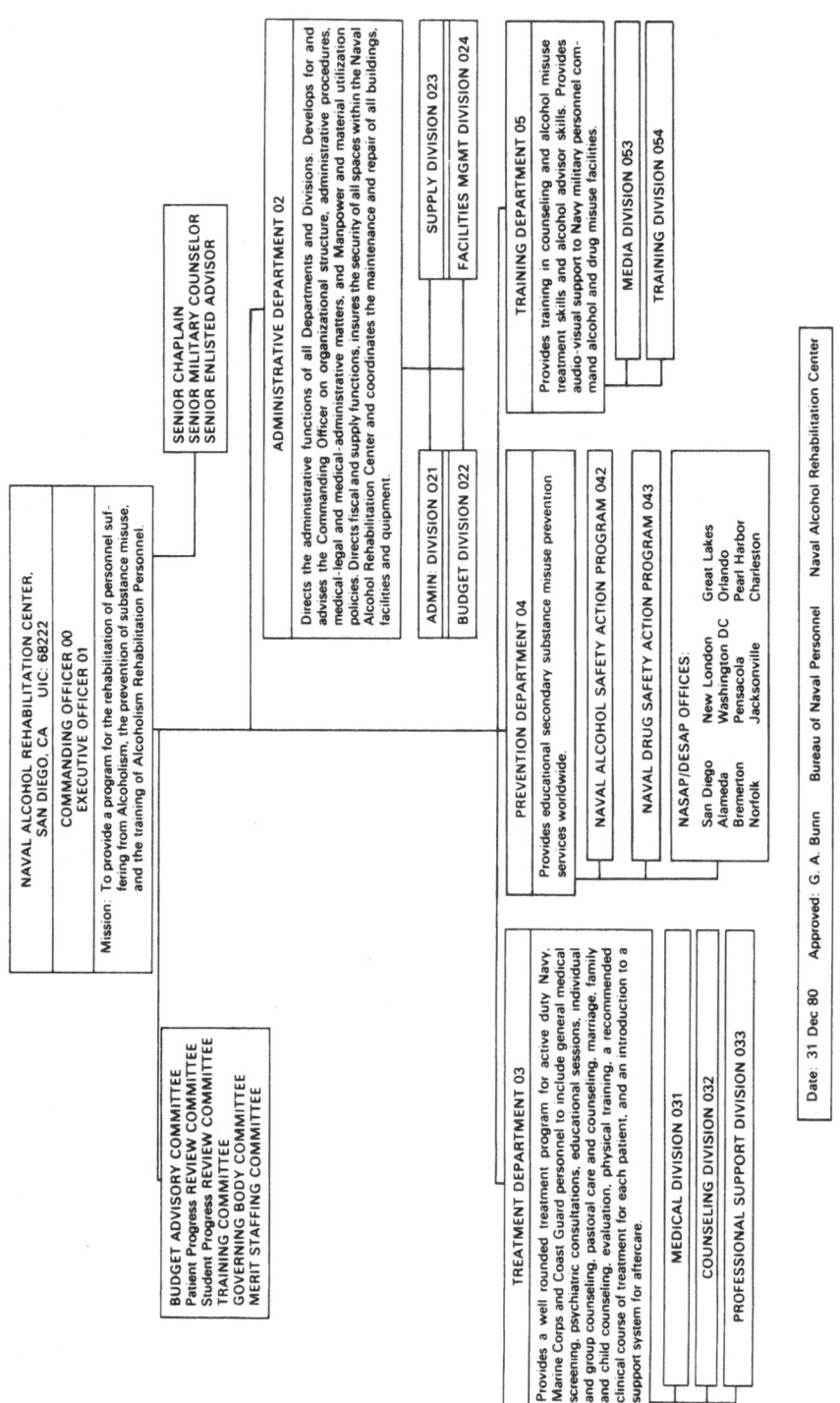

Figure 7.1 Organizational chart

The counselors, by and large, are recovering alcoholics with a minimum of 3 years sobriety but, recovering or not, they are all school trained in the ARC's IAS Course and are subsequently certified as Alcoholism Treatment Specialists (ATS) following a 1 year internship and successful completion of a comprehensive certification exam.

Medical Division

The Medical Division is headed by a Commander, Medical Corps, psychiatrist who is also the administrative head of the Treatment Department. With a staff of three hospital corpsmen, he has total medical responsibility for patient health care, and its documentation. In consort with the Senior Military Counselor and the Professional Support Division Director the development of individual health care plans for follow-on recovery for all patients is also required.

Professional Support Division

A Clinical Psychologist administers the Professional Support Division which entails the services of the Chaplain, Marriage and Family Counselors, and Clinical Interns. The ARC provides graduate and postgraduate internships for several local universities as well as professionals from the US Navy's Health Research Center.

Treatment data

In calendar year (CY) 1981 the ARC statistics for patient demographics, with a maximum bed capacity of 72 beds for males and 10 for females, were as set out in Table 7.1.

Table 7.1 CY 1981 patient throughput

	Officer	Enlisted	Retired	Dependent	Total
USN	14	501	5	16	536
USMC	1	46	0	4	52
USCG	4	19	0	1	24
USA	1	2	0	5	8
USAF	1	3	1	2	7
Other	1	0	0	1	3
Totals	21	571	6	29	628

Inasmuch as the Navy's programme is an occupationally designed effort, it should be noted that while 628 patients completed treatment, 680 were admitted. The remaining 52 patients were terminated from treatment after a minimum of 3 weeks (of a 6 week programme) with a recommendation for release from active duty for refusal to participate in their own recovery. To ensure maximum pressure and support is provided, all patients are visited by parent command representatives, most often their own Commanding Officer. Progress reports are made to parent commands where aftercare responsibility resides.

Residential treatment regimen

The programme is a 6 week effort that entails:

(1) *Initial*
   (a) Orientation and indoctrination
   (b) Physical examination − Antabuse clearance
   (c) Assignment to group
   (d) Phase I restriction − 2 weeks
   (e) Psychological testing

(2) *Elements of treatment*
   (a) Six week residential programme
   (b) Alcoholics Anonymous (AA) − mandatory evening meeting
   (c) Disulfiram (Antabuse)
   (d) Small group counselling
   (e) Individual counselling
   (f) Women's group counselling
   (g) Couple's/significant other group counselling
   (h) Family counselling
   (i) Psychodrama
   (j) Lectures and films
   (k) Physical fitness programme

(3) *Follow-up*
   (a) Continue AA
   (b) Continue Antabuse
   (c) Letter to Commanding Officer
   (d) Letter to CODAA/DAPA.

Figure 7.2 depicts a typical weekly schedule of events. Every hour of the day from 0600 to 2300 is utilized for maximum therapeutic effect.

Treatment evaluation

The US Navy's treatment effort has undergone several evaluative analyses. One was completed in 1979 and encompassed data collected on 16 000 patients[1]. The criteria utilized in this approach were as follows.

(1) Upon completion of treatment, was the individual who had at least 6 months left on active duty able to complete his present enlistment and be recommended for re-enlistment?

WEEK OF 25 JANUARY - 31 JANUARY

TIME	MONDAY	TUESDAY	WEDNESDAY	THURSDAY	FRIDAY	SATURDAY	SUNDAY
0730	DC: LARRY MUSTER/QUARTERS CLEAN UP SICK CALL — CDO: TMC RIPPLE	DC: RICH MUSTER/QUARTERS CLEAN UP SICK CALL — CDO: SSGT GUERRA	DC: JOHN MUSTER/QUARTERS CLEAN UP SICK CALL PATIENT FAREWELLS — CDO: RMI GRIFFIN	DC: RUDY MUSTER/QUARTERS CLEAN UP SICK CALL — CDO: SKC COOK	DC: RON MUSTER/INSPECTION CLEAN UP 0800 SICK CALL/NEW PT CHECK-IN — CDO: SSGT GUERRA	CDO: BMC HATCHER	YMC CONANT CDO:
0830	SMALL GROUP BLDG 261	SMALL GROUP BLDG 261	SMALL GROUP BLDG 261 PROJECTEES MEETING	SMALL GROUP BLDG 261	0830-0945 SMALL GROUP — 0930 ZONE INSPECTION	0930 BLDG 265 MUSTER PHASE 1 — 0945 MOVIE: ROOM 210	0930 MUSTER PHASE 1
0945	0945-1130 PT STATION GYM		0945-1130 PT STATION GYM *1000-1130 WOMEN'S GRP	1230 *SERENDIPITY WOMEN'S			
1000	1000-1200 NEW PT ORIENTATION *1000-1120 WOMEN'S GRP *MANDATORY FOR ALL WOMEN PATIENTS	MEDICAL ASPECTS ROOM 210	*MANDATORY FOR ALL WOMEN PATIENTS	(C). PARK HILL METH. CHURCH. 545 E. NAPLES. CHULA VISTA *MANDATORY FOR ALL WOMEN PATIENTS	1000-1050 GUEST SPEAKER		
1130			1250 GROUP LEADERS MEETING WITH SME		CLOSURE: DUTY COUNSELOR 1130-1200 CLEAN UP		
1250	MONDAY THROUGH PATIENT GROUP THURSDAY MUSTER NEW PATIENT CHECK-IN MON THUR	AA MEETING 1300-1400 SMALL GROUP	1330-1400 SIGNIFICANT OTHERS 1300-1415	LUNCH TRMT DEPT WORK SHOP 1300-1515			
1415	AA TRNG GRP 1300-1415		COUPLES GROUP	FIELD DAY	LIBERTY STAFF		
	REENTRY WORKSHOP	1430-1600	1430-1600	PATIENT PROGRESS REVIEW	1200 FRIDAY		
1600	1430-1600 COUNSELORS TIME	COUNSELORS TIME	GROUP LEADERS TIME 1500 XO SCREENING 1500-1600 COUNSELORS TIME	CAPTAINS MAST 1600-1630	0730 MONDAY		MUSTER
1630	1600-1630 CLEAN UP	1600-1630 CLEAN UP	1600-1630 CLEAN UP	COUNSELORS TIME	PHASE 2 1200 FRIDAY 2300 SUNDAY		
1900	SUN - THUR MUSTER REPORT FROM GROUP LEADERS TO CDO 1900 AND 2300 ARC BLDG NAVSTA 1800 COUPLES GROUP 1830 OUTPATIENT GROUP 2000 DRY DOCK 21 2000 ALANON MEETING	GRP 1 TORRY PINES GRP 2 BERYL STREET GRP 3 MIRA MESA DISCUSSION GRP 4 OCEAN BEACH GRP 5 NO. SHORES GRP 6 SO. BAY GUYS & GALS DISC. 270 C., CV GRP 7 SO. BAY GUYS & GALS DISC. 270 C., CV	GRP 1 CARE & SHARE NO. SHORES GRP 2 CORONADO *GRP 3 PROSPECT GRP 3 HILLTOPPERS GRP 4 SARSIDE GROUP GRP 5 STEP 1 GROUP GRP 7 PT LOMA *ALL ALANON/CO-ALCOHOLICS WILL ATTEND HILLTOP ALANON MEETING WITH GRP 3 WED EVENING	GRP 1 LINDA VISTA GRP 2 VA HOSPITAL GRP 3 E. SAN DIEGO GRP GRP 4 E.V. DOCK 21 GRP 5 SO BAY PIONEERS GRP 6 GRASS ROOTS GRP 7 LA JOLLA THURS. NIGHT (OPEN) *CLAIREMONT WOMEN'S (C) ST MARKS CHURCH 3205 CLAIREMONT DRIVE *MANDATORY FOR ALL FEMALE PATIENTS	PHASE 1 CONTINUE DAILY ROUTINE MUSTER PHASE 1 (1900) AA MTG. BAYSIDE ALANO CLUB. 230 GLOVER ST. CHULA VISTA	SOUTH BAY PIONEERS, 270 "C" ST.. C.V.	PH 1 AA MTG. NO SHORES ALANO. 4861 CASS OR LEMON GROVE COMN CTR ON SCH. LN. NEXT TO FOOD BSKT. MANDATORY FOR ALL PHASE 1 PATIENTS

Figure 7.2 Treatment Department weekly schedule

(2)   What was the frequency of sick call visits and the frequency and length of hospitalizations for a 2-year period before and after treatment?

(3)   How was the individual functioning on the job — as determined by evaluations filled out by the individual's Commanding Officer (CO) at intervals of 6, 12, and 24 months following treatment? (Questionnaires were sent from the facility in which the patient was treated to his present CO to evaluate his present level of functioning. In addition, the CO was asked to determine whether he would recommend the individual for re-enlistment as well as for promotion or advancement.)

(4)   What was the change in psychological test data (i.e., change in anxiety, depression, hostility, trust, and ability to relate to other people)?

(5)   What was the change in drinking habits as measured by self-report questionnaires and evaluations of superiors?

(6)   What were the changes in attitudes toward drinking, drug use, relationships to others (particularly various forms of authority), as measured by attitudinal questionnaires?

(7)   What was the frequency with which the individual has had disciplinary difficulties, before and after treatment?

(8)   What were the discharge rates and types (e.g., honourable) for the patients who have completed treatment?

This study indicated that the overall effectiveness rate (defined as completion of enlistment and recommendation for re-enlistment and advancement) was 72%. When the data were divided into two segments at 24 months (one group 25 years of age and younger, the other 26 years of age and older), the latter group had an 84% effectiveness rate and the former group has a 53% effectiveness rate. A follow-up analysis of nearly 3000 patients' records at 36 months after treatment shows that 83% of the older members and 46% of the younger groups were classified as effective. The weighted average of all those treated was 70%. While these statistics cover patients treated at all Navy inpatient facilities, a comparison between these facilities indicates that ARC San Diego was as effective overall, with its greatest success differential between activities existing in the area of the younger client[2].

Another report formulated by Presearch Incorporated completed on 1 July 1977 clearly established the cost benefits of treating Navy alcoholics. Its major findings and conclusions were as follows.

(1)   Alcohol abuse results in annual economic losses to the Navy ranging between $360 and $680 million per year.

(2)   The alternative of arbitrarily discharging diagnosed alcoholics and replacing them with new personnel is 2.2 times more costly than the present alcoholism rehabilitation initiative. Most important, the advantage in rehabilitating the career personnel group (aged 26 and over) is more than 5 to 1.

(3) With 5077 Navy and Marine Corps personnel afforded resident alcoholism treatment during 1976, the Department of the Navy (DON) spent $22.6 million. To obtain the same number of man years of future service by replacing these personnel, it would have cost the DON $49 million.

(4) Treatment effectiveness for the age 26 and over group (essentially career personnel) is 83%. The present treatment effectiveness for personnel aged 25 and under is 44% based upon a 2-year post-treatment evaluation.

(5) Prior to treatment, alcoholics have a sick-day rate three times higher than the average Navy–Marine Corps service member. Successful rehabilitation returns the sick-day rate to the all Navy–Marine Corps average of 2.7 days per person per year. Considering only the 5077 alcoholics treated in residential facilities during calendar year 1976 (not including the 12 609 alcoholics treated as non-resident or outpatients), this reduction in demand for inpatient health care services in the 2-year post-treatment period equates to a cost avoidance of $5.5 million. Similarly, an additional $2.3 million in outpatient health care resources are made available during the same 2-year post-treatment period.

TRAINING

The Training Department is comprised of two divisions, the Training and Education Division and the Media Division with an overall mission of providing skill training to personnel assigned world-wide to the overall NADAP effort. The training objectives are to provide to both advisors and treatment specialists the necessary knowledge and skills to treat, educate, train, advise and assist other commands in dealing with the multiple aspects of the alcoholism continuum. Educational and training approaches are under continual development in alcohol/drug misuse and addiction for a student population comprised of military personnel and civilian employees primarily from within the Navy Department, as well as other Department of Defense (DOD) employees, foreign military, and additional federal, state, and local government agency personnel on a space-available basis.

Training and Education Division

The Training and Education Division is responsible for the conduct of the Alcoholism Administration, Training, and Advisor (ATA) and the Institute in Alcoholism Studies (IAS) Courses. Figure 7.3 illustrates the training sequence, time line and requirements of those individuals designated.

Alcoholism Administration, Training and Advisor (ATA) Course

The ATA Course is a 2-week intensive course on alcoholism information. The ATA Course has been designed to transfer appropriate knowledge and

PREREQUISITE ⟶ ATA COURSE (2 WEEKS) ⟶ ATA FIELD EXPERIENCE (1 YEAR) ⟶ IAS COURSE (10 WEEKS) ⟶ ATI FIELD INTERNSHIP (9 MONTHS) ⟶ CERTIFICATION AS ATS

ATA COURSE ENTRANCE REQUIREMENTS:

One (1)* year sobriety, if alcoholic

ATA COURSE
(2 WEEKS)

REQUIREMENTS:

a. Be a volunteer
b. E-5 or above

ATA FIELD EXPERIENCE
(1 YEAR)

In field in CODAA roles of:

a. Referral agent
b. Administrator
c. Education Coordinator
d. Program Coordinator
e. designated Naval Enlisted Classification 9521

IAS COURSE
(10 WEEKS)

REQUIREMENTS:

a. Be a volunteer
b. Screened/recommended
c. ATA graduate with one year satisfactory performance in the field
d. If alcoholic, 2 years sobriety
e. E-5 or above
f. Recommendation of Commanding Officer

COMPLETION OF IAS COURSE

IAS Graduation

ATI FIELD INTERNSHIP
(9 MONTHS)

INTERNSHIP

In field in ATS roles of:

a. Screener/Evaluator
b. Counselor
c. Coordinator
d. Consultant

SUPERVISORY AND TRAINING PROGRAMS-AVAILABLE

a. *Advanced Training*
   Provide on-site training and supervision for IAS graduate
b. *Correspondence Courses*
   To advance training and skills developed in IAS
c. *Civilian Schools*

QUARTERLY REVIEWS

Quarterly reviews are provided by Counselor's Supervisor, Commanding Officer and peers

CERTIFICATION AS ATS

REQUIREMENTS:

a. Satisfactory completion of 9-month internship
b. Recommendation by Commanding Officer
c. Passing of worldwide certification exam
d. Award of Naval Enlisted Classification 9519 by Naval Military Personnel Command

ATA: Alcoholism Administration, Training and Advisor
CODAA: Collateral Duty Alcoholism Advisor
IAS: Institute in Alcoholism Studies
ATI: Alcoholism Treatment Intern
ATS: Alcoholism Treatment Specialist

* All times indicated are minimum

Figure 7.3   Training sequence for a Navy Alcoholism Treatment Specialist

skills at a level sufficient to prepare an in-field alcoholism programme advisor known as the Collateral Duty Alcoholism Advisor (CODAA) to initiate the necessary actions to institute, maintain and evaluate an ongoing command level programme in alcoholism prevention.

The following is a position description of the CODAA: The CODAA assists commands in establishing and maintaining a local alcoholism programme under guidelines set forth in NADAP directives. Assists commands in identifying alcoholics and referring them into formal treatment programmes where indicated and supports individuals returning to duty from these programmes in adjusting to their new environment through long term rehabilitation programmes. Conducts alcoholism education, as required, by programme directives or as deemed appropriate to apprise personnel of the facets of alcoholism. (The Navy Enlisted Classification for this position is NEC 9521.)

The ATA Course is designed for personnel assigned to the Naval Alcohol and Drug Abuse Program (NADAP) to familiarize them with (1) the Navy program, (2) the problems of alcoholism and other alcohol misuse among Naval personnel, both military and civilian and (3) the concept of alcoholism as a treatable illness with procedures for recognition and referral.

Throughout the course there is practice in fulfilling the roles of an administrator, referrer, educational coordinator and programme coordinator, which are roles of significance to the CODAA. These basic skills are attained in the class, in group activities, in workshops (practicum experience) and in staff–student and student–student interactions, and in other experiential activities scheduled in the ATA programme. The course aims to provide information and to provide opportunity for practical application so that the student will be better equipped to manage an alcohol programme at his command.

The course runs for 2 weeks, with instruction beginning at 0745 and ending most days by 1630 (4:30 p.m.). The meeting times are scheduled according to instructional content and Alcoholics Anonymous (AA) meeting demands. Homework assignments are made for each day which include, but are not limited to, readings, daily paper assignments, and attendance at AA, Alanon, and Alateen meetings.

Instructional methodology for the course includes didactic instruction, small group and large group activities, and application exercises supported by multimedia instruction. Course content or knowledge areas include the alcohol element within the Human Resources Management Program of the Navy; symptoms and phases of alcoholism, the physical, psychological, and spiritual aspects of alcoholism; recognition and referral of the alcoholic and other alcohol misuser; rehabilitation of the alcoholic; and, continuing recovery programmes such as Alcoholics Anonymous[3] (see Figure 7.4).

Institute in Alcoholism Studies (IAS) Course

The Navy Alcoholism Treatment Specialist (ATS) is one of the essential elements in the NADAP. As shown in the flow chart, Training Sequence for a

NAVAL ALCOHOL AND DRUG ABUSE PROGRAM

Purpose
Structure
Policy
Legal aspects

DISEASE CONCEPT OF ALCOHOLISM

Sociocultural Aspects
Theories of causality
Symptoms & phases
Medical aspects
Psychosocial aspects
Spiritual aspects
Iceberg concept
Living sober

PERSONAL AWARENESS & SUBSTANCE ABUSE

Attitudes
Sociodrama experience
Mental health
Polydrug addiction & misuse
Alcoholism: a family affair
AA, Alanon, Alateen
Communications: dynamic listening & interviewing
Philosophy & modalities of treatment

ALCOHOL PROGRAM MANAGEMENT

Recognition & documentation
Resources
Referral
Re-entry & continuing recovery program
Instructional design

ONGOING PROCESSES: Learning Point Exercises/Applications
Daily Paper Assignments
AA Attendance
Group & Individual Meetings With Staff

RECOVERING ALCOHOLIC— Recognition & documentation
Referral & treatment
Resources & re-entry
Continuing recovery program
AA, Alanon, Alateen

ALCOHOLISM STUDIES FLOW

WHAT: Disease

WHY: Sociocultural aspects
Theory of causality

HOW: ALCOHOLIC— Symptoms & phases
Medical aspects
Psychosocial aspects
Spiritual aspects
Iceberg concept

Figure 7.4 ATA Course content areas

Navy Alcoholism Treatment Specialist (Figure 7.3), most individuals entering the 10-week IAS Course have gained some experience and basic programme knowledge in the field of alcoholism through completion of the ATA Course and 1 year's experience as a CODAA.

At this point, the role of the ATS becomes more specific as it is described in the following position description: ATS assists medical officers and other professional staff personnel in establishing and maintaining formal treatment programmes for active duty, retired and reserve personnel and dependents assigned to Alcohol Rehabilitation Centers, Services and Counseling and Assistance Centers; conducts individual and group therapy sessions during hospitalization/rehabilitation periods; maintains statistical data on patients' progress and prepares summary reports; assists treated personnel in returning to full duty; and assists local commands in establishing alcohol misuse prevention, education, identification, safety, and rehabilitation programmes. (The Navy Enlisted Classification for this position is NEC 9519.)

Based on the above job description, the IAS Course was developed.

The IAS Course has been developed from the same perspective with regard to educational objectives as that which formed the foundation of the ATA Course and both courses within the philosophical parameters of training as defined by Petree[4].

The educational taxonomy can be categorized into the following levels of competence: knowledge, comprehension, application, analysis, synthesis and evaluation.

Basically the ATS is required to perform and demonstrate skills as coordinator, consultant, and counselor. As a programme coordinator, the ATS actively seeks to ensure that administrative and programmatic resources are available for the treatment of alcoholics. In this capacity, he must function as a manager of personnel, coordinator of resources, and even as a supervisor of counselors. As a consultant, he functions as advisor, trainer, and expert resource to a variety of organizations utilizing basic consultant and training skills to assist these organizations in providing access and means for treatment of alcoholics. As a counselor, the ATS provides direct services to alcoholic-dependent persons.

The IAS Course is intended to prepare all ATS students to operate in any and all of these roles and perform specified functions with proper supervision and internship. Although the emphasis of the IAS Course is on counselling skills, the basic skills, competencies and self-understanding required to perform effectively as a counselor are the very same as those required to be an effective manager and consultant. The basic competencies in such areas as dynamic listening, the giving and receiving of feedback, empathetic under-standing of others, along with a degree of comfort with self, are all essential in each of these roles. Consequently, training for each role will support and reinforce the training for the other two. Figures 7.5 and 7.6 depict course objectives and flow.

The successful completion of the IAS Course, which has an attrition rate of 40%, is just one more step up the ladder to becoming a qualified ATS.

ROLE	FUNCTION	SKILL	SKILL AREA
COORDINATOR	Personnel management	Conducts supervisor's performance counseling Session	Supervisoral counseling skills Performance analysis documentation
	Administration	Leadership and management theories	Screening interview Leadership model Problem solving process PO & M Development Organizational relationship Policy-resource Use Case recommendation/decision making
CONSULTANT	Consulting	Consultant intervention	Consulting process Entry process Feedback and planning Training development
COUNSELOR	Interpersonal	Analysis of communication process	Non-verbal behavior indicators Communication skills
	Group leadership	Demonstrate group leadership techniques	Group interventions
	Counseling	Conduct counseling session	Define counseling & therapy Human sexuality & alcoholism ATS capabilities/limitations Counseling behaviors Videotape equipment
	Crisis intervention	Emergency & counseling procedures	Drug symptoms & Emergency treatment Crisis intervention counseling
	Case Management	Summary disposition of clients	Initial interview Treatment recommendation
	Counseling practicum	Conducting individual & group counseling	Narrative summary post-treatment Student counselor performance

Figure 7.5 ATA roles and functions

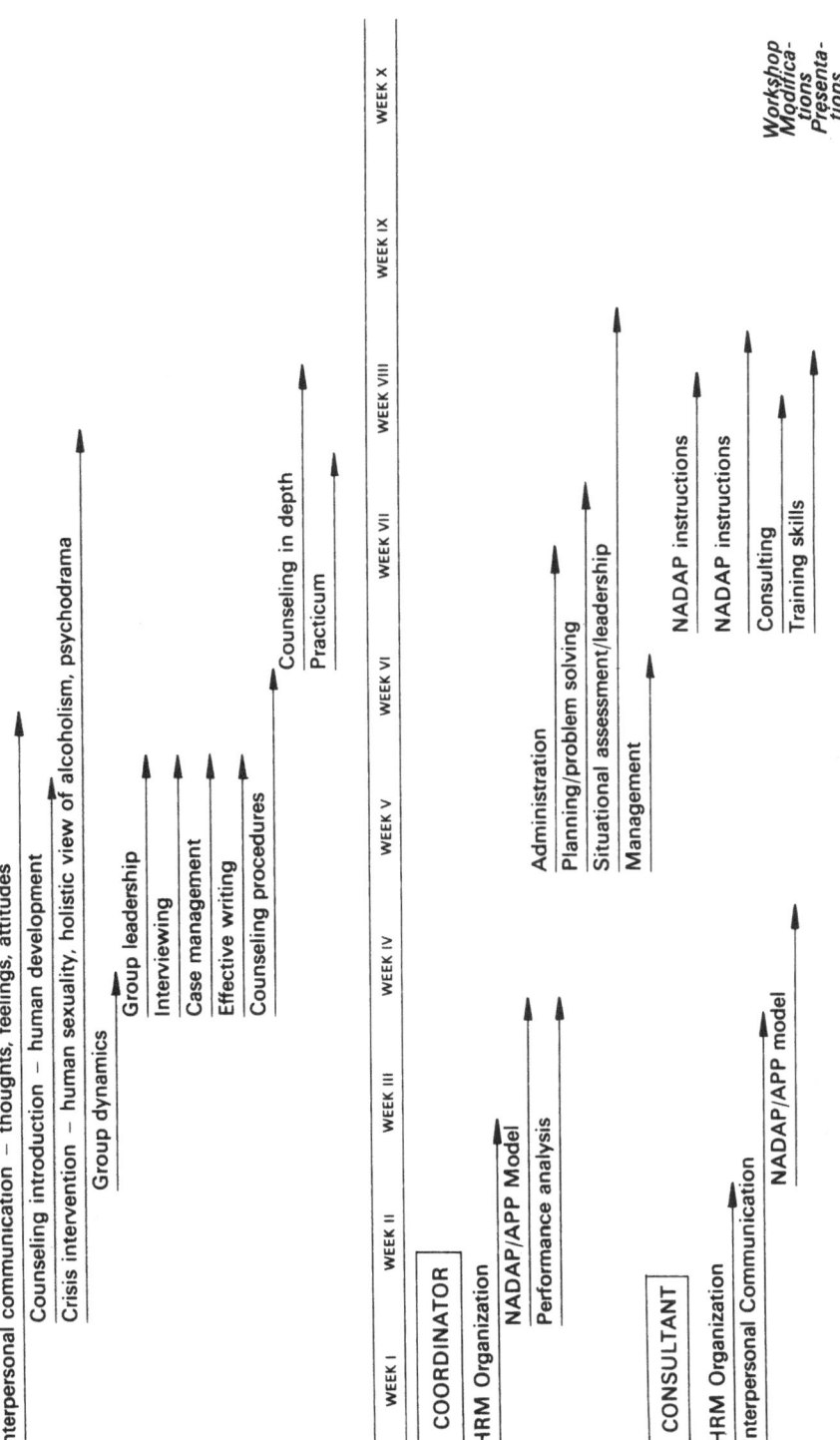

Figure 7.6 IAS Course flow

Following graduation a year of supervised internship is required before the ATI can be recommended by his Commanding Officer, to participate in a comprehensive certification examination. Following successful completion of the examination, the counselor receives the NEC 9519 and title of Alcoholism Treatment Specialist. At present, approximately 70% of those taking the exam succeed on the first try.

Media Division

The Media Division of the Training Department supports the treatment and training programmes of the ARC, San Diego, and provides various assistance and administrative services to Naval Military Personnel Command (NMPC) sponsored NADAP operations and Department of Defense (DOD) drug and alcohol programmes. The Media Division is responsible for the selection of audiovisual hardware, consultation in the evaluation of training material purchases, control and maintenance of media equipment, and in-house production of non-print instructional and educational programmes. Specific functions can be broadly categorized as follows.

Group A/V support

All patient and IAS student group activities within both Treatment and Training Departments are done under 360° camera coverage with taping. Supervision of these functions is accomplished in the main control centre where supervisory remarks can be made on the tape at the time of the actual group process. Through a main switcher console, other supervisory activities are provided to remote stations such as the offices of Commanding Officer, Training and Treatment Department Heads, and the Senior Military Counselor. Figures 7.7–7.10 provide technical information on how this process is accomplished.

A/V library

The ARC, San Diego, houses an instructional resource library accessible to ARC staff, inpatients and ATA students. On an as-available basis, the library will provide short term loans of material to other DOD drug and alcohol programmes in the local area. The library contains a diversified collection of resources on drug and alcohol abuse, treatment practices, counselling strategies, and family and personal relationship development etc. The media ensemble includes playback hardware and over 200 videotape titles, 160 16 mm films, 250 audio cassettes, collection of instructional transparencies, slide/tape programmes and other instructional packages.

Production and media user support

The Media Division produces a bimonthly videotape on a subject pertinent to alcohol and/or drug misuse. This tape is distributed to over 95 activities via the

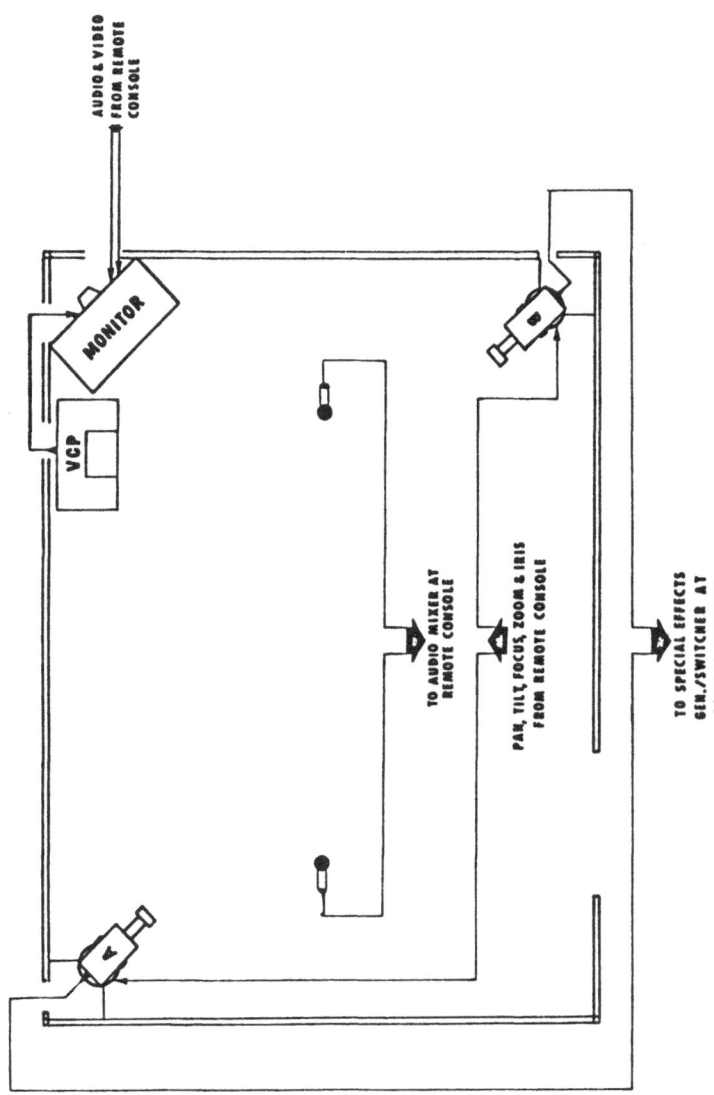

TYPICAL GROUP ROOM

Figure 7-7 Typical group room

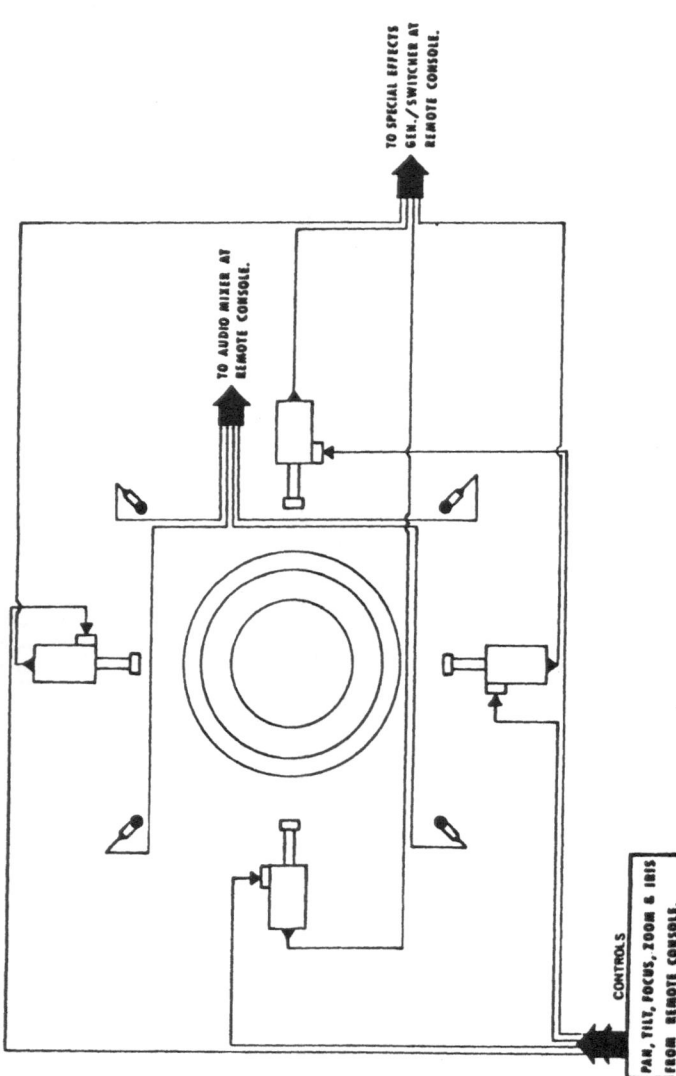

PSYCHODRAMA THEATRE

Figure 7.8 Psychodrama theatre

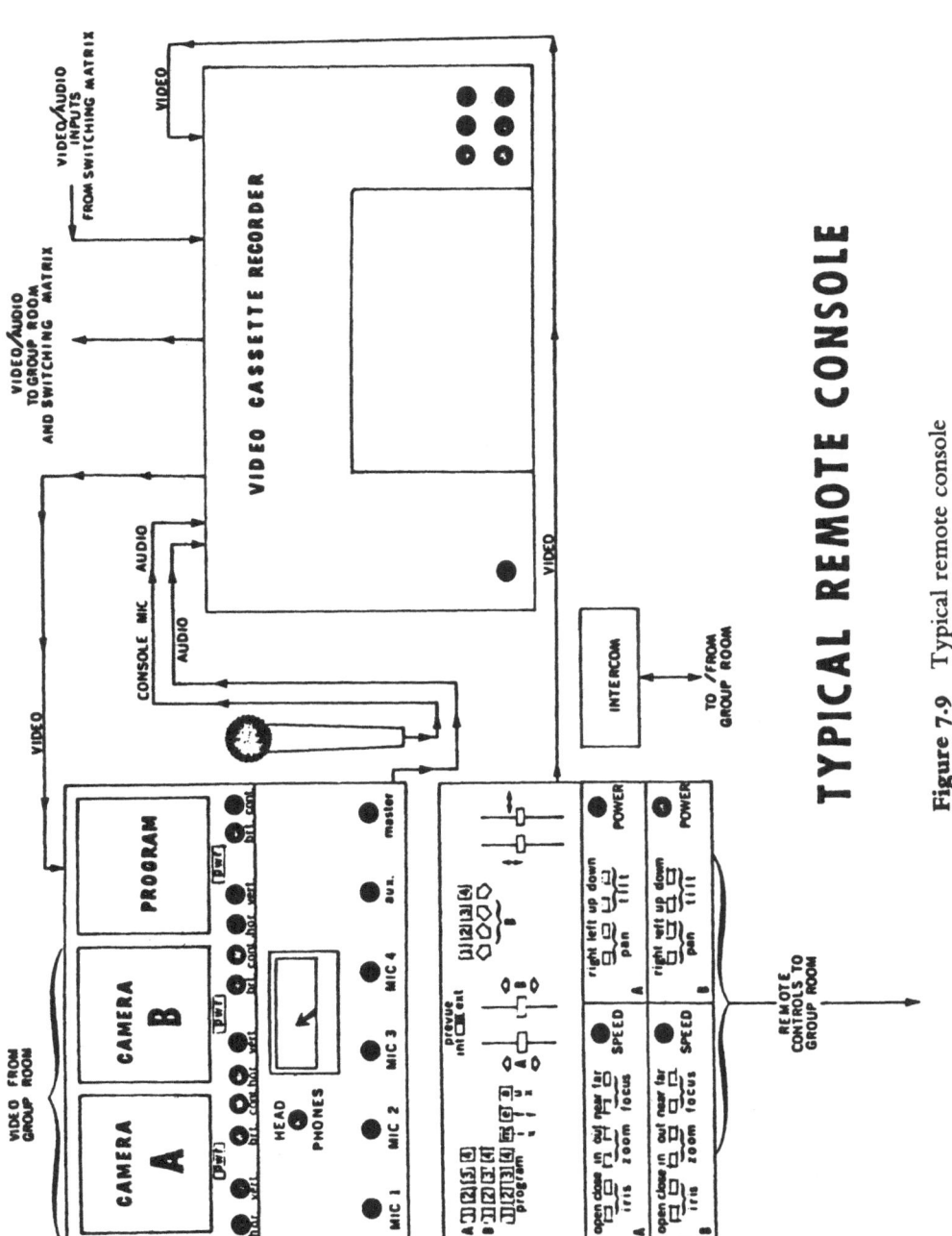

TYPICAL REMOTE CONSOLE

Figure 7.9   Typical remote console

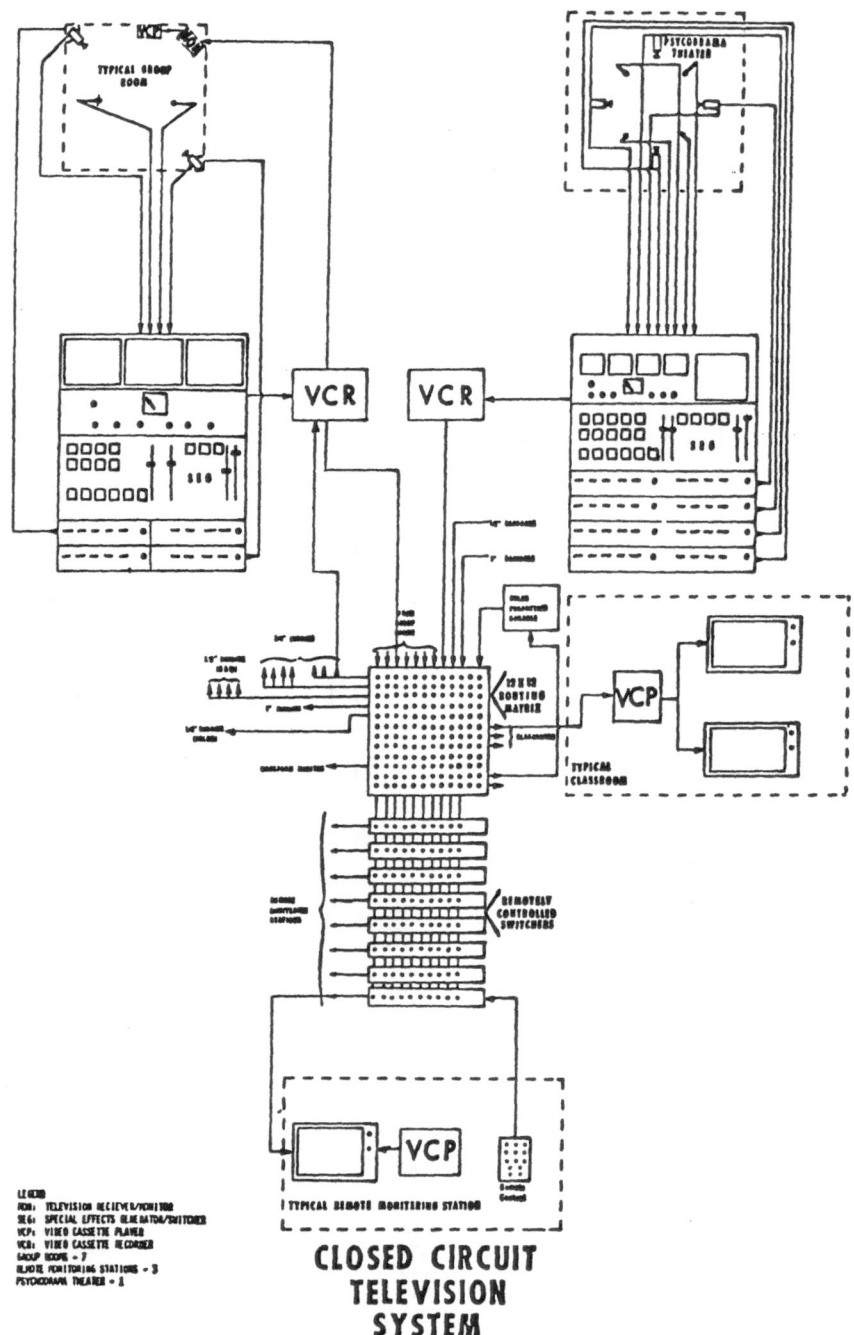

Figure 7.10 Closed circuit television system

Bicycle Program, which was developed in 1976 to provide educational material to NADAP facilities. The production staff duplicates non-copyright video and audio tapes, and dubs transfer films or slide productions to video for distribution to world-wide NADAP installations. Still photography and graphic services are provided for ARC use. Media Division provides facilities, equipment and technical skills for remote camera monitoring and videotaping of inpatient group sessions (728 hours annually), and couple's group (208 hours annually). Support of the IAS Course is furnished by remote camera monitoring and videotaping of growth group (208 hours annually) and supervision group (208 hours annually). The audiovisual taping of these patient/student groups is a vital part of the treatment and training programmes. Audiovisual tapes are made of guest speakers and lecturers for use in the patient and/or student groups. The Media Division staff is responsible for setting up and operating equipment for showing films, slides etc. specifically to the IAS and the ATA Classes, as well as at other times as requested. Instructors from this division are provided training in the use and care of A/V equipment to students of the IAS Course, and they also provide technical support to our sister ARCs and ARSs.

PREVENTION DEPARTMENT

The Prevention Department has as its mission the delivery of actual preventive education programmes to the Navy population as a whole. While the Training Department develops skilled workers who then deliver their services to other commands for use with people, the Prevention Department does this and goes beyond by interfacing with the end product, i.e., fleet personnel themselves. This department has three divisions: Navy Alcohol Safety Action Program (NASAP), Navy Drug Safety Action Program (NDSAP), and Field Office Division.

NASAP

In 1974 the NASAP[8] commenced operations with its mission being alcohol misuse prevention. The purpose was to provide a consistent mechanism through which Navy personnel involved in alcohol-related problem situations occurring within the legal and medical systems could be identified at the earliest indication of alcohol misuse or alcoholism and referred to appropriate levels of education or treatment. This mission is accomplished with as much uniformity as the system will allow and yet with the flexibility to meet local requirements. The NASAP effort attempts to reach people at the earliest point on the continuum, hopefully prior to the addictive phase. The system can be entered either voluntarily or non-voluntarily (as shown in Figure 7.11).

The US Navy began its prevention effort following an extensive nationwide examination of existing programmes beginning with the federally-funded ASAP efforts. NASAP developed and accepted several basic

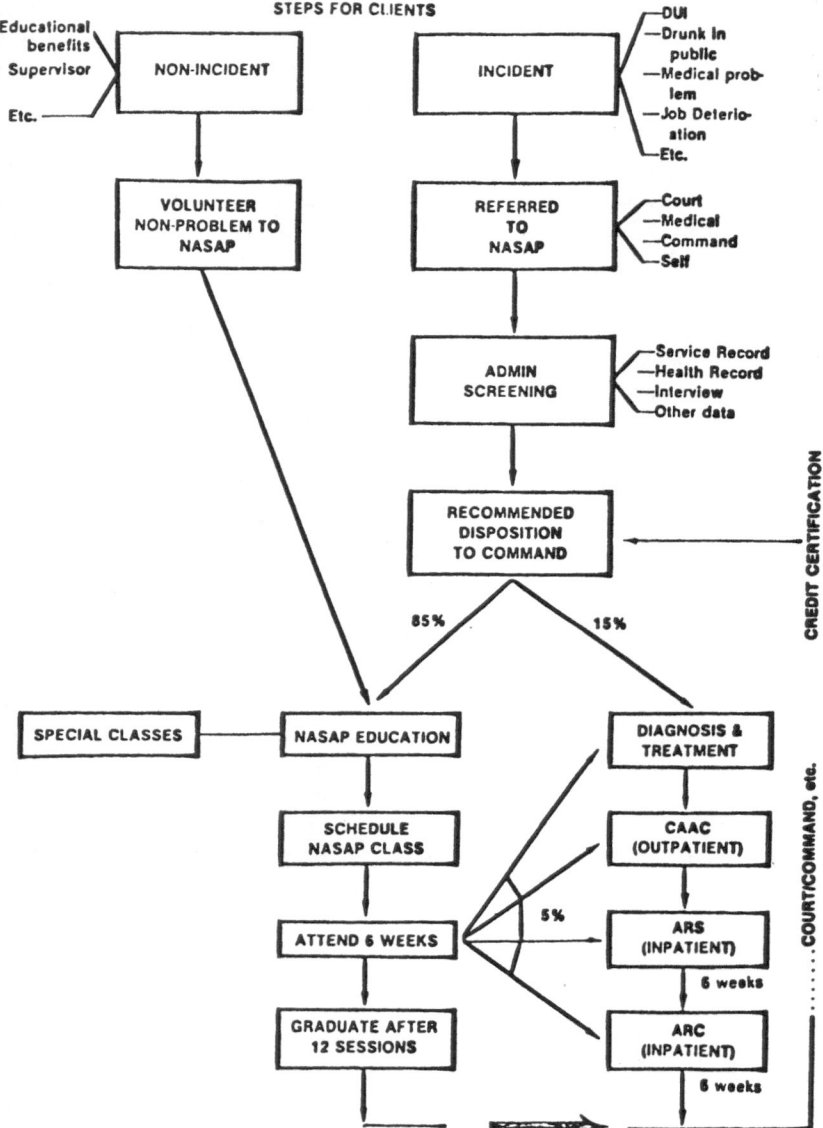

Figure 7.11 NASAP system approach (client flow)

hypotheses which, when validated, became tenets of the approach to the problem. Prevention is one of those tenets.

The purpose of prevention is to increase the individual's understanding of personally and professionally destructive alcohol-related behavior. The Navy Alcohol Safety Action Program is aimed at reducing the number of persons whose potentially existing alcohol-related behaviour adversely affects the way they carry out everyday living.

Prevention activities take place at three levels: primary, secondary, and tertiary.

(1)   Primary prevention includes all activities that reduce the number of new cases with initial alcohol-related disabilities. It is based on an individual's formation of values, attitudes, and beliefs and occurs principally in the formal education of K−12 (from kindergarten to end of twelfth grade) or in the home − generally areas out of direct control of the Navy.

(2)   Secondary prevention efforts are directed to people who have non-addictive drinking-related behaviours such as those which often result from inappropriate use or occasional overuse of alcohol. This requires facilitating the change of existing values and attitudes of the individual − a NASAP process which can occur at any time.

(3)   Tertiary prevention refers to activities concerned with people who have several alcohol-related behaviours. These persons are diagnosed as alcoholics. Therefore, screening and evaluation at the outset become key elements of the programme. Individuals who show a need for more extensive care are referred for clinical diagnosis and treatment.

Because all Navy personnel are over the age of 17, the focus has had to be on secondary prevention. Studies indicate that 45% of the Navy recruits[9] reported heavy drinking prior to enlistment and 27% reported trouble with the law (at least one civil arrest) involving alcohol within the 3 years prior to enlistment. The fact remains that the average age for the commencement of drinking was 16 or under. In a survey of 16 000 patients in Naval hospitals 74.2% fell into this category!

NASAP, as the Navy's secondary prevention effort, is designed to identify and reduce the problems caused by alcohol misuse and/or alcoholism. NASAP's efforts focus on addressing problems at the earliest possible stage, when they are first identified through civilian law violations, work-related accidents, military offences and hospital emergency room or sick call records.

Generally, NASAP's basic entry point occurs upon notification of a crisis or traumatic event that an individual misusing alcohol or, in fact, alcoholic, may be experiencing. The traumatic event could be due to alcohol-induced medical or legal complications that cause the individual to undergo personal discomfort or pain. This expanded identification includes the use of alcohol-related accidents, fights, unauthorized absences, excessive sick calls and hospital treatment, recreational accidents, decreasing job performance and family difficulties. Any such incident or combination thereof can be a signal to the supervisor of the need to get the individual into some form of education or treatment programme. It should also be noted that more than 20% of the participants are now 'walking in' to take the course solely for the information or college credits offered.

The next step in the system is the administrative screening which includes participant completion of a short biographic computer information sheet used for the Navy Alcohol and Drug Information System (NADIS).

The interview is neither a confrontation nor a counselling session, but merely an opportunity to gather information. It also is the optimum time to give the participant positive reinforcement for his taking action.

It must be stressed here that individuals who volunteer to attend NASAP for purely academic reasons undergo no screening except for the completion of the short NADIS information sheet. If, however, during the course, they or the staff recognize a problem that needs further attention, it will be dealt with in the previously described manner.

Once the individual enters the NASAP educational portion of the system (Figure 7.11), he is afforded 36 hours of course material that is designed to do, among other things, the following.

(1) To educate people in recognizing the early symptoms of a developing alcoholic person or misuser.

(2) To provide preventive education to participants, law enforcement officials, supervisors, club managers, medical personnel, dependents, and others who may simply be interested in increasing their own awareness.

(3) To address safety needs by educating safety officials and others on the impact of alcohol and its cause and effect relationship to injuries, deaths and material losses.

(4) To participate as a full partner with the civilian community in addressing common needs with respect to the community's alcohol problems.

(5) To diminish the emotionalism surrounding alcohol and the stigma associated with alcoholics − replacing the negativism with realization that alcoholism is both preventable and treatable.

(6) Finally, to provide commanding officers, law enforcement officials and medical officers with complementary or alternative measures in dealing with sociological or medical complications resulting from alcohol, while still emphasizing personal accountability and responsibility.

NASAP, however, as an educational programme that deals with basic attitudes which affect the whole person is, in its application, in no way restricted to those experiencing alcohol-related difficulties. Its use has been of equal value in the training and development of human behaviour in supervisors, accession point candidates, medical personnel and others. Attitudes regarding alcohol and its use on a personal basis most often reflect the posture of others with whom an individual might have contact such as a supervisor, medical care practitioner, family member, friend or peer. If the attitudes of such persons are based on the many myths or misconceptions prevalent in society, they will be ill-equipped to help those who come within their sphere of influence.

NASAP utilizes a systems approach featuring the meshing of two chains of command which operate side by side and yet independently. The Navy has primary responsibility for the overall management of the programme. To accomplish this mission, each site has an experienced Officer in Charge (OIC) supported by several enlisted personnel.

The principal responsibility of the Navy staff is to effect liaison between NASAP and fleet commanders, courts, other civilian agencies, medical units and treatment facilities. The Navy staff ensures that credibility of NASAP as a Navy resource is maintained, for the staff is best equipped to gain access to the information required to make accurate assessments of personnel and fleet needs. All action relative to the steps taken between NASAP and fleet needs, Naval facilities or civilian judicial systems is the Navy's responsibility.

The second chain of command is that of the University of Arizona (U of A), Tucson, Arizona, which is currently responsible for delivering the educational product through a task-oriented, non-personal service contract. The initial academic institution that helped develop NASAP was the University of West Florida (UWF), Pensacola, Florida. For 7 years, the team effort of the USN with the UWF produced a product that is being mirrored all over the world. This excellent record and team effort is presently being advanced by the U of A where the NASAP/NDSAP effort is organized under the School of Medicine, Department of Family and Community Medicine. All activities relative to educational screening, classroom coordination, education records and facilitation of the actual classes are the responsibility of the Program Director of U of A. The selection, training, and management of the University employees is exercised through the local representatives. Once a participant is referred through the Navy's side of the NASAP system as a candidate for education, it becomes U of A's responsibility to screen, schedule, educate, and then return the participant to the Navy side for final disposition back to command or court. If, during any phase of operations under the control of the U of A, it is considered that the participant is not appropriate for education, he is returned to the Navy part of NASAP for referral to clinical screening and possible formal treatment. Figure 7.12 provides an overview of the system.

Field Office Division

In order to provide the services to the Fleet in a consistent manner, the ARC directly manages 12 NASAP/NDSAP sites and maintains quality control over the programmes that exist at an additional 12 sites ashore and 14 aircraft carrier programmes afloat. The Field Office Division holds responsibility for the coordination effort required for budget, manning, resource procurement and the assistance visits for this world-wide effort. The principal focus of this process is to ensure educational quality growth and consistent programming world-wide. Table 7.2 enumerates site data.

Since NASAP's inception in 1974, over 100 000 participants have been referred. Currently more than 3000 per month are entering the system.

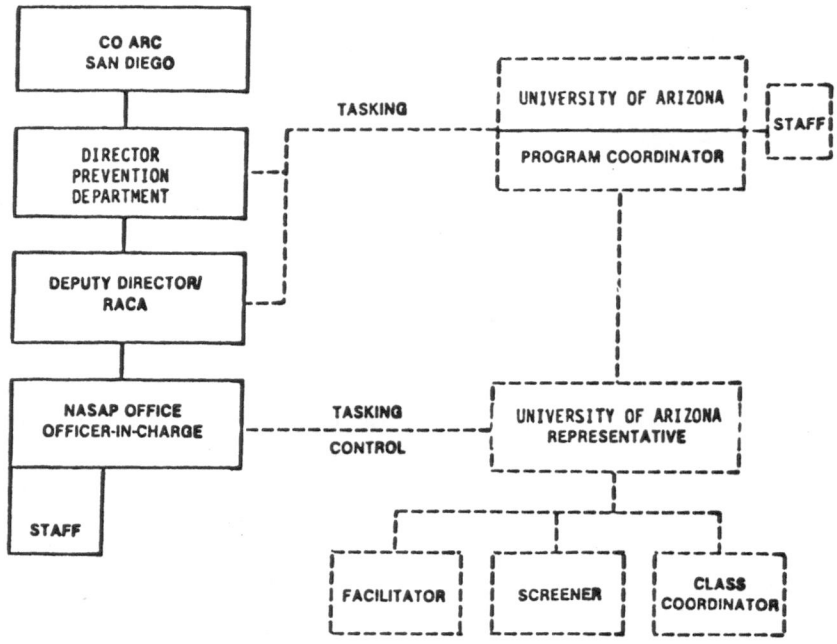

Figure 7.12   NASAP system

Several evaluative efforts have been made including one that indicated that 93 % of NASAP graduates received good or excellent evaluations on work performance, military behaviour, leadership, adaptability and military appearance 6 months after participation. Eighty-six per cent had not required any subsequent disciplinary action, 89 % were recommended for re-enlistment and 80 % were recommended for promotion. When matched with a control group the differences ranged from 3.1 to 5.7[1].

An additional comparison study brought about similarly favourable results when NASAP was compared with other programmes[5]. Also, in the civilian setting of an 'honour camp' for alcohol offenders where a NASAP pilot was utilized, a decrease of annual recidivism from 30 % to 3 % was reported[6]. The current research projects include development and field testing of a predictive model of substance use within the Navy, outcome evaluation of NASAP from 1979 and ongoing outcome evaluation from 1980 and later of the NDSAP. The latter two studies include a matched pairs design comparing the former NASAP and NDSAP models to the current lifestyle education packages. The final study investigates facilitator characteristics and effectiveness in terms of student outcomes. These three efforts are being managed by Dr Barbara Hartman, U of A, in coordination with the Naval Personnel Research and Development Center and the Naval Health Research Center, both in San Diego, California.

Table 7.2 NASAP site data (to 31 December 1981)

Site	Date opened or scheduled	Referrals	Education	Treatment
Bremerton, WA	4—77	5 628	5 178	450
Charleston, SC	7—77	3 834	3 644	190
Corpus Christi, TX	8—80	280	268	12
Great Lakes, ILL	7—79	3 268	3 027	241
Holy Loch, Scotland	4—78	1 626	1 341	285
Jacksonville, FL	2—79	10 826	7 666	3160
Lakehurst, NJ	2—80	803	551	252
Naples, Italy	1—80	370	325	45
New London, CT	12—76	12 725	11 685	1040
Norfolk, VA	1—76	10 610	8 821	1789
Memphis, TN	6—80	418	374	44
Meridian, MS	11—80	416	414	2
Orlando, FL	9—77	6 948	6 514	434
Okinawa, Japan	2—81	119	115	4
Paxtuent River, MD	10—78	400	362	38
Pearl Harbor, HI	3—77	8 082	6 398	1676
Pensacola, FL	9—74	3 659	3 180	479
Philadelphia, PA	4—80	465	446	19
Port Hueneme, CA	2—80	554	554	0
Rota, Spain	9—77	1 297	1 223	74
San Diego, CA	10—76	9 600	8 921	679
San Francisco, CA	8—77	4 823	4 688	135
Subic Bay, R.P.	9—77	2 858	2 656	202
Washington, DC	4—77	2 286	2 066	220

NDSAP

In 1980, as the direct result of the success of NASAP and the direct immediate need to deal with drugs other than alcohol, the Navy Drug Safety Action Program (NDSAP) was developed. Its purpose was twofold also: firstly as an *intervention* programme for the non-addicted user and secondly as a *prevention* programme for the non-user. The NDSAP pilot effort commenced in San Diego, California, Norfolk, Virginia, and Jacksonville, Florida, and lasted one entire year. It readily became apparent that the NASAP and NDSAP efforts were being affected by societal attitudes that separated drugs (other than alcohol) and alcohol for many reasons including:

(1) Legality: Drugs are illegal; alcohol is not.
(2) Drug subculture: Bonding for protection (we/they).
(3) Counterculturing: General society has tolerated a certain degree of drug *use* while USN demands zero tolerance.

(4)   Disease versus crime: Alcoholism is a disease where recovery is possible. Drugger is a sociopath/criminal and should be rejected.

However, the pilot effort processed 2500 referrals and a short term evaluation indicated statistically significant improvements in the area of behaviour, attitudes and potential for continued Naval service[7] (see Table 7.3). The pilot effort, having been proven of value to the Fleet, and following the Chief of Naval Operations' review, was approved for total expansion. Table 7.4 lists the sites of current and future operations.

Table 7.3   Comparison of supervisor ratings before and after attending DSAP among identified drug users

Intial rating (before)	Rating after participation					Percentage showing improvement
	Poor	Marginal	Average	Good	Excellent	
Poor						
Behaviour	43	29	—	29	—	57
Attitude	17	17	17	50	—	83
Potential	42	8	17	17	17	58
Marginal						
Behaviour	4	13	44	35	4	83
Attitude	7	20	17	40	17	73
Potential	4	25	36	25	11	71

ADMINISTRATIVE DEPARTMENT

ARC San Diego presents a wide spectrum of activities devoted to dealing with the alcohol problem continuum and thereby accentuating the need for clear and strong central management. The creation of a health systems environment wherein creative talents can flourish as well as sick personnel can gain health is the core responsibility of the Administrative effort. The Navy uses the systems approach, wherein policy needs are met through centralized command and control which is exercised strongly at ARC. The Commanding Officer, as the focus for decisions necessary to meet the shifting and blending nature of the continuum, relies upon the Executive Officer (XO) and Administrative Department to deal with the manpower, budget and resource requirements which allow the other departments to perform their tasks with a minimum of extraneous administrative chores. The role of the administrators is not only to ensure the availability of the tools to perform each task but also to interact with parent commands, higher authority and outside agencies in order to orchestrate continuing follow-up regarding patients or students with the widest possible spectrum of interested parties. To

Table 7.4   NDSAP: sites of current and future operations (data to 31 December 1982)

Site	Date opened or scheduled	Referrals	Education	Treatment
Jacksonville, FL	4–81	403	248	10
Norfolk, VA	3–81	509	239	25
San Diego, CA	10–80	2075	1176	104
Bremerton, WA	12–81			
Charleston, SC	2–82			
Corpus Christi, TX	6–82			
Great Lakes, ILL	2–82			
Holy Loch, Scotland	4–82			
Lakehurst, NJ	7–82			
Naples, Italy	4–82			
New London, CT	1–82			
Memphis, TN	3–82			
Meridian, MS	6–82			
Orlando, FL	1–82			
Okinawa, Japan	5–82			
Paxtuent River, MD	3–82			
Pearl Harbor, HI	12–81			
Pensacola, FL	2–82			
Philadelphia, PA	6–82			
Port Hueneme, CA	6–82			
Portsmouth, NH	7–82			
Rota, Spain	4–82			
San Francisco, CA	12–81			
Sasebo, Japan	5–82			
Subic Bay, P.I.	5–82			
Yokosuka, Japan	5–82			

accomplish this mission, the ARC has management responsibility for the following.

Administrative Division

The Division covers:

Management responsibility for manpower distributed as follows:

Headquarters, San Diego		World-wide sites
11	Officer	9
20	Enlisted	24
19	Civil Servants	7
20	U of A Associates	700

Armed Services Medical Regulating Office (ASMRO) liaison (Medevac System)
Patient administration
Word processing, central files, correspondence
Legal and discipline.

Budget Division

The Division handles:

$4,900.00 annual budget − FY 82
Contracts manager ($7 300 000) multi-year contracts
ARC operation.

Supply Division

The Division deals with:

Purchasing
Plant property accounting
Pre-expended stores

Facilities Management Division

The Division deals with:

Building maintenance
Public works and grounds
Vehicle control

Management matrix

It is within the overall responsibilities of the principal managers, i.e., Commanding Officer, Executive Officer and Department Heads, that the key policy issues are decided. Central core issues include:

The mix of recovering staff with 'non-recovering'
The interaction of professional and paraprofessional staff
Use of cross-staff assignments
The blend of the primary recovery AA plan and other modalities
Advanced training of staff
Patient responsibilities
Patient termination
Student deselection
Treatment plan modifications
Training curriculum development
Five-year plans
Budget calls
Personnel replacement

World-wide inspection visits
Staff papers, publications and convention publications
Discipline and legal matters
Policy recommendations to higher authority
Liaison with civilian and military community.

The combined results of the ARC from 1973 to date are:
5245 patients admitted
4354 patients returned to duty
3965 ATA students graduated
416 IAS students graduated
98 187 NASAP referrals
2764 NDSAP referrals.

Key personnel travel throughout the world on a continuing basis to ensure quality growth and the widest possible information dissemination. The ARC has become the benefactor of patients and students on a continuous basis from Canada, Australia, and individual graduates from New Zealand and Britain with visitors from many additional countries.

Following a 2-week visit to the ARC recently, a renowned physician commented that while the Treatment, Training, and Prevention Departments represented the best there was in their respective areas, the fact remained that proper management was the key. ARC San Diego is part of a larger human resource effort that responds to a central leadership dedicated to mission readiness with an overall emphasis on personal pride and professionalism.

CONCLUSION

Officially the US Navy has, by edict of the Secretary of the Navy, as early as 1972, stipulated:

'The Department of the Navy recognizes that the disease, illness, or condition known as alcoholism is preventable and treatable, and requires the application of enlightened attitudes and techniques by command, supervisory, and health service personnel. Prevention is the responsibility of the individual . . . an individual must actively seek and cooperate in treatment or rehabilitation efforts or he may be determined to be unsuitable for further military service or employment and may be separated.'

This policy received further delineation a year later when the Chief of Naval Operations spelled out in further detail:

'Alcohol abuse and alcoholism to any degree constitutes an unacceptable loss to the Navy in training investment and operational efficiency and a high cost in resources and human suffering.'
'Alcoholism is an illness for treatment and rehabilitation purposes.'
'Alcoholism is not compensable for disability purposes.'

'While the basic individual responsibility for prevention and treatment is recognized, commands are responsible for identifying alcoholic persons and ordering them into rehabilitation whether or not they first seek or volunteer for treatment.'

'Commands must make every effort to confront and eliminate the stigma which has long been associated with alcoholism.'

As it can be seen, the joint responsibility, shared between the command and the individual, is clear. Stated otherwise, while an individual may not be responsible for contracting the disease of alcoholism, once treated, he is responsible for his own recovery. At the same time, the misuse of alcohol is also an issue of individual accountability with commands retaining educational responsibility relative to responsible use.

The statement of policy and its uniform application form the key to the Navy's effort, but the Navy has gone further than most agencies by creating indigenous treatment programmes as well as training programmes supported by considerable number of personnel and millions of dollars. This effort is characterized by its total immersion within the system. Patients and students are dealt with within the organizational melee from which they come thus preserving the organizational involvement from identification, referral and follow-up. Treatment personnel come from the Fleet and return to the Fleet, thereby preserving the common bond of professional identity between patient and counselor. Training personnel also are not only from the Fleet but themselves are trained counselors who are current with patient demographics.

Not content with this, the Navy has made a tremendous commitment to the field of prevention, long before it was fashionable and during the time when treatment and rehabilitation captured most of the attention and resources. In the past, the disease model of alcoholism demanded an obsession with the alcoholic, literally ignoring warning signs until the addicted phase was firmly established. The Navy has often described treatment as an ambulance at the bottom of the cliff collecting casualties after their fall. However, through NASAP, initially, and now NDSAP, fences are being built at the top in the hope of interrupting the more destructive processes. In addition, the massive retention and follow-on successful careers of those personnel treated, trained or educated, mutes most effectively the age-old issue of stigmatization.

Currently, the Navy, through the leadership of its current Chief of Naval Operations, Admiral Thomas Hayward, is undergoing a revitalization, with emphasis on pride and professionalism being the focal point. Just as low self-worth and lack of self-esteem have been one of the identifying symptoms of the alcohol-afflicted person, pride and personal credibility are the hallmarks of those individuals who either work in the Navy's alcohol and drug programme or who have become the product of one of its many services. The ARC and its sister organizations located throughout the world represent not only the largest single system devoted to alcohol continuum, but it also remains a leader in the continuum of care.

Acknowledgments

This paper represents the experiences, thoughts, and the realization of the dreams of many truly dedicated program people from the past like Capt Jim Baxter, USN (Ret.), Capt Stu Brownell, USN (Ret.), Cdr Chuck Sapp, USN (Ret.), Cdr Bill Jernberg, USNR-R, Mr Ken Allison, LCdr Burt Frazier, USN (Ret.), Ms Mary Bergman, Mr George Gilpin, PNC Carl Samples, USN (Ret.), and countless others the author worked with and learned from while assigned to the Navy's Alcohol Office in Washington, DC. Many others from the other branches of the military such as LtCol Karen Wheeler, USMC (Ret.), LCdr Mike Bell, USAF, Col Dave Carney, USA, and from the Department of Defense itself Mr Bob Stein and Dr John Mazucchi also contributed greatly to our efforts. Fellow ARC Commanding Officers, Cdr Steve Stevenson, USN, and Capt Tom Glancy, USN are a source of inspiration.

Here at ARC, San Diego my long-time associates – Mr Pete Petree, MGYSgt Frank Moran, USMC, Mr John McGary, LCdr Tully Lale, USN, Lt Tom Burden, USN, Mr Carroll Stroud, Mr Steve Knight, AMHC Fred Sipe, USN, Mr Bob Remillard, YN1 Diane Henderson, USN, Mr Bill Burns, Cdr Walt Welsh, USN, Mrs Dolores Harris, Mrs Barbara Baylon, BMCM 'W.' 'T.' Monroe, USN, Mrs Mildred Casad, MGYSgt Carl Mullen, USMC, YNC Tom Conant, USCG, Still McKerley, our 'major domo' Mrs Judy Brown who tried to bring order out of chaos, and all the *other truly* dedicated staff members in Treatment, Training, Prevention and numerous NASAP/NDSAP sites worldwide from the past to the present including Capt Jerry Tappan, USN (Ret.), Mr Bill Albertson, USN (Ret.), Cdr Howard Petty, USN, and Capt Clarence Priddy, USN (Ret.), who made learning such a challenge. A great deal of leadership and constructive thought was and is generated by Capt Hal Taylor, USN, Capt Jack Taschian, MC, USN, and Mr Daryl Kreglo from the Naval Drug Rehabilitation Center (NDRC), Miramar, CA. The contributions within the research and evaluation efforts of LCdr Steve Bucky, USNR-R, Mr Ed Thomas and Mr Doug Kolb were significant. I also must not forget the contributions of my 'brother' Paul for they were many. Many others deserve to be mentioned and I beg their forgiveness but time and space preclude this.

References

1 Bucky, S. F. (1979). *The 1978 Evaluation of the Navy's Alcohol Rehabilitation, Alcohol Safety Action (NASAP), and Alcoholism Counselor Training Programs.* (San Diego: Naval Alcohol Rehabilitation Center)

2 Borthwick, R. B. (1977). *Summary of Cost-Benefit Study Results for Navy Alcoholism Rehabilitation Programs.* (Technical Report No. 346) (Arlington: Presearch Incorporated)

3 Bunn, G. A. (1980). *Training—Developing a Navy Alcoholism Treatment Specialist.* (San Diego: Naval Alcohol Rehabilitation Center)

4 Petree, C. L. (1980). *Development of An Alcoholism Counselor Training Program: The Navy Model.* (San Diego: Naval Alcohol Rehabilitation Center)

5 Kolb, D. (1980). *Comparison of Navy Alcohol Safety Action Program with Other Alcohol Rehabilitation Programs.* (San Diego: Naval Health Research Center)
6 Simmons, D. (1978). *Recidivism in Camp Viejas.* (An unpublished report) (San Diego: County Probation Department)
7 *Navy Drug Safety Action Program, Preliminary Assessment of Pilot Course.* (1981). (San Diego: Navy Personnel Research and Development Center)
8 Bromley, P. E. and Bunn, G. A. (1980). *NASAP: A Family of Winners.* (San Diego: Navy Alcohol Safety Action Program Headquarters)
9 Dunning, K. P. and Jansen, E. (1975). *Problem Drinking and Attitudes Toward Alcohol Among Navy Recruits.* (Report No. NPRDC TR 76−21) (San Diego: Navy Personnel Research and Development Center)

APPENDIX: SPECIAL NOTES

(1)   The opinions expressed herein are those of the author and do not necessarily express the views of the United States Navy.
(2)   The use of the pronoun, he, as used throughout this paper, does not necessarily indicate male, nor exclude female. It is used for brevity and clarity purposes when referring to individuals not specifically or necessarily identified as male or female.
(3)   For additional copies of this report, or for copies of any of the other Navy evaluations listed below, contact: Commanding Officer, Naval Alcohol Rehabilitation Center, Naval Station, Box 80, San Diego, CA 92136. Phone: (619) 235-1437.
(4)   Navy evaluations available:

(a)   Evaluation of Alcohol Treatment Programs
(b)   Effectiveness of Treatment for Navy Enlisted Men in Alcohol Rehabilitation Centers and Units
(c)   A Note on Hospitalization and Discharge Rates of Men Treated at The Navy's Alcohol Centers
(d)   Primary and Secondary Benefits from Treatment for Alcoholism
(e)   Prognostic Indicators for Black and White Alcoholics
(f)   Anti-social Histories in Young Alcoholics
(g)   A Search for Bias in Evaluating Job Performance in Rehabilitated Alcoholics
(h)   Measuring Cost Effectiveness of Employee Alcoholism Programs
(i)   The 1976 Evaluation of the Navy's Alcohol Rehabilitation Programs
(j)   Prediction of Post-treatment Effectiveness in Navy Alcoholics
(k)   Reported Drinking among Post-treatment Alcohol Abusers
(l)   Outcomes for Recidivists in Navy Alcohol Rehabilitation Programs
(m)   Summary of Yearly Reports Statistics for All Alcohol Facilities Submitted Data during the Reporting Period 1 January 1976 to 31 December 1976
(n)   The 1977 Evaluation of the Navy's Alcohol Rehabilitation, Alcohol Safety Action (NASAP), and Alcoholism Counselor Training Programs
(o)   Predicting Treatment Outcome for the Female Alcoholic
(p)   Alcoholism Treatment Effectiveness for Naval Officers
(q)   Pre-treatment Outpatient Visits for Alcoholics in the US Navy
(r)   The Impact of Paraprofessional Alcoholism Counselor Training
(s)   Recidivism in Navy Alcoholism Treatment
(t)   A Comparison of the Comrey Personality Scales Scores for Two Subpopulations of Navy Personnel
(u)   Comparisons of the Navy Alcohol Safety Action Program with Other Alcohol Rehabilitation Programs
(v)   Psychodrama with an Alcohol Misuser Population

(w)   Training — Developing a Navy Alcoholism Treatment Specialist
(x)   NASAP: A Family of Winners
(y)   Casual Factors in Alcohol Rehabilitation Success or Failure
(z)   Participants' Evaluation of the Navy Alcohol Safety Action Program
(aa) Winning — The Story of NASAP

(5)   The following studies were completed by graduate students during their internship at the Naval Alcohol Rehabilitation Center. Copies of these evaluations also are available by contacting the Naval Alcohol Rehabilitation Center.

(a)   Modification of Anxiety by Means of Biofeedback in Treatment of Alcoholism
(b)   Effect of Biofeedback on Treatment for Navy Alcoholics
(c)   Effect of a Power Motivation Program on Locus of Control of Navy Alcoholics
(d)   Evaluating the MMPI as an Assessment Tool at an Early Stage in an Alcoholism Rehabilitation Program
(e)   Counselor Interpersonal Style and its Effects in Alcoholism Treatment
(f)   Social Skills and Communication Training in the Treatment of Navy Alcoholic Patients
(g)   Alcoholic Depression and its Effects on Spouse and Family

8
The Henwood programme – treating the whole person

J. MEDDINGS

According to the literature there is no distinctive personality profile of the alcoholic. However at Henwood, an inpatient treatment centre in Alberta, Canada, funded by the Alberta Alcoholism and Drug Commission, we do hold that there are certain assumptions or beliefs which we can make about our clients. These we present to them on admission in the form of a discussion or lecture, thus setting the stage for their treatment, and explaining the reasons why our programme is designed as it is, and attempts to touch on all areas of their lives. The feedback we receive from doing this is that it is reassuring to them, and that it makes sense and fits.

Briefly, our assumptions or beliefs are as follows:

(1) We recognize that many may be feeling dubious or pessimistic about the outcome of treatment, both because of their previous unsuccessful attempts to abstain, and from the very prevalent attitude that alcoholism is difficult to treat successfully. We therefore need to emphasize our very real optimism, and our belief from years of experience that none are too old, too set in their ways or too hopeless to make very real changes in their lives. In fact, the entire staff work from that basis and are convinced that change is possible if they want it.

(2) We assume that someone has made the judgment that the way they use alcohol is destructive to them, or they would not be in treatment. However, we do not yet know whether this is their own belief, or merely reflects the pressure applied by families, doctors, employers, friends or lawyers. We are prepared, provided they have an open mind, to give them some time to come to a decision, but stress that it must soon be their opinion that they do have a problem with alcohol, as it is usually not possible to stay sober to please others for long. Thus, although we are interested in the circumstances of their referral, our main concern is

to ascertain if they, themselves, consider their drinking is destructive, and if so, do they want to do something about it.

(3)   We believe that most come with a very negative self-concept, brought about by the losses and failures alcoholism causes, and therefore our programme is very personal and probing to encourage a realistic self-awareness, and increase self-esteem, and so they can expect us to touch on all areas of their lives.

(4)   We believe, (and this is usually met with almost unanimous agreement) that for a long time, most have felt very much alone and very much misunderstood. This of course comes about partly because of the strange behaviour caused by drinking and blackouts, and by the incomprehension of others, and often of themselves, at their repeated destructive behaviour.

(5)   We believe that they have a very strong defence system, and that the defences they have used to protect the drinking, which in itself may have originated as a defense against perceived inadequacies, may now stand in the way of treatment. We will therefore be encouraging them to examine their defences to ascertain if they are now working in their best interests.

(6)   We believe that partly because of this defence system, many have very incomplete knowledge about alcoholism and its effects, and we will therefore attempt to give good information so that they are better equipped to make decisions about their addiction.

(7)   We also believe that many have for a long time been very out of touch with their feelings, and have in fact escaped from guilt, depression and anxiety, by taking another drink, and in escaping the negative feelings, have also lost touch with good feelings, thus living in a 'grey' world. They can expect from us an emphasis on feelings, and an attempt to help them to reintegrate awareness of feelings into their lives. We emphasize that awareness of feelings can often give early warning of possible relapse into drinking, and also that the inability to deal with anger in a constructive way, or failure to deal with guilt or resentments are frequent causes of relapse. We will also be encouraging them to live in the present instead of regretting the past or worrying about the future.

(8)   Lastly we acknowledge that alcohol has been very important in their lives, and state our belief that it is not possible to remove something which in the past has met so many needs, without substituting other ways of attaining these good things. Thus they can expect to establish with us the ways alcohol has benefited them and find alternative methods of achieving these positive effects.

This explanation of our position, together with our assessment of each client, sets the stage, we feel, for an acceptance of our programme.

Assessments are done with each client by the counsellor working with them, and covers first his readiness for treatment, that is his motivation, previous treatment experiences, and the reason for seeking help at this time. Secondly we look at the risk his addiction is causing him — that is the type and severity of his addiction and the effects it is having on all areas of his life. Thirdly we assess with him his rationality, his emotional state, his impulsiveness or propensity for violence, noting especially depression or suicidal tendencies which need treatment. Fourthly we look at the relationships he has with others, both past and present. Lastly we assess with him his resources such as his skills, his career, his family, his interests, on which he can build to help overcome his present problems. With this information we can establish an individual treatment plan dealing with both short and long term objectives.

We have found that there is benefit in having a multidisciplinary treatment staff, and a programme where all areas of a person's life are at least touched on, realizing that for each individual the emphasis will need to be different. Thus at Henwood we look at physical health with a team of doctors and nurses, and an excellent dietary staff, realizing that it is difficult, if not impossible, to deal optimistically with life if one is in poor physical condition. We have 21 counsellors and a psychologist on staff coming from a wide range of academic backgrounds, but all having optimism, the ability to confront with gentleness and caring, the ability to model a healthy lifestyle, and the skill and experience to work in individual, group and family counselling. As counsellors we help our clients to understand and express their feelings, and gain self-esteem and self-awareness. We work on the ways they relate to others and encourage more positive ways. The area of sexuality is often beset with problems for the alcoholic and we believe frank discussion is important. We have an excellent programme for the families where they live at Henwood and engage first in information sessions, and later are involved in the regular programme with the client. Our belief in the necessity of involving the families cannot be stressed enough. We believe family members need to look at their own part in this family illness, and realize how it has affected them and what changes they need to make, for although the feeling our clients have of being alone and misunderstood can quickly change with the warmth and understanding experienced at Henwood, it is really from the significant others in their lives that they need this understanding. Family involvement is necessary for this to happen.

We believe that for some an opportunity to examine spiritual concerns is important, and we therefore have, on staff, counsellors with the background to facilitate this. We believe the AA programme to be the best follow-up programme for our clients, and therefore have AA counsellors on staff to give support, encouragement, and information.

Lastly we have an excellent recreation programme, because we believe the ways our clients use leisure time is very important to their sobriety. In fact it is our contention that many of the good things alcohol has accomplished in the past for our patients can also be achieved (although perhaps not so quickly) by leisure activities. Thus if alcohol was facilitating social interaction, so can recreational pursuits. Feelings of self-confidence can be gained by proficiency in sports or crafts. Relief from tension follows many sports. Boredom and empty time can be eliminated by recreational interests. Because we find alcoholics have rarely learned to enjoy life away from alcohol, and have a real tendency to become 'workaholics' if sober, we stress all forms of recreation not only to fill the hours previously used in drinking, but also to meet the very real needs formerly met through drinking. Relaxation training is also taught.

In addition, the lack of knowledge is rectified by lectures and films, dealing with all aspects of alcoholism. Working as a team, the staff attempt to monitor clients' behaviour and progress. Thus for example, if clients are very aggressive on the volleyball court, we ask if this is a behaviour common to the rest of their life, and if so, does it work for them. If they are withdrawn and always sit by themselves in the cafeteria, we will discuss it with them, and if they want to change, give support and encouragement. Fortunately in an inpatient treatment centre there is opportunity for this observation and also more support to practise new behaviours. We are also fortunate in the fact that Henwood is located in a country setting, and affords a real opportunity to escape the pressures of everyday living, thus giving every opportunity to make changes. Our optimism is in fact justified by both our programme and success rate.

9
A social–psychological approach to alcohol use and abuse

M. DIDIER C.

As the awareness of the importance of cultural factors in alcoholism grows[1], the need for a model of how they influence alcohol use increases. Such a model could help us to understand the common features of different drinking styles typical of cultures in which alcoholism rates are either high or low, and the features that differentiate cultures which differ in such rates.

This paper puts forward a model of the phenomenon of 'cultural alcohol use patterns' and the implications of such a concept for research and action in the field of alcohol abuse and alcoholism.

THE MODEL

People who share similar positions within the same culture, class or group seem to use alcohol in similar ways. This regularity is achieved by a common socialization about alcohol use, through the influence of the family[2], peers[3] or the mass media[4]. Even so, within a country several alcohol use patterns can be found, especially where immigration is frequent or where a conquering and a conquered culture have managed to coexist rather than merge.

The socialization process results in the acquisition of a *cultural pattern of alcohol use* by most of its members. Knowledge of this pattern is necessary to understand how, and why, alcohol is used and abused in a given population.

In order to describe an alcohol use pattern, two types of variables must be considered: (1) the functions of alcohol and (2) the social norms regarding the ways in which alcohol can or must be taken.

Functions of alcohol

Functions can be defined as the uses alcohol is given within a culture: which effects can be expected from it if taken in the prescribed ways. These functions

145

are assigned according to:

(1)   How alcoholic beverages affect the physiological functioning of the drinker, specially through the effect upon both nervous systems.

(2)   The expectations about the effects of the substance, induced through a cultural conditioning. Psychologically speaking, expectations act as a cognitive framework for the interpretation of the effects of alcohol upon bodily functioning. The evidence seems to support the importance of expectancies about the effects of alcohol on the subjective experience and even physical reactions of the drinker[5].

Functions usually assigned to alcohol can be grouped in four categories: social, emotional, homeostatic and religious.

We say that social functions are assigned to alcohol when a culture or subculture prescribes drinking for social purposes. These can be achieved through the use of the substance as a symbol (of friendship, confidence or intimacy) or through the effects of alcoholic beverages on the social behaviour of drinkers, especially by disinhibiting usually hidden feelings and increasing emotional expression.

Emotional functions are given to alcoholic beverages when they are used to modify one's mood, especially to manage feelings like anxiety, frustration, yearning and so on. People are encouraged to manage such aversive emotions through forgetfulness or by fleeing from a painful (real) situation to a pleasurable (fantasy) one through alcohol use.

In certain cultures or groups, alcohol is used to maintain or recover a sense of physical well-being, avoiding hunger or cold, preventing or curing illness[6, 7]. In such cases, alcohol fulfils homeostatic functions.

Finally, some societies or groups within them use alcohol as a vehicle of communication between man and God or the Cosmos[8]. In these cases, religious functions are said to be given to alcohol. Though this seems typical of more primitive cultures, they survive nowadays in syncretic religious expressions of 'folk religiosity' in many places in Latin America[6].

Functions assigned to alcohol seem to relate to those needs a culture usually fails to satisfy. Maloff and her associates[9] point out that in many cultures where the expression of sexual or aggressive impulses is usually inhibited, alcohol seems a trigger for their expression in a most uncontrolled way. Classical anthropological research carried out in the 1940s which relates inebriety to subsistence anxiety seems to provide further support for this idea.

The functions assigned to alcohol in a culture can help us to predict alcohol abuse. Usually, the most dangerous patterns seem to be those where alcohol is used to manage emotional strain and suffering[3]. This is especially so since, when someone drinks in order to relieve anxiety or depression, the first drinks usually bring him the state of euphoria he is looking for. This feeling will disappear if the drinking proceeds. This causes the drinker to increase his intake in order to regain the original state of artificial happiness, a useless attempt[10]. Furthermore, as the causes of emotional distress do not disappear, or rather have been intensified, the person will relapse over and over again[11].

Social functions, nevertheless, can be as dangerous, particularly when alcohol use, especially in excessive doses, is considered a symbol of group identification or solidarity. In such groups, abstainers are traitors to their peers, and quickly become social outcasts. Some working-class alcoholics we have met in Chile report awareness that treatment success depends on their refusing to meet their old friends and fellow workers in order to avoid pressures towards drinking.

Norms

In any culture or subculture where alcohol has been used for some time, attempts are made to integrate use to normal life. This is achieved by means of a set of social norms which shape the ways in which alcoholic beverages are to be taken. These norms vary from group to group and from culture to culture, in the degree they are respected and enforced, and in their content itself.

An important group of norms refers to those members of the culture who are considered potential users of alcohol. They can be defined according to demographic criteria, like age or sex, or to social characteristics, like profession, income level, religious affiliation among others. Some of these rules are formalized, like the laws that regulate the minimum age for buying alcoholic beverages. Others may be informal, but considerable pressure can be brought to bear on the deviant. In Chile, for example, certain groups of workers, like garbage collectors and bakery workers, are said to have high rates of alcoholism due to their tradition of associating drinking after – and sometimes before and during – work hours with belonging to the group.

Another group of norms regulates the context of alcohol intake. This can be a physical or a social context, or the occasions on which drinking is mandatory, allowed or forbidden.

The importance of the physical context of use seems to relate with the existence of cues in the physical environment which promote or inhibit drinking. Furthermore, it usually interacts with the social context of ingestion. If by physical context we understand the place where people drink, by the social context we mean the people present at the moment of use, whether drinking or just watching[12]. It seems that drinking at home and with the family (specially the nuclear family) promotes moderate drinking, while drinking in a bar with peers of the same sex tends to produce excessive intake.

Many patterns accept excessive drinking on certain occasions, but declare other occasions 'dry'. Others seems to allow drinking in moderate amounts on almost any occasion, but restrict excessive use to exceptional cases only. Research which is being carried out now by the author in the Chilean middle class shows a pattern of drinking being related to no special occasions, but usual with meals. On the other hand, working-class drinkers seem to have some occasions on which alcohol is frequently abused, like Independence Day and New Year's Eve. In addition, pay day seems to be another occasion strongly related to heavy drinking[11].

The type of alcoholic beverages preferred in different groups or cultures makes a difference in a drinking pattern, too. Some drinking patterns favour the use of drinks with low alcohol content, like beer or wine, while others prefer spirits, alone or mixed. Wine seems specially related to food, as does beer but not spirits.

Introduction of a new type of alcoholic beverage can disrupt habitual patterns of alcohol use. Lomnitz[13] describes the role of spirits of poor quality given to the native Mapuche in the conquest of the south of Chile. The Mapuche pattern, built to manage the use of drinks with little alcohol like fermented fruit juices, was unable to protect the drinkers against stronger drinks. This, in turn, made the conquest easier.

A final set of rules relates to the optimum dose of a given beverage to be taken by a given user in a certain context. These rules govern the amount of drinking considered fit for a situation. In some cases, drinking moderately is considered adequate, while in other patterns it is considered cowardice or not masculine. Some groups reject drinking itself, like some Protestant churches. Others approve moderate but not excessive drinking, as traditionally the Jewish culture has done. In contrast, yet others ridicule abstainers and moderate drinkers.

Functions and norms

In the interaction of functions and social norms, a complex set of combinations shapes the alcohol use pattern of a culture. For example, in different groups the same functions may be assigned to alcohol, but they are achieved by use guided by different norms. In Chile, for example, alcohol is mainly used for social purposes in all socioeconomic levels. Nevertheless, middle-class drinkers usually drink in the family and do so in a moderate way most of the time. Working-class drinkers drink with the peer group, away from the family and, sometimes, with the stated purpose of getting drunk.

There are norms which protect certain members of the culture from alcoholism and favour alcoholism in others. One such example is the case of the traditionally lower alcoholism rates for women compared with men's rates. In Chile, female alcoholism represents a phenomenon different from that of male problem drinking. If among men there are four intermittent alcoholics for each inveterate one[14], women show a different pattern: two inveterate alcoholics for each intermittent one[15]. Pathology seems to be twice as frequent among alcoholic women than among their male counterparts[15].

ALCOHOL USE PATTERNS AND RESEARCH AND PRACTICE IN ALCOHOLISM

I shall devote this last section of this paper to addressing some implications of the model I have stated above (summarized in Table 9.1) for research and practice in the field of alcoholism.

First, let us see how alcohol use patterns can explain some problems in

Table 9.1   Components of a cultural pattern of alcohol use

Functions	Social norms
Pharmacology + expectancies	Integration into cultural lifestyle
Social: Symbol Effect on user	*Users*: Demographic criteria Social criteria
Emotional: Management of aversive feelings	*Context*: Physical occasions Social occasions
Homeostatic: Use as Food Use as medicine Against cold	*Type of beverage*: Alcohol content Combinations
Religious: Relation between man and God or the Cosmos	*Optimum dose*: Minimum or Maximum

personality research. Many authors have looked for, and failed to find, an alcoholism-prone personality. This may be due to the fact that, given different alcohol use patterns, different people are prone to become alcoholics. For example, introverted, socially isolated people are alcoholism-prone in cultures which emphasize the management of feelings of depression or loneliness, but not in those where alcohol is taken only on social occasions. In this case, extroverted, socially active people are likely to be more troubled by alcohol abuse. A psychopathic personality is alcoholism-prone in cultures where norms stress moderate drinking and peer pressure points there. If peer pressures aim towards excessive drinking, such traits as caring little for rules and the feelings of friends can protect someone against such problems.

In the field of treatment, the long controversy between moderate drinking and total abstinence as therapeutic aims can benefit from the consideration of cultural variables. If the patient's group favours moderate drinking and disapproves excessive use, the moderate use alternative must be preferred, when viable, to the total abstinence approach. But if the client belongs to a group where heavy drinking is central and enforced through group pressures, total abstinence seems the only indicated treatment approach, since peer pressures will work against any attempt to drink moderately while others drink in excess. In Chile, some respect for patients in treatment has been detected, if they try to abstain arguing they are taking medicine or disulfiram (Antabuse). If they start drinking, nevertheless, they are no longer allowed to drink moderately.

The idea that prevention must promote responsible drinking rather than total abstention is another field in which cultural variables must be considered. Such campaigns are basically attempts to change existing drinking patterns. In many cases, the training of people who can promote a new, safer drinking style on the part of persons who drink in a way that may be dangerous to themselves may be a new approach to prevention. Promoting safer ways to drink among the young, for example, may be a useful alternative to presenting drinking as evil, and its avoidance as the only possible solution.

Cultural change, however ambitious as an aim, may be the only way to prevent alcohol abuse in some societies. It should be attempted if many people are to be saved from developing alcoholism and associated problems.

References

1 Heath, D. B. (1981). Determining the sociocultural context of alcohol use. *J. Stud. Alc.,* *Suppl.* **9**, 9

2 Armor, D. J., Polich, J. M. and Stambul, H. B. (1978). *Alcoholism and Treatment*. (New York: Wiley)

3 Wilkinson, R. (1970). *The Prevention of Drinking Problems*. (New York: Oxford UP)

4 Didier, M. (1981). Patrones de ingestion de alcohol en la publicidad televisiva chilena. *Rev Chilena Psicol.*, **4**, 49

5 Donovan, D. M. and Marlatt, A. G. (1980). Assessment of expectancies and behaviours associated with alcohol consumption. *J. Stud. Alc.*, **41**, 1153

6 Barros, G. (1980). *Religiosidad Popular y Alcoholismo*. Mimeographed Research Report, School of Social Work, Catholic University of Chile

7 Dallairac, D. (1971). *Dossier: Alcoolisme*. (Paris: Laffont)

8 Klausner, S. Z. (1964). Sacred and profane meanings of blood and alcohol. *J. Soc. Psychol.*, **64**, 27

9 Maloff, D., Becker, H. S. Foranoff, A. and Rodin, J. (1979). Informal social controls and their influence on substance abuse. *J. Drug Issues*, 161

11 Didier, M. (1982). Cultural pressures towards excessive alcohol consumption and the treatment of drinking problems. In Golding, P. (ed.) *Alcoholism: A Modern Perspective*. (Lancaster: MTP)

12 Tomaszewski, R. J., Strickler, D. P. and Maxwell, W. A. (1980). Influence of social setting and social drinking stimuli on drinking behavior. *Addict. Behav.*, **5**, 235

13 Lomnitz, L. (1976). Alcohol and culture: the historical evolution of drinking patterns among the Mapuche. In Everett, M. W., Waddell, J. O. and Heath, D. B. (eds.) *Cross-cultural Approaches to the Study of Alcohol*. (The Hague: Mouton)

14 Bello, S., Salinas, M. J. and Ruiz, A. M. (1979). Evaluacion de un programa de prevencion secundaria del alcoholismo. *Rev. Med. Chile*, **107**, 1047

15 Kattan, L. *et al.* (1973). Caracteristicas del alcoholismo en la mujer y evaluacion del resultado de su tratamiento en Chile. *Acta Psiqiatr. Psicol. Am. Lat.*, **19**, 104.

10

Field-independence–dependence and levels of logical reasoning as predictors of programme completion in the treatment of alcoholism

J. E. ERWIN and J. J. HUNTER

INTRODUCTION

According to Hunt, Barnett, and Branch[1], 60–70% of patients addicted to cigarettes, heroin, or alcohol relapse during the first 3 months after completion of treatment. This is illustrated in Figure 10.1. They suggest that the majority who relapse may be distinguishable from the minority who continue to recover by some personality correlate. One clue pointing to the identity of such a variable is empirical evidence indicating that alcoholics as a group are significantly more field-dependent than controls[2], and that field-independent alcoholics are more likely to maintain abstinence than field-dependents[3]. Another clue was given by informal clinical observations that suggested to us that alcoholics who are capable of hypothetico-deductive thought have a higher probability of recovery than those only capable of concrete reasoning.

This study constitutes a test of the hypotheses that (1) field-independence–dependence and (2) level of logical reasoning predict outcome status in a typical programme for the treatment of alcoholism.

MATERIALS AND METHODS

Eighty subjects participated in the study. All were inpatients at a private hospital in a ward that specializes in the treatment of alcoholism. All had been

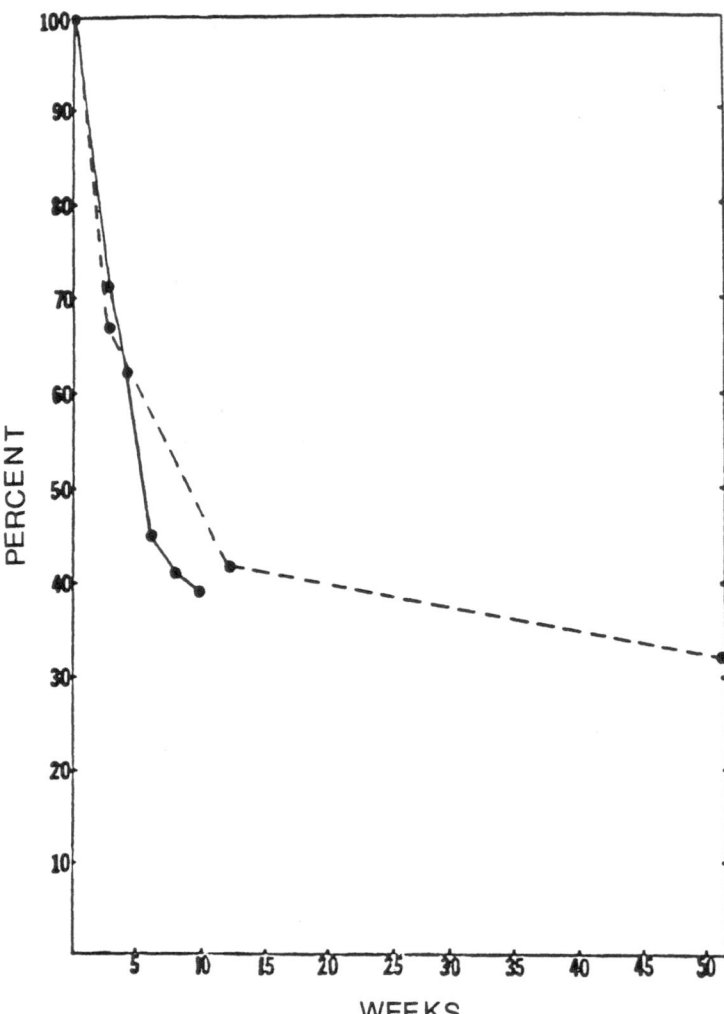

Figure 10.1   Percentage of patients sober 2 weeks, 3 months and 12 months after completion of treatment (after Hunt, Barnett and Branch[1]), and percentage of patients remaining in outpatient treatment 2, 4, 6, 8 and 10 weeks following completion of inpatient treatment (present study). ● – – – – – – ● = Hunt, Barnett and Branch[1]; ●————● = present study

hospitalized with a primary diagnosis of alcoholism. Fifty-three were males, 10 were black (two females), and 36 were married. Age ranged from 18 to 77. All but ten had a record of recent employment in occupations that ranged in prestige from professional/managerial (27.5 %) to clerical/labourer (31.25 %).

Depending upon the terms of their contracts, the subjects were inpatients for either 3 or 4 weeks. Following that, they were required to attend at least one of three weekly outpatient sessions for 10 weeks. Treatment outcome was measured by the number of weeks outpatient sessions were attended.

Three psychological tests were administered to each subject during the third week of treatment. The Embedded Figures Test (EFT) is a measure of field-independence—dependence. The Plant Problem and Pendulum are tests of level of logical reasoning.

Scores on the EFT were expressed as mean time in seconds to solve the first 12 cards of Form A. Trials that exceeded 4 minutes were terminated and the time was recorded as 240 seconds. The Plant Problem and Pendulum were administered in the usual manner and subjects' responses were noted in shorthand. Verbatim transcripts were rated independently by two trained judges for level of logical reasoning.

RESULTS

Inter-rater agreement

The two judges agreed on their ratings of level of logical reasoning a high proportion of the time. Rho (78) = 0.91 and 0.96 for Pendulum and the Plant Problem. Both results are significantly beyond the 0.01 level.

Relationships among tests of logic and field-dependence

Logic tests

Scores on the Plant Problem and Pendulum correlate positively and at a significant level (rho (78) = 0.88, $p < 0.01$). The two tests appear to be highly redundant and may be considered equivalent operations for defining level of logical reasoning.

Logic and perceptual tests

Rank order correlation coefficients indicate that field-independence (low mean EFT score) is significantly related to abstract reasoning (high logic test score); rho for EFT and Pendulum (78) = -0.79, $p < 0.001$, and rho for EFT and Plant Problem (78) = -0.81, $p < 0.001$.

Test scores as predictors of programme completion

The relationships of the field-independence—dependence and logic test scores are displayed in Figure 10.2. All three tests predict programme adherence and dropout status effectively. These tests account for 36% of the variance of treatment outcome. Of the subjects who scored below the median on the EFT (field-dependent) or who scored preoperational or concrete operational on the logic tests, only 10–20% completed treatment. Correlations between test scores and the number of sessions completed also reflect a high degree of relationship (rho (78) = 0.49, $p < 0.001$ for Pendulum, and rho (78) = 0.59, $p < 0.001$ for Plant Problem, and r (78) = −0.50, $p < 0.001$ for EFT). (Table 10.1)

DISCUSSION

The magnitude of the correlations of field-independence–dependence and logic test scores suggests that all three tests measure similar cognitive abilities. This convergence has been noted before. Rubinstein[4] and Muzio[5] showed that field-independence correlates highly with level of logical reasoning in normal adolescents and adults.

Why field-independence–dependence and logic scores are so effective in predicting treatment outcome is an issue for theoretical speculation. An adherent of Witkin's model of cognitive style would assert that field-dependent patients drop out of treatment because they are not able to discriminate internal from external sources of anxiety and therefore continue to rely upon alcohol as a panacea. According to this account, the field-dependent personality is defective in his or her sense of self-non-self segregation. The anxiety inherent in living must be reduced. Having little sense of precision in analysing problems, the global personality embraces a global solution.

Piaget's theory offers a different perspective. Logical sophistication is identified by the possession of suppositional or hypothetico–deductive thought. Higher levels of logical reasoning are marked by the ability to imagine what would happen if a different state of affairs were to prevail.

The results of this study indicate that most preoperational and concrete operational patients drop out of treatment. Unlike formal-operational patients, they are not able to anticipate conditions in their private lives following treatment. Two verbatim quotations exemplify this difference.

The first quotation is that of a preoperational and field-independent patient responding to a therapist's request to imagine a sober day in the future.

I really don't know what it will be like. You don't know something that hasn't happened yet. I will know after it happens. I don't know that I won't drink. I don't have any desire anymore — that's gone. The doctor took it away when he told me what the alcohol was doing to my body. [The therapist asks the patient to try to imagine a day next month.] I'll just go to work and when the other guys drink on their lunch hour, I'll go read a newspaper. [The therapist asks for another example.] On payday I'll go home and watch TV instead of going out with the guys. [The therapist asks

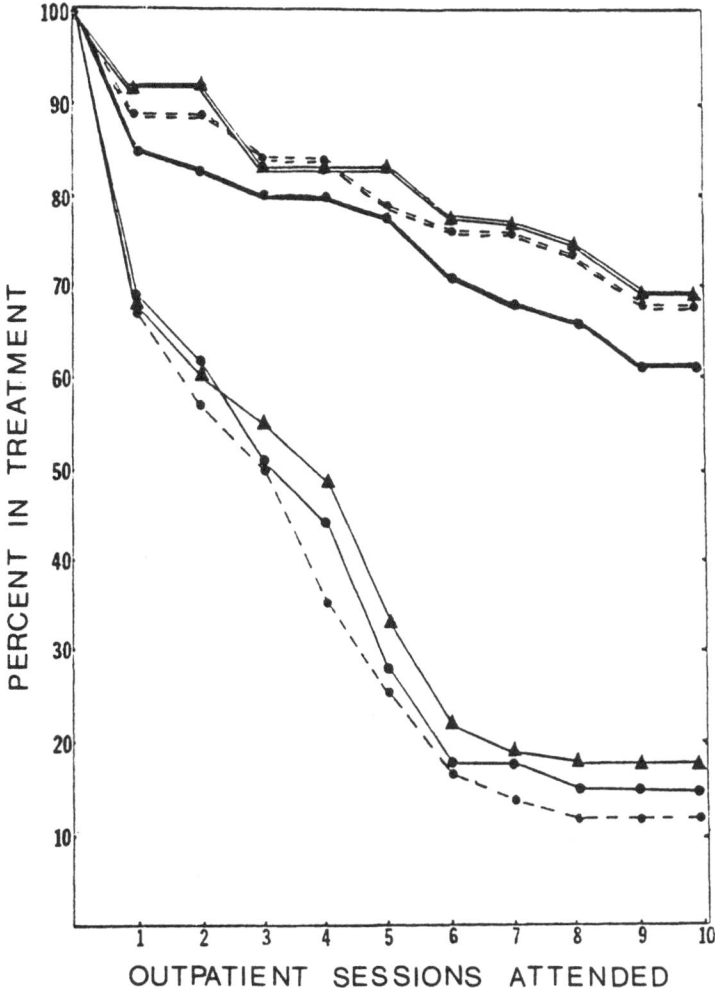

Figure 10.2 Percentage of patients remaining in outpatient treatment in each of 10 weekly sessions, classified by high and low scores on Pendulum, Plant Problem and EFT. •————• EFT < median: •════• pendulum levels 3 & 4; ▲═══▲ plant, levels 3 & 4; •————• EFT > median; •————• pendulum, levels 0, 1, 2; ▲————▲ plant levels 0, 1, 2

if the patient usually drank while watching TV. The response was yes.] Probably I'll go out with them a little so they won't think I'm stuck up, but I'll probably say 'No, thanks' if they offer me a drink. This assignment isn't helpful because I can't say what I will do before it happens.

The second quotation is that of a formal-operational and field-independent patient answering the same question:

Table 10.1   Correlation matrix of cognitive tests and sessions attended

	Plant problem rho	Pendulum rho	Number of sessions attended rho	r
Plant problem		0.88*	0.59**	
Pendulum			0.49**	
EFT	−0.81**	−0.79**		−0.50**

  * $p < 0.01$
** $p < 0.001$

If it is a work day, I will probably have no problem during working hours, as I did not drink during that time period. However, I get off work at 4:00, and that was my favourite time to begin the 'happy hour'. I think that for at least a few months it will be necessary for me to plan on being in special alcoholic group activities during those difficult hours. I've found several groups that meet at that time, and have visited two of them − one is near where I work, so I could go there straight from work. I've also considered what are the times when I think I *have* to drink. It is generally when I am very uptight physically, and when I'm lonely. I am really working on the relaxation exercises and have found a group, which one of the nurses referred, that works with relaxation. It meets on Thursday nights, and isn't far from where I live. I may need that group for at least 6 months − and it is a way to meet more people so I won't be so lonely. One of the reasons I was lonely was because I didn't want to risk meeting people, but working on my alcoholism has given me a common denominator so that I'm not so afraid.

Although this is admittedly anecdotal evidence, the difference in cognitive ability is obvious.

Finally, in view of the dramatic difference in dropout rate between field-independent, formal operational patients and field-dependent, concrete or preoperational patients, it seems reasonable to conclude that the treatment of alcoholism in hospitals as it is now practised is effective only for the former group. This could easily be because the treatment programmes are designed and administered by field-independent, formal-operational professionals who are unable to detect and adapt to cognitive differences. Perhaps this is true because alcoholic denial is a form of transductive logic even among formal-operational alcoholics. If we are to improve our effectiveness in the treatment of addictive disorders, we must begin to take the cognitive properties of our patients into account.

References

1 Hunt, W. A., Barnett, L. W. and Branch, L. G. (1971). Relapse rates in addiction programs. *J. Clin. Psychol.*, **27,** 455

2 Karp, S. A., Witkin, H. A. and Goodenough, D. R. (1965). Alcoholism and psychological differentiation: Effect on achievement of sobriety on field-dependence. *Q. J. Stud. Alc.*, **26,** 580

3 Kissen, B., Platz, A. and Su, W. (1970). Social and psychological factors in the treatment of chronic alcoholism. *J. Psychiatr. Res.*, **8,** 13

4 Rubinstein, R. A. (1980). Field-dependence and Piagetian operational thought in northern Belize. *Child Stud. J.*, **10,** 67

5 Ehri, L. C. and Muzio, I. M. (1974). Cognitive style and reasoning about speed. *J. Educ. Psychol.*, **66,** 569

11
Diagnosis and treatment of drinking problems in health centre patients suffering from anxiety states, phobias and psychosomatic symptoms

V. G. LOKARE

Recent interest in alcoholism has intensified efforts to develop more effective treatment strategy. Implementation of treatment strategies is complicated by the fact that aetiological factors involved in chronic abusive drinking appear to be extremely complex. Although speculation and theorizing abound in the alcoholic field these factors have not as yet been delineated. The lack of knowledge seems directly related to the paucity of factual information on the causes of abusive drinking. In spite of this, numerous theoretical models have been proposed to explain alcohol abuse and in turn treatment projects based upon these theories have been devised and are being implemented.

The disease model initially proposed by Jellinek[1] views alcohol abuse as a progressive irreversible disease though no specific aetiological factors have been demonstrated to be pathognomonic for alcohol abuse. 'Loss of control' or disease concept leads to difficulty in treatment strategies. The recovering alcoholic is often not given credit for relapses during which he consumes just one or two drinks, terminates drinking and then remains sober once again. Experimental tests of the 'loss of control' notion was reported by Marlatt, Demming and Reid[2], ' . . . The amount of beverage consumed has not influenced the outcome even when alcohol was being consumed if the subject believed that he was drinking a non-alcoholic beverage.' The authors relate their findings to the importance of cognitive variables in determining 'loss of control'. Sociological models such as proposed by Miller and Eisler[3] describe three major factors related to substance abuse. These include the availability of the drug, the context within which it is used and the sanctions imposed upon its abuse. Others like Bandura[4] claim that there is evidence to support the notion that patterns of abuse are transmitted within a family group by means of social role modelling. Again this model creates difficulties for treatment strategies as one finds that alcohol abuse still takes place in States and countries that prohibit the use of alcohol and when one finds that all members of a family do not necessarily become alcoholics. Physiological models range from . . . alcohol abuse is related to a basic nutrient deficiency which is genetically determined . . . to . . . a popular belief of alcohol abuse that it is an inherited disorder. The evidence for the hereditary theory is far from conclusive. Maybe there is an indirect link in terms of physiological predisposition.

Lokare[5] reports that attempts to identify alcoholic personality, MMPI, types in the hope of providing means of determining those at risk in the population proved to be of little help. The findings met with the same fate as did the results of the MMPI and the subscales derived from the MMPI which were used by MacAndrew and Geertsma[6], MacAndrew[7], Rosenberg[8] and Hoffman et al[9]. Most of the scales, while identifying pre-scale alcoholics, also misclassified a substantial number of controls, suggesting that the differences found were probably due primarily to general maladjustment rather than to alcoholism or alcoholic personality[10].

Attempts to compare MMPI profiles of alcoholics with drug addicts and a group of delinquents, however, showed some interesting differences. The drug addicts generally showed higher scores on scales for F, D, PD and SC and in the pathological range compared with normals and the alcoholics, whereas the alcoholic's profile was much nearer to the normal controls, except that it still showed elevation on the Depression Scale and only marginally in the pathological range of the PD and the PT scales. In general these characteristics go with neurotic tendencies described by Eysenck[11] on the dimensionality scales. This was further confirmed by Lokare's[5] results of the EPQ, as all the alcoholics tended to show high scores on the Neuroticism scale. Those who accepted help and were able to co-operate on programmes tended to be neurotic introverts (compatible with the high scores on the MMPI, on the Depression and the PT scales) and those who dropped out without completing the treatment programme tended to be neurotic extroverts (compatible with high scores on the PD scale of the MMPI). Therefore, in one sense they tended to be different from the normals but similar to neurotics who suffered from various emotional problems and reported symptoms such as depression, anxiety states, phobias, psychosomatic symptoms etc. as reported by Lokare[12].

Theories as to the aetiology of alcoholism are numerous though alcoholics do not form a homogeneous group and no single causal agent has been identified. Attempts to divide the alcoholics into subgroups for purposes of estimating aetiological contributions, prognosis and treatment still continue. One approach based on learning theory suggests that alcohol is reinforcing because it results in a reduction of tension and anxiety. It is claimed that alcohol is drunk for its anxiolytic properties. Marks et al.[13] report two alcoholics and two barbiturate abusers in a group of 38 phobic patients.

Quitkin *et al.*[14] report ten cases of phobic anxiety syndrome exaggerated by drug dependence and alcohol abuse. They show concern with the fact that drug or alcohol abuse becomes a focus and the basic problem, namely phobic state, tends to be overlooked and this leads them to advocate that clinicians should suspect the phobic anxiety syndrome in all patients abusing sedative use or alcohol. Woodruff and co-workers[15] claim 25% of the anxiety neurotics were heavy drinkers, 15% were alcoholics and 10% were suffering from symptoms of phobic avoidance.

The Report of the Special Committee of the Royal College of Psychiatrists[16] states that 'the severe anxiety state or some form of situational anxiety such as agoraphobia or claustrophobia' frequently underlie alcoholism. Mullaney and Trippett[17] in a recent report state that 68.7% of an alcoholic population were found to suffer from agoraphobia and/or social phobia to either a mild or serious degree. The present study was originally conceived on the basis of impressions prior to the publication of the Report of the Special Committee of the Royal College of Psychiatrists[16] and the paper by Mullaney and Trippett[17]. In view of this, part of the work was diverted to attempt to confirm or otherwise the findings of these reports.

MATERIALS AND METHODS

Apart from the study of severe anxiety states and/or situational anxiety such as agoraphobia, social phobia etc. among the alcoholics, the study also looks at patients who presented symptoms of anxiety phobias and psychosomatic symptoms without reporting alcohol abuse. This was the more difficult bit because information regarding drinking habits was not available when the referral was received nor had it previously been considered relevant to the problems. There was the practical difficulty of identifying the alcohol abuse, as questionnaires like the Hilton Drinking Questionnaire[18] could not be routinely dished out to these patients because there was every chance that this would offend an overwhelming majority of them. However, if their co-operation was asked for as part of a controlled study for research purposes, a fair number would naturally have opted out and it was possible that some of those who opted out would have even withdrawn from accepting help with their problem for which they originally attended the clinic, because this kind of procedure sometimes puts a dent in their confidence and rapport with the clinician. There was also the danger that some of those who would not complete the questionnaire might be from the minority group with the drinking problem as well, as it is well known that the drinker hides the extent of his drinking from himself and also from those around him reasonably successfully at times. In addition, in the study of these groups not only was one dealing with the problem of consumption of drink, which may be the effect or the cause or both or neither, but there was a clinical problem for which the patient was seeking help.

The final sample of subjects included in the study are one batch of 100 alcoholics who had voluntarily accepted treatment in the Alcoholism Unit, and one batch of 93 patients suffering from anxiety phobia, psychosomatic symptoms sometimes accompanied by mild depression, who were referred for treatment for these conditions by the general practitioner. The second batch of patients had no recorded history of alcoholism and there was no suspicion that drinking had anything to do with the symptoms at the time of referral by the GP. In respect of the 100 alcoholics included in the study, the information reported was collected systematically from the time of contact and they were followed-up after their discharge and are part of a larger study. The second batch of 93 patients are, however, a mixed bunch. In the cases of those who admitted alcohol abuse during the investigation of the other conditions for which they were originally referred, systematic information was collected regarding their condition and they were systematically followed up. However, the others who did not reveal alcohol abuse during the course of investigation and treatment consisted of those on whom a retrospective study was carried out and also those who were part of a planned systematic study.

RESULTS

The patients from the first group who were seeking help for alcoholism as their primary problem and were admitted for treatment at the alcoholism unit did mention some other problems during the course of their stay in the special unit for alcoholism. Looking at Table 11.1, it can be seen that 48 % gave no obvious reasons for alcohol abuse. Of the remaining, 17 % reported various phobic types of anxiety symptoms, 13 % referred to social and marital problems as the cause for their drinking while 12 % reported mixed nervous symptoms and the remaining 10 % gave some vague reasons which are classified as miscellaneous. It must be pointed out at this stage that nearly half of those who gave some reasons for their drinking did so in a haphazard way. This was particularly true of men, while women tended to give reasons for

Table 11.1 Group of 100 alcoholic patients treated for alcoholism in a special unit

Category	Description of category	Number
1	No obvious reasons	48
2	Phobic anxiety symptoms (mild and severe)	17
3	Social marital problems	13
4	Mixed nervous symptoms, anxiety states, psychosomatic symptoms etc.	12
5	Miscellaneous (death of relative, conflict at work etc.)	10
		100

drinking much more easily and at times related specific incidences in their life as the starting point of their alcoholic drinking.[19]

Table 11.2 presents the treatment outcome at 9 months follow-up after the alcoholic was discharged at the completion of treatment for alcoholism. Looking at these results it is obvious that, of all those who stayed abstinent after treatment, the overwhelmingly larger number came from Category 1 and those in Categories 2, 3, 4 and 5 are in descending order. Among those who stayed mainly dry, those in Category 1 seemed to have benefited most and then those in Categories 2 and 3 are identical in number and 4 and 5 in descending order. The figures for readmission show that the largest percentage readmitted were from Category 1 and then in descending order from Categories 2 and 4, and Categories 3 and 5 were identical. Among those with whom contact was lost, although the total number is small the largest number came from Category 1, from Categories 2, 3 and 5 an identical number were involved, whereas the smallest number came from Category 4.

Table 11.3, which presents data of Table 11.2 in a different form, shows what is happening within each category as to what percentage remain abstinent, stayed mainly dry, were readmitted or were those with whom contact was lost, and its effect within each category. There do not seem to be significant differences between Categories 1 and 2 when one looks at the figures for those who benefited fully or partially or for that matter for readmissions and those with whom contact was lost.

Table 11.4 presents the same data slightly differently. It helps to compare Category 1, namely the alcoholics who cited no obvious reasons for their drinking with all the other categories who cited some reasons for their drinking. Here there are no longer differences between the two groups. In fact, those who do not cite reasons for their drinking benefit from the treatment for alcoholism to the same extent as those who had cited some reason for their drinking when treatment is directed to their drinking problem. This becomes obvious if one looks at the combined figures in this table for those who were abstinent and those who stayed mainly dry for Category 1 and the other categories.

The contents of Table 11.5 show the analysis of patients' problems at referral and the problem of alcohol abuse which was discovered during the course of investigations and treatment of their original problems. Only 15 of the 93 patients had shown alcohol abuse as one of the major problems but they had concealed this fact from the GP and in some cases from other specialists to whom they had been referred on earlier occasions for similar conditions. The number of people who show alcohol abuse as one of the problems is significantly smaller than the proportion in the alcoholic group who show symptoms such as phobic anxiety, social/marital problems, mixed nervous symptoms such as psychosomatic symptoms etc.

An analysis of the outcome of results of treatment for those patients who were originally referred by the GP from the Health Centre for treatment of anxiety state, phobia, psychosomatic symptoms etc. with no indication of a drinking problem, and who were found after investigation to have been

Table 11.2. The treatment outcome at 9 months follow-up of group of patients mentioned in Table 11.1

Categories*	Abstinent		Stayed mainly dry with occasional lapses but recovered with little or no help		Readmitted but failed to benefit		Lost contact		Total number
	No.	%	No.	%	No.	%	No.	%	
1	15	53.57	16	43.24	11	50.00	6	46.16	48
2	5	17.86	6	16.22	4	18.18	2	15.38	17
3	3	10.71	6	16.22	2	9.09	2	15.38	13
4	3	10.71	5	13.51	3	13.64	1	7.70	12
5	2	7.15	4	10.81	2	9.09	2	15.38	10
	28	100.00	37	100.00	22	100.00	13	100.00	100

* For description of categories see Table 11.1

Table 11.3 Treatment outcome at 9 months follow-up within each category

	Categories*				
	1	2	3	4	5
Abstinent	31.25	29.41	23.08	25.00	20.00
Stayed mainly dry with lapses but recovered with little or no help	33.33	35.29	46.16	41.67	40.00
Readmitted but failed to benefit	22.92	23.53	15.38	25.00	20.00
Lost contact	12.50	11.77	15.38	8.33	20.50
Total	100.00	100.00	100.00	100.00	100.00

* For description of categories see Table 11.1

Table 11.4 Comparison of treatment outcome at 9 months follow-up for the alcoholics who gave no obvious reasons for their drinking and all the others who gave some reasons for their drinking

	Category 1 Alcoholics who gave no obvious reasons for their drinking		Categories 2—5 Alcoholics who gave some reason for their drinking	
	No.	%	No.	%
Abstinent	15	31.25	13	25.00
Stayed mainly dry with lapses but recovered with little or no help	16	33.33 ⎭ 64.58%	21	40.39 ⎭ 65.39%
Readmitted but failed to benefit	11	22.92	11	21.15
Lost contact	6	12.50	7	13.46
		100.00		100.00

abusing alcohol, is presented in Table 11.6. It is interesting to note that these symptoms at referral bear a strong relationship to the abuse of alcohol, almost suggesting an aetiological link-up, namely that alcohol abuse seems to be the primary problem and the other symptoms to be the result of alcohol abuse. Even when the treatment was directed solely to their alcohol problem, these patients showed improvement with regard to their other problems such as anxiety state, phobia, psychosomatic symptoms etc. It is interesting to note that these findings are similar to those reported in Table 11.4 for the alcoholics who sought help voluntarily for their alcoholism, were found later on to have other symptoms, but who received treatment mainly for their alcoholism.

Table 11.5 A group of 93 patients referred by the GP from the Health Centre for treatment of anxiety state, phobia, psychosomatic symptoms, etc. with no indication of a drinking problem

Reasons for referral	Alcohol abuse	No alcohol abuse	Total
1 Agoraphobia, travel phobia and social phobia	9	29	38
2 Anxiety tension	3	27	30
3 Mixed neurotics	3	22	25
	15	78	93

DISCUSSION

The results indicate that among the alcoholics treated in the Voluntary Special Admission Unit for Alcoholism, about half the patients claim no obvious symptoms of neurotic illnesses as reasons for alcohol abuse and so do not in any way see a causal connection. However, of the remainder, 17 % claim phobic anxiety symptoms and 12 % acute anxiety states and psychosomatic symptoms as aetiological factors in their alcoholism. For argument's sake, if one feels like conceding to the argument that those who claim to have anxiety and social phobia as causal factors in alcoholism, the number in the current sample is much smaller in that only 30 % claim any such connection. This figure is obviously a very much lower figure than what has been worrying other workers in this field who report a higher percentage in their samples. One such recent study by Smail[20], which claims half of the alcoholic population reporting phobic anxiety and social phobic symptoms, goes on to suggest that phobic anxiety plays a role in initiating alcohol dependence. This of course is going a bit too far and jumping to conclusions. If there was an aetiological connection in that if these phobic conditions caused alcoholism, then these alcoholics would not have benefited from a regime of treatment directed towards their alcoholism without special treatment for their phobic condition.

The fact remains that in the sample of 100 alcoholics, not only did treatment directed towards their drinking problem bring about relief of this condition to varying degrees, but there was reciprocal relief of phobic symptoms though no specific treatment was directed towards these symptoms. Again, if the various phobic conditions were aetiologically responsible for alcoholism, then one would have expected a substantial percentage from the 93 patients who are referred for the treatment of phobia and other neurotic symptoms to have shown alcohol dependence. This is not borne out by the facts. Only 15 out of the 93 patients revealed alcohol dependence and these patients not only did not connect their phobic conditions to their alcoholism, they also failed to acknowledge alcoholism as one of their

Table 11.6 Outcome of results of treatment directed mainly to alcohol abuse in patients referred by the GP from the Health Centre for treatment of anxiety state, phobia, psychosomatic symptoms etc. with no indication of a drinking problem

Reasons for referral	Abstinent and lost symptoms for which originally referred	Stayed mainly dry, occasional lapses, but recovered with little/no help, mostly lost symptoms for which originally referred	Continued abusing alcohol, not much change in other symptoms for which originally referred
1 Agoraphobia, travel phobia and social phobia	3	4	2
2 Anxiety tension	1	1	1
3 Mixed neurotics	1	1	1
	5	6	4

problems and it had never crossed their mind that their phobic and other symptoms could have been the result of their drinking and dependence on the drug. Once again the treatment results would suggest that even in this group of patients who were seeking help for their phobia and neurotic symptoms originally but were found to be alcohol dependent, treatment and help directed towards the drinking problem resulted in alleviating the neurotic symptoms. This makes it almost impossible to accept that phobic anxiety and other neurotic symptoms are in any major way connected aetiologically with the problem of alcoholism.

References

1 Jellinek, E. M. (1960). *The Disease Concept of Alcoholism.* (New Haven: College & University Press)
2 Marlatt, G. A., Demming, B. and Reid, J. B. (1973). Loss of control drinking in alcoholics: An experimental analogue. *J. Abstr. Psychol.*, **81,** 233
3 Miller, P. M. and Eisler, R. M. (1977). Alcohol and drug abuse. In Craighead, W. E., Kazdin, A. E. and Mahoney, M. J. (eds.) *Behavior modification: principles, issues, and applications.* (Boston: Houghton Mifflin)
4 Bandura, A. (1969). *Principles of Behavior Modification.* (New York: Holt, Rinehart & Winston)
5 Lokare, V. G. and Roach, F. (1982). Self-labelling and personality factors in alcoholism. In Golding, P. (ed.) *Alcoholism: A Modern Perspective*, pp. 489–502. (Lancaster: MTP)
6 MacAndrew, C. and Geertsma, R. H. (1963). An analysis of responses of alcoholics to scale 4 of the MMPI. *Q. J. Stud. Alc.*, **24,** 23
7 MacAndrew, C. (1965). The differentiation of male alcoholic outpatients from non-alcoholic psychiatric outpatients by means of the MMPI. *Q. J. Stud. Alc.*, **26,** 238
8 Rosenburg, N. (1972). MMPI alcoholic scales. *J. Clin. Psychol.*, **28,** 515
9 Hoffman, H., Loper, R. G. and Kammeier, M. L. (1974). Identifying future alcoholics with MMPI Scales. *Q. J. Stud. Alc.*, **35,** 490
10 MacAndrew, C. and Geertsma, R. H. (1964). A critique of alcoholism scales derived from the MMPI. *Q. J. Stud. Alc.*, **25,** 68
11 Eysenck, H. J. and Eysenck, S. B. G. (1975). *Manual of the Eysenck Personality Questionnaire.* (London: Hodder & Stoughton)
12 Lokare, V. G. (1971). Neuroticism, extraversion and the incidence of depressive illness in children. In Annell, A. -L. (ed.) *Depressive States in Childhood and Adolescence*, pp. 142–148. (Stockholm: Almqvist & Wiksell)
13 Marks, I. M., Birley, J. R. T. and Gelder, M. G. (1966). Modified leucotomy in severe agoraphobia, a controlled serial inquiry. *Br. J. Psychiatry*, **112,** 757
14 Quitkin, F. M. *et al.* (1972). Phobic anxiety syndrome complicated by drug dependence and addiction, a treatable form of drug abuse. *Arch. Gen. Psychiatry*, **27,** 159
15 Woodruff, R. H., Guze, S. B. and Clayton, P. J. (1972). Anxiety neurosis among psychiatric outpatients. *Compr. Psychiatry*, **13,** 65
16 Special Committee of the Royal College of Psychiatrists (1979). *Alcohol and Alcoholism.* (London: Tavistock Publications)
17 Mullaney, J. A. and Trippett, C. J. (1979). Alcohol dependence and phobias, clinical description and relevance. *Br. J. Psychiatry*, **135,** 565
18 Hilton, M. R. and Lokare, V. G. (1978). The evaluation of a questionnaire measuring severity of alcohol dependence. *Br. J. Psychiatry*, **132,** 42
19 Dahlgren, L. (1978). Development and pattern of problem drinking. *Acta Psychiatr. Scand.*, **57,** 325
20 Smail, P. A. (1981). Alcohol Dependence and Phobic States. *Dissertation for MSc*, University of Surrey

12
Is neuro-electric therapy of possible use in alcohol misuse?

K. SCHMIDT and M. CAMERON

INTRODUCTION

Having become familiar with acupuncture (to which the approach presented here is related) during his work over many years in south-east Asia and in the South Pacific, one of us (K.S.) at the same time had also encountered 'alcohol free' societies. In the course of his duties he collected transcultural data in South Pacific cultures, and comparing them with south-east Asian cultures, presented them to the 28th International Congress on Alcoholism and Drug Dependence in Sydney in 1972[1]. At the same time, viewing alcohol misuse as a cultural problem, a management programme was developed by the author in two South Pacific territories, the Melanesian New Hebrides and French Polynesia (Tahiti)[2]. From data received since some measurable success was noted.

The president of the International Society for Electro-stimulation (I.S.E.S) Dr F. Wagender, Department of Anaesthetics, University of Graz, at two conferences drew the senior author's attention to the use of electro-stimulation (ES) with alcohol problems (as well as with drug problems, sleep disorders etc). At the same time Dr Margaret Patterson[3] had presented her approach to alcohol and drug problems by neuro-electric therapy (NET) at the I.S.E.S. 5th International Symposium in Graz, Austria, in 1978.

What started us on the approach presented here, however, were two conferences Dr Patterson organized in October and December 1980 at the Royal Society of Medicine in London[4]. She also presented her approach on television. She taught us her approach with the Shackman – Patterson Neuro-Electric Stimulator when she joined our team at Yeovil District Hospital for 1 month in 1981. We now also use the Spembly 9000 neuro-electric stimulator which was developed originally for treatment of pain by transcutaneous neuro-electric nerve stimulation (TENS). As regards alcohol (and drug) problems it must be emphasized that little can be hoped for if this approach is not complemented by an intensive, well-structured rehabilitation programme. We have presented our experience with the treatment, on a small series of cases, to the Third World Congress of Biological Psychiatry in Stockholm in June 1981, and a larger series to the Sixth International Symposium on Electro-Stimulation in Albena, Bulgaria in September 1981. Both papers dealt with a fairly wide spectrum of conditions where the approach finds application.

METHODS

In the present paper we have extracted the 14 cases with alcohol problems (and a fifteenth case which we did not treat) out of our total series of 36 cases. We are an acute psychiatric unit in a modern district general hospital and treat the whole spectrum of psychiatric disorder with a fair loading of psycho-geriatric disorders – in other words we are *not* especially geared to alcohol problems.

One of the main reasons for taking up the presently described approach – apart from our dissatisfaction with our then management of alcohol problems – was a number of hard-drug addicts where we have been very successful.

Neuro-electric therapy

The approach is twofold. Prior to starting treatment, the usual clinical and biological investigations are carried out (F.B.C., L.F.T.) On day 1 of the intensive 1-month programme – with longitudinal follow-up *ad infinitum* where possible – the patient is fitted with one of the two stimulators, either the Shackman–Patterson or the Spembly 9000 with two electrodes fitted behind the ears after shaving areas 2 inches (5 cm) in diameter. He is taught how to turn the 'On' dial and the 'Output' dial after a demonstration of the expected sensation first on the fingers ('Oh yes, I can feel it now').

The range goes up to 35 V.

The frequencies of the 0.22 ms square wave with which we work in alcohol problems is either 70 or 110 or 500 Hz per second – whichever frequency is most comfortable for the particular patient. The range of frequencies for the various conditions has been established empirically by Dr Margaret Patterson and in general we follow her Training Manual. During NET therapy daily blood sugar estimations are made to exclude hypoglycaemia with its attendant risk of convulsion.

The patient is connected to the portable stimulator from his two electrodes behind the ear via leads. He wears the apparatus on his belt or in a supplied bag over his shoulder. The Shackman–Patterson Stimulator which contains the rechargeable battery has to be charged twice daily from the machine by a charger for 10 minutes approximately, a light indicates when the apparatus is fully charged. The stimulator is disconnected for these two short periods only but is otherwise worn for 24 hours for 10−14 days. The Shackman−Patterson stimulator has a frequency range of 0−2000 Hz/s.

The Spembly 9000 is worked by ordinary batteries available from stores. They have to be changed every 70 hours or so. Its frequency output is within a much smaller range, i.e. between 15 and 200 Hz. This obviously somewhat limits it − though there is a good chance that the firm will bring out an apparatus with a wider range (they also have a two-channel one). The aim of the electro-stimulation here is to detoxify the patient, which the apparatus does very successfully, and to take away the craving. This is achieved equally successfully, and very speedily.

The mechanism by which it works is thought to be mobilization of the endorphin−encephalin groups of neurotransmitters with the aim (usually achieved) to get the patient quickly out of the state of dysphoria, anhedonia or dysthymia. For ratings employed see Table 12.1.

Table 12.1

Ratings Degree	Social impairment No.	Anxiety/depression
Total	6	6
Severe	5	5
Marked	4	4
Moderate	3	3
Minor	2	2
Minimal	1	1
None	0	0

Rehabilitation programme

Also on Day 1 starts the detailed hour-by-hour programme after a contract has been signed (Consent Form for Neuro-Electric Therapy). It is similar to the consent form for the so-called e.c.t. in outline (and as regards counter-signature). The programme outline starts at 8 a.m. and includes at 9 a.m. the first of four prescribed daily readings from 'Twenty-four Hours'. This is followed by a set of yoga exercises: four introductory ones, ten standard ones and five replacement ones according to the date (and to introduce some degree of diversity). The patient is given the sheet with the 'Contract' and taught by K.S. − though a nurse trained in the exercises in fact reads them out. This is followed by 20 minutes' meditation according to Gestalt therapy − of which a procedure sheet is also attached to the contract. This again is taught by K. S., though a nurse or sometimes another patient reads it out and keeps time. Later in the morning there is prescribed reading of approximately 5 pages from

Presnall's *The Search for Serenity* and occupational therapy (O.T.). The afternoon continues with the third prescribed reading from the *Big Book* (Alcoholics Anonymous) followed by a session of O.T. and group counselling or individual psychotherapy. The programme continues with the afternoon yoga exercises, meditation and reading from *Day by Day*. The aim of this part of the programme is a change of the frame of reference and taking responsibility. In other words our approach is a biological and psychological one. Whilst under active treatment and rehabilitation — and hopefully forever after — the patient also takes part in a family therapy group once a week and attends AA. He is also offered counselling by one of the ministers of religion of all denominations on our panel.

Also attached to the contract is our evaluation sheet with its various parameters (and of course in the case-notes is the schedule of the frequencies employed). Table 12.2 gives a summary of the outcome.

Table 12.2   Summary of outcome to date

Category	Number
'Recovered'	8
One relapse — recovery	2
Two relapses — recovery	1
Doubtful	1
Failure	2
Not treated	1
Total	15

3. RESULTS

Table 12.3 shows that, of the 14 cases treated for alcoholism, eight have been 'successes.' Bearing in mind that alcoholism is a chronic and recurrent disorder it is probably not surprising that there have been the failures quoted.

Case reports

Four cases are cited.

Case 1

B.R., male, 42 years, started NET therapy on 25 June 1981. He was a confirmed alcoholic for 20 years or more and had just completed therapy with rifanol with the chest physician for pulmonary T.B. He was in exceedingly poor physical condition, also he had suffered much social degradation, having lost job, wife and family. After admission, during the period of assessment before going on NET he suffered a severe and prolonged series of *grand-mal*

Table 12.3 Assessments

Drinking outcome	Period of follow-up (months)	Age	Sex	Anxiety/depression						Social impairment					
				Prior to NET	End of NET	1/12 y after	3/12 y after	6/12 y after	12/12 y after	Prior to NET	End of NET	1/12 y after	3/12 y after	6/12 y after	12/12 y after
(1) L.V. recovery	10	24	F	4	0	1	2	1		3	0	0	1	1	
(2) B.I. relapse recovery	10	39	M	5	1	3	2	2		4	0	3	1	1	
(3) B.R. recovery	9	42	M	5	1	1	0	0		6	3	2	1	0	
(4) H.G. doubtful	8	41	M	5	3	3	4	2		5	3	3	3	2	
(5) L.J. recovery	8	49	F	3	3	2	1	0		4	1	0	0	0	
(6) W.N. relapse but recovery	7	34	M	4	2	2	4	1		4	1	2	3	0	
(7) C.M. several relapses	6	56	M	4	3	2	1	1		5	2	2	3	2	
(8) C.E. recovery	5	40	F	3	2	2	1			4	2	2	0		
(9) I.S. recovery	5	35	M	3	0	0	0			4	0	0	0		
(10) B.G. total failure	5	42	M	3	0	2	1			4	3	4	4		
(11) M.A. total failure	5	51	M	4	3	3	3			4	3	3	4		
(12) E.S. recovery	4	31	M	5	3	2	1			4	2	1	1		
(13) O.H. recovery	2	57	F	5	2	2				4	2	3			
(14) P.L. recovery	1	29	F	5	2	1				5	3	2			
(15) H.J. refused treatment	0	45	M	2	NA					4	NA	NA			

attacks when he bit his tongue severely, and a cardiac arrest call had to be made to give him emergency treatment for his alcohol withdrawal symptoms by i.v. diazepam.

After going on NET he progressed satisfactorily and at the end of therapy became a completely different person. He is now working in London. His own family were supportive. The social services provided him with ample convalescence. There was liver damage in his case. He attends AA.

Case 2

W.N., male, aged 34 years. He is an anxious person with longstanding alcohol addiction. He is a local government officer. He started a course of NET therapy on 4 September 1981. The future of his job and marriage were dependent on his giving up alcohol. The treatment was successful. After discharge he had one relapse, but recovered again and is now fully functional as a planning officer attending AA.

Case 3

M.A., 51 years. This man was treated with NET from 19 December 1981 as an inpatient. He was a model patient but a confirmed alcoholic of long standing and had undergone many treatments in alcoholic units with no success. He was not really motivated, but was pushed by his wife to undergo NET therapy. In the end after improving greatly in health he started coming onto the ward smelling of alcohol. It was arranged for him to go to an alcohol unit locally. He did not turn up and was found drunk heavily again. He has again approached this local unit for admission. He had an unusually meek manner which covered resentment and lack of self-esteem.

Case 4

H.J., male, 45 years. This man has been a confirmed alcoholic for many years. He shows basically a personality disorder of the sociopathic type. He was a well-to-do farmer but has squandered his heritage somewhat now, and his family have suffered severely. He has had many attempts to help him — reforms but always relapses to drinking again. He refused to have NET and when a treatment contract was offered by us, wanted immediately to return once more to one of the more expensive private alcoholic units in another part of the country. Was he afraid of being 'cured'?

DISCUSSION

The best conception we have so far of our approach is that of weeding a field. Whether the weeds will grow again depends on the efficiency with which the nursing team can be won over to supervise and enforce the rehabilitation programme. Unashamedly one has to state that in a private facility this can be assured. In the British National Health Service where the consultant usually works in a number of different settings (in my case (K.S.) — I work in seven different places, not counting the crisis intervention visits, or the ordinary domiciliary visits, or the committees, or teaching) and with the continually changing nursing teams (we have lost the charge nurse but now have at least two, changing shift-wise — a great drawback in the authors' view), this is less assured.

This author (K.S.) can see no future in Britain for a broad epidemiological approach to the problem in terms of a change of alcoholism that is a drastic reduction in incidence or prevalence, and I am looking forward to the evaluation of educational campaigns promised at this conference. On the other hand, I know of societies where this has happened, largely by a change of national consciousness, group cohesion, and a work ethos, religious reawakening and fostering of personal responsibility, something so badly lacking in Britain today where public encouragement of egotism and demand for immediate personal satisfaction are fostered and propagated in all mass media.

As regards *prognosis*, the success of this (and probably other approaches to alcoholism) will hinge on the question: Does he really want to change? (or even in some cases: Why should he?) — in other words it hinges on motivation. If there is a family we manage to rope in for the group therapy process where we offer an identification group, a church, an employer, a friend, the prognosis is improved. The prognosis is further improved (but not necessarily bringing about change by itself) if the gains from abstinence are high, such as wife or child returning and the offer of a job (as in our cited Case 1, above) or the resumption of marriage and an open door to the house as well as maintenance of a good job (in our cited Case 2, above). The stability he has or has not shown in his previous personality and the strength of reactive factors 'justifying' drinking, as well as the family history with or without absence of alcoholism and other psychiatric disorder, underlying other psychopathology — and of course the duration of alcohol misuse and organic damage of the liver, the c.n.s., and c.v.s. — are all factors which are taken into account as regards prognosis.

As regards further *research* we have invited the appropriate departments at both Bristol and Bath Universities to help us with outside evaluation. We also have made new approaches to a number of research centres in this country and abroad to help with measurements of endorphin—encephalin changes in the blood serum (as opposed to the c.s.f.). We already have assurances from the Karolinska Institute in Stockholm and the NIMH in Bethesda, Maryland, USA that they will help if all else fails. At the same time we are studying how we can increase our own motivational skills.

Lastly, in our psychotherapeutic counselling we follow the 'Six-stage Programme in Managing the Alcoholic' proposed by G. L. Lloyd[7].

Acknowledgements

We are grateful to the Somerset Area Health Authority, especially to Dr A. Parry-Jones, Area Medical Officer, for facilitating the approach described and for sanctioning it. Equally we are grateful to Dr. Margaret Patterson for all we learned from her, especially whilst she was a member of our team. We are also grateful to our nurses for in principle accepting another new form of treatment with all the question marks about it — especially for the help of the Nursing Officer, Mr K. Mooniaruck, for smoothing out numerous tight situations. Our thanks are also due to the postgraduate tutor, Mr J. Slater, FRCOG, through whose offices we obtained the first stimulator, to the League of Friends of Yeovil District Hospital as well as the Inner Circle for the others — and to the Hospital Administrator, Mr Roy Pritchard, and the engineers, Mr Watson and his team, for their patience and help. Lastly I wish to thank our ever-patient secretary, Mrs B. Martin, for her help at all times.

References

1 Schmidt, K. (1971). The drug-and alcohol misuse situation in South Pacific territories to-date. Presented at the *28th International Congress on Alcoholism and Drug Dependence*, Sydney
2 Schmidt, K. (1973). Preventive Psychiatry with Emphasis on Primary Prevention in the South Pacific, pp. 64. et sqq., p. 96. (SPC Monograph) (Noumea, New Caledonia: South Pacific Commission)
3 Patterson, M. (1978). The significance of current frequency in neuro-electric therapy (N.E.T) for drug and alcoholic addictions. In *Report of the 5th International Symposium of I.S.E.S.*, p. 285. (Graz: University Press)
4 Patterson, M. (1975). *Addictions Can be Cured.* (Berkhamsted: Lion Publishing)
5 Schmidt, K., and Cameron, M. (1981). Neuro-electric therapy, a preliminary report. Presented at the *3rd World Congress of Biological Psychiatry*, Stockholm
6 Schmidt, K. and Cameron, M. (1981). Neuro-electric therapy (N.E.T), the widening spectrum of its application. Presented at the *6th International Symposium on Electro-Stimulation*, Albena, Bulgaria (Report, p. 50 et sqq.)
7 Lloyd, G. L. (1982). A six-stage programme in managing the alcoholic. *Mod. Med.*, **27,** 50

13

Alcoholics as a problem of alcohol control policy

S. AHLSTRÖM

INTRODUCTION

The harmful consequences of excessive drinking are emphasized by the sorry plight of the alcoholic. It is only natural that those who are professionally involved in controlling alcohol problems should be very interested in alcoholics. Nevertheless, a measure of controversy exists about how alcoholism should be viewed. There are two main arguments. On the one hand, those who hold that control measures should be liberalized and the public encouraged to adopt moderate drinking habits maintain that the alcoholic is beyond redemption. Alcoholics are addicted to drink, must and will have it, and lie outside the scope of alcohol control policy. Those who believe that alcohol should be subject to strong measures of control, on the other hand, contend that sufficiently thoroughgoing steps will affect even the pathological drunk.

Can one influence the drinking habits of alcoholics? And if one can, is it likely that limiting the availability of alcohol will prove efficacious? These questions are central to alcohol research and before attempting to answer them, we shall first have to know what the drinking habits of alcoholics actually are.

If one were to ask a social scientist and a layman about the pathology of alcoholism, one might well receive two very different answers. Something is, however, known about the way in which the alcoholic drinks. There is a clear, consistent, well established body of evidence, based on clinical models of the alcoholic and the hypotheses of the AA movement (though these tend to be bound up with its therapeutic aims). Simplifying matters somewhat, we might say that the drinking habits of the alcoholic are generally thought to be very different from the 'normal' use of alcohol. It is usually held – especially in spirits countries – that the alcoholic's inability to control his drinking leads to lengthy drinking bouts, to large amounts of alcohol being ingested on single occasions, to heavy annual consumption and, inevitably, to impaired health. This, however, does not really say much about how alcohol policy measures affect alcoholics.

The belief that alcoholics are diametrically opposed to the rest of the population has had a marked bearing on Finnish alcohol policy. Indeed, whenever alcohol control policies are discussed, it is the figure of the down-and-out on the city streets which first comes to the minds of the general public and the authorities alike. The label 'alcoholic' is often thought to apply to skid-row bums only. The whole question of the difference between the alcoholic and the 'normal' drinker has attracted more attention in recent years: empirical evidence now suggests that alcohol control policies leave a mark on both overall consumption and the drinking habits of the public at large[1].

Furthermore, alcoholics account for a disproportionately large share of the overall consumption of alcohol. Though the argument is a weak one, it might be maintained that since there is not much qualitative difference between the drinking habits of the alcoholic and the 'normal' drinker, alcohol control policies must have some effect on alcoholic drinking.

ALCOHOLIC DRINKING AND EMPIRICAL EVIDENCE

It used to be thought that the alcoholic's drinking and the drinking habits of the general public had very little in common. The alcoholic, first of all, was considered to be prone to prolonged drinking bouts. These recurrent periods – interrupted by spells of abstinence – were thought to be due to the alcoholic's inability to drink on one day only. Moderate drinking and alcoholic drinking were held to be diametrically opposed. Moreover, it was maintained that alcoholics would spend a great many days drinking in the course of a single year and that, being unable to drink in moderation, they would also tend to consume a great deal of alcohol each day. It was also believed that the annual quantities drunk by alcoholics were so great that their health inevitably suffered.

Drinking bouts

There are very few studies of the drinking habits of alcoholics. Nevertheless, a series of investigations employing uniform methods has been conducted in seven different locations – Japan, Switzerland, Italy, New York, Brazil, California, and France[2-8]. The aim of the research was to ascertain the classes of beverages consumed by alcoholics and the drinks which they preferred. The definition of the term 'alcoholic' used unfortunately varied from one location to another, and this makes it somewhat difficult to compare the seven sets of findings. If one makes allowances for this inconsistency, however, some interesting points come to light.

Instead of focussing on the frequency of drinking, most social studies of alcoholism tend to concentrate on continuity – one of the most 'alcoholic' aspects of the alcoholic's drinking habits. In the series of seven studies referred to above, the interviewees were asked how long their drinking bouts usually lasted. With the exception of the wine-drinking countries where alcoholics drink daily, the results were remarkably consistent. Between 45% and 58% of the alcoholics interviewed stated that the average duration of their drinking bouts was not less than 7 days.

My own study of Finnish alcoholics[9] aims at describing alcohol use in terms of drinking bouts (and uses methods which are similar to the ones used in studies of the general public which tend to concentrate on the characteristics of drinking occasions). I found that the average length of a drinking bout was 12 days, but that it was by no means uncommon for the alcoholic to limit his drinking to a single day on occasion. My study did not support the hypothesis that alcoholics are compelled to indulge in prolonged drinking bouts: whilst there were drinking periods of considerable length, these were often interspersed with drinking occasions limited to a single day. Some of those single days coincided with events which Finnish society recognizes as excuses for drunkenness and even condones – weddings, funerals, May Day, Midsummer and New Year. Some had foreshadowed prolonged drinking bouts whilst others had been isolated instances.

Sober spells

Many alcoholics experience periods of sobriety, but this is an aspect of the behaviour of alcoholics which research has tended to overlook. Wiseman's study demonstrates that some alcoholics have periods of drunkenness when they are only vaguely aware of the passage of time, and yet experience spells of sobriety when they live according to precisely regulated timetables[10]. Ludwig has actually measured the duration of this sobriety: in a follow-up study of alcoholics which spanned 18 months, sober periods were found to last for 4 months on average [11]. Very few of the alcoholics studied by Ludwig drank continuously during the 18 months when they were under observation; the majority drank periodically, sober spells alternating with drinking bouts.

My study of Finnish alcoholics[9] also looks at sobriety, but from a slightly different point of view. As well as examining voluntary periods of sobriety, it notes the periods when the subjects were forced to remain sober during the 12 months immediately preceding the interview. Alcoholics are at times compelled to do without alcohol, and it is obvious that these spells affect the frequency of their drinking. Whenever an alcoholic is imprisoned, undergoing treatment, hospitalized and so on, he will be prevented from satisfying his desire to drink. My findings indicate that every other alcoholic living in Helsinki had experienced compulsory periods of sobriety; the corresponding figure for alcoholics who lived in the countryside was a mere 15%. All in all, approximately 40% of the interviewees had remained sober by choice at one time or another. Indeed, one of the most important results of the methods which the study used was that it made it evident that sober spells are a salient aspect of the alcoholic's drinking habits.

Frequency of drinking

The frequency with which alcoholics drink is a subject which has tended to escape attention. In general, studies have contented themselves with noting that the alcoholic's drinking occasions are less interspaced with periods of sobriety than the moderate drinker's. The alcoholic, in effect, is usually seen as likely to drink daily. The annual drinking frequency of the general public can be estimated with comparative accuracy by measuring the period between the two previous drinking occasions or through data on how often an individual drinks each week or month. But it is much more difficult to estimate how frequently the alcoholic drinks — imprisonment, hospitalization and so on obscure the general picture[9]. Charting drinking occasions over a week — or even a month — will fail to give a reliable impression of how often the alcoholic drinks over the course of a year[12].

Amount drunk

Similarly, not many studies have interested themselves in the quantities of alcohol which alcoholics use[13]. Furthermore, most of the few estimates which are available tend to be curtailed to single drinking occasions — though it is true that many of these occasions continued for a whole day and night.

A study was made by the Swedish physician, Berglin[14], which gave figures on the amounts of alcohol consumed by 455 alcoholics who received aid from the Social Welfare Board of the City of Gothenburg between 1948 and 1954. Berglin was not interested in estimating annual — or even daily — consumption, however; he aimed at ascertaining the largest amount of alcohol ingested in one day. His findings, which he believed 'medium serious' cases of alcoholism, indicated that the mean value of a single 24-hour period maximum intake was 24 cl of absolute alcohol.

Two of the seven connected studies which we mentioned earlier estimated the daily alcohol consumption of alcoholics[2, 8]. French alcoholics were found to have an average daily intake of 34 cl of absolute alcohol, 73 % of which was wine. These estimates were based on information about the day and night immediately before the interview. The Japanese alcoholics were found to drink considerably less daily: the average daily intake was 16 cl of absolute alcohol.

Lelbach[15] has computed estimates of the amounts which heavy drinkers and alcoholics consume daily; his figures are a compilation of the findings of various studies. No clear division separates the moderate drinker from the alcoholic; the daily intakes overlap. Nevertheless, the consensus of informed opinion is that heavy drinkers drink at least 11 cl of absolute alcohol a day. Lelbach's study also includes data on the quantities of alcohol which patients undergoing treatment for alcoholism are in the habit of drinking daily. The amounts varied between 24 and 30 cl of absolute alcohol, and the nationality of the patient seemed to make little difference.

Finnish alcoholics[9] tend to consume 20–24 cl of absolute alcohol a day. Alcoholics living in the other Nordic capitals consume similar amounts, and the Finnish alcoholic's intake corresponds with the figures which Lelbach gives as the daily consumption of German, Austrian, Canadian and Australian alcoholics. French alcoholics[16], however, tend to drink a great deal more – some 34 cl of absolute alcohol each day. Research indicates that whilst the Finnish alcoholic often begins a drinking bout by drinking a great deal, his consumption falls as the bout comes closer to its end.

As we have seen, the amount which Finnish alcoholics and other Scandinavian heavy drinkers consume during a drinking period is smaller than the daily intake of the French alcoholic. Before drawing comparisons, it should be emphasized that different studies define alcoholism in different ways, and that this must affect matters. Furthermore, the measurements by which estimates are arrived at and the reliability of the results also vary. Nevertheless, it is evident that the French attitude towards alcohol, coupled with the Gallic habit of drinking wine with meals, leads to higher daily consumption than in the Nordic countries. And it would appear that this tendency is true of both the general public of the two countries[17] and the French and Finnish alcoholic as well.

Finnish alcoholics and the alcoholic type

One often hears it said that there are several types of alcoholic. 'Periodic drinkers' and 'French-type alcoholics' are familiar phrases. The best known description of alcoholic types was given by E. M. Jellinek[18]. The treatment of alcoholism is often based on the assumption that there is either one single alcoholic type, or that there are several alcoholic types, each of which has its own particular hallmarks.

My study of Finnish alcoholism[9] suggested that whilst there would appear to be no readily distinguishable alcoholic types, alcoholic drinking clearly does exist. Alcoholic drinking, furthermore, tends to be matter of separate drinking bouts rather than the alcoholic's drinking history over a period of, say, 1 year. The alcoholic is able to drink like other people at times. Kiviranta[19], looking at the pathology of alcoholism, also finds that there is no common denominator applicable to alcoholics as a whole.

ALCOHOLICS AND CHANGES IN DRINKING HABITS

Whilst it would not be true to say that drinking habits have not been studied at all, most of the work which has been done has taken the form of cross-sectional research. Most studies have aimed at describing a particular subgroup's use of alcohol or at evaluating the specific characteristics of a given group's drinking habits. Changes in drinking habits have not attracted a great deal of attention.

There has, however, been a recent upsurge of interest. This has been due to two reasons. First of all, modern life causes people's habits in general to change so rapidly that it seems reasonable to assume that some modification must take place in drinking habits as well. And secondly, it is difficult to implement alcohol policy if one has no way of assessing its effects. Taking a broader view, it would also seem that the growth of interest in change is a reflection of changing attitudes towards research in general: historical studies are winning ground and the cross-sectional approach losing favour.

One might say that there are two types of research into changing drinking habits. To begin with, the changes which take place in a person's drinking habits at different times in his life are undeniably interesting in their own right. Many studies have addressed themselves to determining how age influences drinking patterns. Economic and social activity, social ties, and health all vary with age and obviously play a part in the way in which drinking habits change.

Secondly, an especially close watch has been kept on any changes which might take place in drinking habits when the availability of alcoholic beverages has undergone change. In general, most fluctuations in the availability of alcohol are the result of deliberately planned measures, but matters have altered spontaneously on occasion, too.

Life cycle and the use of alcohol

Studies which are specifically addressed towards changes in the drinking habits of alcoholics are few and far between. Moreover, the majority of samples which are intended to represent the general public have not included many heavy drinkers.

There are a few studies which relate changes in drinking to the amount of alcohol consumed, but it would be a mistake to regard as heavy drinkers the subjects which are found by these studies to drink the most. Very little research has been conducted into the subject of how the drinking habits of heavy drinkers and alcoholics alter with the passage of time. Whenever the manner in which the drinking habits of alcoholics change has been looked at, the underlying aim has been to evaluate the efficacy of different approaches to the treatment of alcoholism. Simple, forthright cures have tended to be emphasized – abstinence, making drinking less frequent, helping the alcoholic achieve mental and emotional equilibrium and so on. Even when drinking habits have been directly observed, the findings have been too vague to allow one to assess any changes which might have place.

Don Cahalan is probably the only person who has paid close attention to changes in the drinking patterns of the problem drinker. Cahalan's Hartford study[20] comprises two sets of measurements, made within $2\frac{1}{2} - 3$ years of each other, and uses two indices: changes in the index of intoxication based on the volume of alcohol ingested on each drinking occasion, and the escape or relief cited by respondents as a reason for drinking. Since Cahalan's findings are based on indices, they do not give any knowledge of changes in individual drinking patterns. Nevertheless, he noted that 'there is a substantial turnover in the drinking and the heavy drinking populations' as 'indicated by the finding that a fairly large proportion, about one fourth, of the population showed a shift in drinking habits or reasons for drinking within the relatively short period of three years'.

Another study by the same author[21] is a nationwide investigation of the correlates of problem drinking. The index used, besides shedding light on drinking habits themselves, also scrutinizes the problems which psychological addiction to alcohol brings about. This later study is also based on two sets of interviews, one made in 1964–5 and the other in 1967. Each respondent was scored on a combined index for psychological dependence and frequency of intoxication and classified as either 'high' or 'low' on both counts. Whilst Cahalan's later findings are also not applicable to changes in drinking habits themselves, some 15% of the interviewees were found to have switched between 'high' and 'low' scores inside the short space of 3 years. Cahalan's findings are supported by earlier evidence[20, 22] which suggests that age and social and psychological factors play a large part in effecting change in drinking habits.

Drinking patterns and supply

Two factors influence the availability of alcoholic beverages: supply and price. The term 'supply' includes both off-licence retail sales of alcohol and beverages sold for consumption on licensed premises. The consequences of experimental modifications in availability and spontaneous changes in supply have attracted wide interest. It has proved more difficult to study the effect of changes in the price of alcohol.

Spontaneous changes in supply

The Swedish alcohol monopoly, the Vin- och Spritcentralen, was hit by a strike in 1963 which made it necessary to regulate the distribution of wine and spirits. Whilst the strike was in progress, it was particularly difficult to obtain spirits. The effects of the strike were surveyed[23]; some 70 'normal' drinkers and 60 problem drinkers were interviewed in Stockholm. Both groups were interviewed several times in order to shed light on the changes which had taken place before, during and after the strike. Moderate drinkers seemed to be very little affected; their consumption remained uniformly low throughout the whole of the period studied. Problem drinkers, however, drank less often and drank slighter amounts, despite the fact that the strike had no effect at all on the availability of beer and ale.

A similar event took place in Finland in the spring of 1972 when the staff of the State Alcohol Monopoly's retail outlets (ALKO shops) went on strike. The strike lasted for 5 weeks, during which time the most important channel for the distribution of alcohol was completely closed. The strike, however, had no effect on restaurants and the distribution network for medium beer.

The effect which the strike had on drinking patterns was shown by the number of arrests made for drunkenness: the average daily frequency of arrests fell 52 %[24]. The strike had its greatest effect on the socially integrated, but even homeless alcoholics experienced a 'drying-out' period. Records of the number of patients who were treated while under the influence of alcohol at two Helsinki polyclinics were examined after the strike[25], and the behaviour of homeless alcoholics in the City of Tampere was studied through participant observation[26]. The data for Helsinki and Tampere seem to indicate that the strike affected homeless alcoholics in two ways: whilst a significant proportion stopped drinking when the normal supply of alcohol ceased, others found refuge in substitutes for alcoholic beverages. The data on arrests for drunkenness also demonstrate these trends. And whilst fewer homeless alcoholics were arrested for drunkenness during the strike, the number of skid-row bums arrested for using substitute alcohol increased dramatically[24].

Summing up the strike's overall effects, Mäkelä[27] noted that it had a far-reaching influence on the drinking of inveterate alcoholics — an observation which is at variance with the hypothesis that the alcoholic is psychologically predestined to become addicted to alcohol and that his drinking habits are little affected by the norms of society in general.

Experimentally modified supply

A new Alcohol Act was passed in Finland in July 1968; it came into force the following year. The revised legislation had two effects on the availability of alcoholic beverages. First, it made ALKO shops' monopoly of the sale of medium beer a thing of the past and permitted grocery stores and cafés to sell medium beer. And secondly, it provided for the establishment of ALKO shops and licensed restaurants in the countryside — facilities which had previously only been available in cities and towns.

The slackening of the control of medium beer had some effect on the drinking habits of the alcoholic[9]. Alcoholics living in Helsinki began to drink more medium beer, though their consumption of it rose less than the average for the total population of the Province of Uusimaa. Medium beer is slightly cheaper than strong beer but is more expensive than other alcoholic beverages if the price is computed in terms of absolute alcohol. Alcoholics tend to be very conscious of the value they receive for their money and, since alcohol is readily available in Helsinki, the new legislation did not prompt the alcoholics of Helsinki to buy much more medium beer. Alcohol, however, is far less readily available in the countryside, and alcoholics who lived in rural areas did begin to drink more medium beer. Nevertheless, whilst alcoholics' consumption of medium beer rose proportionally more than the average for rural districts, the life of the alcoholic in the countryside was not much changed by the ready availability of medium beer. The reasons for this are obviously that medium beer is relatively costly and that alcoholics prefer to take their alcohol in the form of strong beverages which it is easy to carry around.

The State Alcohol Monopoly conducted an experiment of closing ALKO shops on Saturdays. The experiment lasted for 8 months and a follow-up study[28] indicated that the trial closure reduced overall alcohol consumption, lessened the incidence of public disorder and lowered the number of arrests for drunkenness.

The price of alcohol and drinking patterns

The seven interconnected studies[2-8] which we have already mentioned demonstrate that alcoholics do not have a marked preference for a particular type of beverage. Neither do alcoholics tend to remain faithful to any one given class of drink. The bottle which the alcoholic buys does, however, display a connexion between price and alcoholic strength. Some studies, for instance, have paid attention to the stated preferences of the alcoholic and the beverages which alcoholics tend to favour in practice. Generally speaking, the number of those who say that they are most fond of, say, whisky, will be far greater than the number of heavy drinkers who actually buy bottles of whisky. Few alcoholics state a preference for inexpensive drinks, but the number of heavy drinkers who purchase inexpensive beverages is far higher. The data for California[7] provide a case in point: some 63 % of Californian alcoholics would drink spirits if they had the chance, but a mere 29 % said that they mainly relied on strong alcoholic beverages. Correspondingly, 16 % of the heavy drinkers interviewed said that they would drink wine if they were able to pick up a glass from a table where every conceivable type of beverage was on offer, but virtually every other alcoholic tended to buy more wine than whisky. This tendency seems to have little to do with national traits – whilst the majority of Swiss and Brazilian[3, 6] alcoholics drink spirits, the Swiss and Brazilian prices of strong alcoholic beverages offer the best value for money in terms of absolute alcohol.

Our Finnish study[9] also seemed to indicate that alcoholics keep price uppermost in their minds when choosing which beverage to buy. Indeed, price is probably more important than cultural factors. The beverages which French alcoholics use are very dependent on the area in which the alcoholic lives and the types of beverage which are locally available[8]. And in Switzerland[3], the alcoholics of a French-speaking, wine-drinking canton drank 'snapps' because wine cost more.

The longer a drinking bout lasts, the more important price becomes[6, 9]: the alcoholic runs out of money towards the end of a drinking bout and is forced to buy the cheapest drinks.

There is also evidence to suggest that price affects the alcoholic's drinking habits under experimental conditions. Experiments which vary the cost of drinking have found that cost influences both the amount which the alcoholic drinks and the times at which he drinks[29]. And these experimental findings are especially interesting since the alcoholics were subject to a measure of control.

Later 'happy hour' experiments[30] indicate that price is important to the casual user and the heavy drinker as well. 'Happy hour' subjects tended to drink as much in the experiments as they did under normal conditions, whereas 'non-happy hour' subjects drank less than was their wont.

SUMMARY AND DISCUSSION

It is usual for alcohol policy to divide the general public into three categories: young people, who have to be protected from the harm wrought by alcohol; moderate drinkers, people who know their limits; and alcoholics, who invariably drink as much as they can and cannot be affected by control policy. Every time new alcohol policy measures are proposed − when, in other words, individual freedom is curtailed − the distinction between the moderate drinker and the alcoholic engenders controversy. It is often held that the moderate drinker should be allowed to buy a few bottles for the weekend and even become drunk without upsetting his finances. Price increases are said to only penalize the moderate drinker, it being 'well known' that alcoholics always consume a given amount of alcohol a year regardless of how much money they have and how much alcohol costs. It has even been suggested that a special kind of cheap 'alcoholic booze' should be marketed as this would spare the alcoholic's family from some of the consequences of price increases.

Whilst it is easy to distinguish between young people and the rest of the population, it is not as easy to draw a line between the alcoholic and the moderate drinker. There are no obvious criteria. The drinking habits of alcoholics and moderate drinkers are not so very different, nor does the alcoholic lack all control. It may even be that the quantity of alcohol which an alcoholic drinks over the space of 1 year will be no greater than the annual consumption of a 'respectable' drinker who only uses alcohol in moderation but has something to drink each day. Heavy drinkers are not always labelled alcoholics − and those who are labelled as alcoholics are not always heavy drinkers. Furthermore, new empirical evidence seems to suggest that the alcoholic's drinking habits can be modified through social influences[31]. If true, the generally accepted picture of an alcoholic − a person whose drinking cannot be controlled − is obviously inaccurate. To use Room's[32] phrase, maybe we should say 'farewell to alcoholism'.

The increase in overall consumption which is a characteristic of modern society makes it still harder to distinguish between the moderate drinker and the alcoholic. In Finland, for instance, people did not usually drink on many days in the year; in the past, how likely a person was to continue drinking on more than one successive day formed a measure of his dependence on alcohol. Nowadays, however, so many people drink small amounts each day that one should define the 'probability of continued drinking' anew. It would be better to assess how dependent a person is on alcohol on the basis of how likely he is to remain drunk over an extended period.

We do not know much about the drinking habits of alcoholics. The little information which is available, therefore, should be utilized as much as possible. First of all, the treatment of alcoholism should take the periodicity of drinking into account. Instead of aiming at lifelong abstinence, the goal might be the maximizing of sober periods and the minimizing of drinking bouts. Secondly, since it is known that the alcoholic attaches a great deal of importance to price when he decides which drink to buy, the pricing of various beverage classes ought to take this into consideration. Some beverages have less harmful effects in the long run than others, and it would be sound policy if the least harmful beverages were the cheapest. Heavy drinkers should be thought of as a special group when price increases are planned. The alcoholic's choice of drink is heavily influenced by economic considerations, and it seems likely that the several months' advance warning of price increases in Finland which was given in 1974 and 1975 encouraged heavy drinkers to drink as much as they could while alcohol was still cheap. Heavy drinkers also tend to buy in cheap stocks of alcohol before price increases come into effect, and this pushes consumption up as well.

The alcoholic is affected by how liberal alcohol policy is. The alcoholic is nowadays able to melt into the crowd on many occasions. Finnish wet weekends and Bank Holidays provide the alcoholic with ample 'cover'. There are a host of times when heavy drinking excites little comment: the more easily the heavy drinker is able to indulge himself, the greater the risk to his health becomes.

It would seem that the alcoholic does not drink steadily; rather, he tends to have periods when he drinks heavily, and others when he uses alcohol in relative moderation. There also seems to be no way of foretelling how violently a particular individual's life will be upset by heavy drinking[33]. Furthermore, the alcoholic's consumption is influenced by external factors: whilst he will drink more at one time than the moderate drinker, the amount which he consumes over a year depends on the frequency of his drinking. And there are clear links between the frequency of drinking occasions and the availability of alcohol.

This chapter has discussed the alcoholic from the point of view of alcohol policy, but it has not analysed the part which policy plays in the gestation of alcoholism. Virtually the only thing which is certain is that making it easier to become drunk will not help to prevent or cure alcoholism.

References

1 Bruun, K., Edwards, G., Lumio, M., Mäkelä, K., Pan, L., Popham, R. E., Room, R., Schmidt, W., Skog, O.-J., Sulkunen, P. and Österberg, E. (1975). *Alcohol Control Policies in Public Health Perspective*. Helsinki, Finnish Foundation for Alcohol Studies, Vol. 25

2 Ando, H. and Hasegawa, E. (1970). Drinking patterns and attitudes of alcoholics and nonalcoholics in Japan. *Q. J. Stud. Alc.*, **31**, 153

3 Devrient, P. and Lolli, G. (1962). Choice of alcoholic beverage among 240 alcoholics in Switzerland. *Q. J. Stud. Alc.*, **23**, 459

4 Lolli, G., Golder, G. M., Serianni, E., Bonfiglio, G. and Balboni, C. (1958). Choice of alcoholic beverage among 178 alcoholics in Italy. *Q. J. Stud. Alc.*, **19**, 303

5 Lolli, G., Schesler, E. and Golder, G. M. (1960). Choice of alcoholic beverage among 105 alcoholics in New York. *Q. J. Stud. Alc.*, **21**, 475

6 Parreiras, D., Lolli, G. and Golder, G. M. (1956). Choice of alcoholic beverage among 500 alcoholics in Brazil. *Q. J. Stud. Alc.*, **17**, 629

7 Terry, J., Lolli, G. and Golder, G. M. (1957). Choice of alcoholic beverage among 531 alcoholics in California. *Q. J. Stud. Alc.*, **18**, 417

8 Sadoun, R. and Lolli, G. (1962). Choice of alcoholic beverage among 120 alcoholics in France. *Q. J. Stud. Alc.*, **23**, 449

9 Ahlström-Laakso, S. (1975). *Drinking Habits Among Alcoholics.* Forssa, Finnish Foundation for Alcohol Studies, Vol. **21**

10 Wiseman, J. P. (1972). Sober time: The neglected variable in the recidivism of alcoholic person. Presented at the *Second Annual Alcoholism Conference of the National Institute on Alcohol Abuse and Alcoholism,* sponsored by the National Institute of Mental Health, 1–2 June, Washington, DC

11 Ludwig, A. M. (1972). On and off the wagon. Reasons for drinking and abstaining by alcoholics. *Q. J. Stud. Alc.*, **33**, 91

12 Diderichsen, A. and Skyum-Nielsen, S. (1969). *Om brug og misbrug af alkohol.* (About the use and abuse of alcohol.) Copenhagen, Socialforskningsinstituttet, Publication **36**

13 Goldberg, L., Bjerver, K. and Neri, A. (1965). Alkoholkonsumtionens fördelning på olika alkoholvanegrupper. (The distribution of alcohol consumption among different groups of alcohol users.) *In Alkoholkonflikten 1963,* Medicinska verkningar. (Norstedt, Stockholm: Wenner-Gren Center)

14 Berglin, C. -G. (1960). Dryckesvanor hos 455 alkoholister (Drinking habits among 455 alcoholics). *Alkoholfrågan,* **54**, 66

15 Lelbach, Werner K. (1974). Organic pathology related to volume and pattern of alcohol use. In Gibbins, R. J. et al. (eds.) *Research Advances in Alcohol and Drug Problems.* (New York: Wiley)

16 Sadoun, R., Lolli, G. and Silverman, M. (1965). *Drinking in French Culture.* (New Haven: Rutgers Center of Alcohol Studies)

17 Ahlström-Laakso, S. (1976). European drinking habits: A review of research and some suggestions for conceptual integration of findings, in Everett, M. W., Waddell, J. O. and Heath, D. B. (eds.) *Cross-cultural Approaches to the Study of Alcohol,* pp. 119–132. (The Hague: Mouton)

18 Jellinek, E. M. (1960). *The Disease Concept of Alcoholism.* (New Haven: College & University Press)

19 Kiviranta, Pekka (1969). *Alcoholism syndrome in Finland.* Helsinki, The Finnish Foundation for Alcohol Studies, Vol. **17**

20 Cahalan, D. (1968). *Correlates of change in drinking behavior in an urban community sample over a three-year period.* PhD Thesis, George Washington University. (Ann Arbor, Michigan: University Microfilms)

21 Cahalan, D. (1970). *Problem drinkers.* (San Francisco: Jossey-Bass)

22 Williams, J. J. (1967). Waxing and waning drinkers. Presented at the *Annual Meeting of the Society for the Study of Social Problems.* 27 August, San Francisco

23 Bjerver, K. and Neri, A. (1965). Alkoholkonsumtionens förändringar våren 1963 hos måttliga alkoholförtärare och hos personer med alkoholproblem. (Changes in alcohol consumption in the spring of 1963 among moderate drinkers and persons with an alcohol problem.) In *Alkoholkonflikten 1963,* Medicinska verkningar. (Norstedt, Stockholm: Wenner-Gren Center)

24 Säilä, S. -L. (1973). *Lakkosäilöönotot* (Drinkers taken into custody during the Alko strike). Reports from the Social Research Institute of Alcohol Studies No 67. Mimeograph. (Helsinki)

25 Mäkelä, K. (1974). *Alkon lakko ja alkoholiin kytkeytyvät hoito- ja huoltopalvelukset.* (The Alko strike and treatment and welfare services connected with alcohol.) Reports from the Social Research Institute of Alcohol Studies No 75. Mimeograph. (Helsinki)

26 Murto, L. (1973). *Alkon myymälälakko ja Tampereen asunnottomat alkoholistit.* (The Alko

strike and the homeless alcoholics of Tampere.) Reports from the Social Research Institute of Alcohol Studies No 61. Mimeograph. (Helsinki)

27 Mäkelä, Klaus (1974). *Types of alcohol restrictions, types of drinkers and types of alcohol damages: The case of the personnel strike in the stores of the Finnish Alcohol Monopoly.* Reports from the Social Research Institute of Alcohol Studies No 77. Mimeograph. (Helsinki)

28 Säilä, S. -L. (1978). A Trial closure of ALKO retail outlets on Saturdays and its effects on alcohol consumption and disturbances caused by intoxication. Presented at the *24th International Institute on the Prevention and Treatment of Alcoholism*, 25 June–1 July, Zürich

29 Bigelow, G. and Liebson, I. (1972). Cost factors controlling alcoholic drinking. *Psychol. Rec..*, **22**, 305

30 Babor, T. F. and Mendelson, J. H. (1980). Empirical correlates of self-report drinking measures. In Galanter, M. (ed.) *Currents in Alcoholism. Vol. 7. Recent Advances in Research and Treatment*, pp. 161–168. (New York: Grune & Stratton)

31 Caudill, B. D. and Lipscomb, T. R. (1980). Modeling influences on alcoholic's rates of alcohol consumption. *J. Appl. Behav. Anal.*, **13**, 355

32 Room, R. (1981). A farewell to alcoholism? A commentary on the WHO 1980 Expert Committee Report. *Br. J. Addict.*, **76**, 115

33 Roizen, R., Cahalan, D. and Shanks, P. (1978). 'Spontaneous remission' among untreated problem drinkers. In Kandel, D. B. (ed.) *Longitudinal Research on Drug Use*, pp. 197–221. (Washington, DC: Hemisphere Publishing)

14

Impact of mandated alcohol abuse referrals on outpatient treatment agencies in New York State

M. CORBIN

INTRODUCTION

Alcohol related offences in the United States have begun to be treated from a health/legal approach rather than as civil or criminal justice matters. In response to this movement, the New York State Alcohol and Drug Rehabilitation Programme was put into operation in the Autumn of 1975. Motorists convicted of Driving While Intoxicated (DWI), with a blood alcohol concentration of 0.10 % or more, or Driving While Ability Impaired (DWAI), 0.08 % or 0.09 % blood alcohol concentration, may enter an education/rehabilitation programme. This programme can last from 7 weeks up to 8 months. Most motorists are then eligible for a conditional driver's licence. If the convicted driver chooses not to enter the programme, the first offender's driving licence is then revoked for 3–6 months.

In New York State, as in most areas of the United States, there is no effective public transportation system. Consequently, the great majority of the population depends on daily, independent automobile travel. Having a driver's licence seems like a basic 'right' to most citizens. Therefore, any legislation and enforcement concerning this privilege draws great attention.

There is a high correlation between alcohol use, highway deaths and serious injuries in the United States. The major conclusions from the 1978 Alcohol and Highway Safety Review are that:

(1) nearly 50 % of all fatally injured drivers have a blood alcohol concentration over 0.10 %,

(2) the risk of being involved in a serious crash is much greater with a blood alcohol concentration over 0.10 % than with no alcohol,

(3)   basic behaviour related to driving is impaired in most individuals at a blood alcohol concentration or 0.10% or greater.

Blood alcohol concentration, Table 14.1, can best be understood in terms of actual consumption. The level of 0.15% is reached when a 180-pound man (nearly 13 stone, 81 kg) has drunk eight 12-oz glasses of beer (4½ imperial pints, 2.5 litres) within 2 hours. Studies have shown that the majority of social drinkers reach a blood alcohol concentration of 0.07% at cocktail parties.

A number of factors contribute significantly to the highway safety situation. First is the frequently demonstrated impairment of reaction time, which impedes one's split-second safety decision-making ability. The second is visual impairment, both in depth of field perception and in light distortion. Night vision is especially affected in this manner. The third, and perhaps most important, is judgement. Many drivers do not believe that they are in any way impaired while under the influence of ethyl alcohol. On the contrary, they believe that they are better drivers!

Table 14.1 Blood alcohol concentration

Drinks in 1 hour	Body weight in pounds							
	100	120	140	160	180	200	220	240
1	0.04	0.03	0.03	0.02	0.02	0.02	0.02	0.02
2	0.08	0.06	0.05	0.05	0.04	0.04	0.03	0.03
3	0.11	0.09	0.08	0.07	0.06	0.06	0.05	0.05
4	0.15	0.12	0.11	0.09	0.08	0.08	0.07	0.06
5	0.19	0.16	0.13	0.12	0.11	0.09	0.09	0.08
6	0.23	0.19	0.16	0.14	0.13	0.11	0.10	0.09
7	0.26	0.22	0.19	0.16	0.15	0.13	0.12	0.11
8	0.30	0.25	0.21	0.19	0.17	0.15	0.14	0.13
9	0.34	0.28	0.24	0.21	0.19	0.17	0.15	0.14
10	0.38	0.31	0.27	0.23	0.21	0.19	0.17	0.16

Information needed to calculate B.A.C.: (1) body weight, (2) amount of alcohol consumed, (3) time span
One drink equals: 1½ oz 80° liquor, 12 oz beer, 4 oz table wine
Liver oxidization rate: approximately 0.02% B.A.C. per hour
New York State law: DWAI = 0.08% B.A.C. DWI = 0.10% B.A.C.

With the plan to educate convicted motorists and change this myth, New York State offers a basic education programme of 16 hours, in a 7-week period. This is a series of classroom presentations designed to provide information to the social drinker, the beginning problem drinker and the alcoholic. The long term health goal of the Drinking Driver Programme in New York State is to assure that all drivers who are convicted and in need of professional assistance for alcohol related problems will be referred into and will receive treatment.

The primary safety goals of the alcohol and drug rehabilitation programme must be clearly stated:

(1)   reduce alcohol related highway crashes in the client population,

(2)   reduce alcohol related traffic arrests and convictions in the client population,

(3)   prevent clients from displaying problem drinking which is potentially harmful to themselves and others.

Other community programmes are now developing to work with offenders and mandate them into treatment. One such which attempts to rehabilitate and educate rather than punish is Pretrial Diversion. Designed to work with Youthful Offenders, persons between 16 and 19 years, it helps to avoid criminal records, if possible. These young people are often in need of drug and/or alcohol programmes and can be mandated into treatment.

The New York State Probation Department also has a goal, a focus on alcohol treatment for offenders, where appropriate. Recent data have shown that as high as 45% of the legal charges which put people on probation supervision in New York State are alcohol related.

The New York State Department of Motor Vehicles, in concert with the New York State Division of Alcoholism, has established the only State-wide programme with built-in treatment. The Drinking Driver Programme, once agreed to by the motorist, is an alternative to total loss of licence. Licence sanction, enforcement and adjudication are carried out co-operatively by the Department of Motor Vehicles, the police and the courts.

Research has been built into this Programme since its inception. This chapter will discuss data gathered from the 61 Drinking Driver Programmes and the 83 outpatient treatment agencies who serve most of their clients. The purpose of this paper is to examine the Drinking Driver Programme, the rationale for its existence, the impact of these mandated patients on the alcoholism treatment agencies and how the Drinking Driver Programme affects community health and safety.

THE NEW YORK STATE ALCOHOL AND DRUG REHABILITATION PROGRAMME

Organization of the Programme

The New York State Drinking Driver Programme is a progression of steps as in Figure 14.1. Many of them are legal and clerical. The three major components described here are: (1) the 16-hour education component, (2) the clinical evaluation and (3) the clinical treatment phase. This model integrates several systems into a total programme with separate modalities and goals.

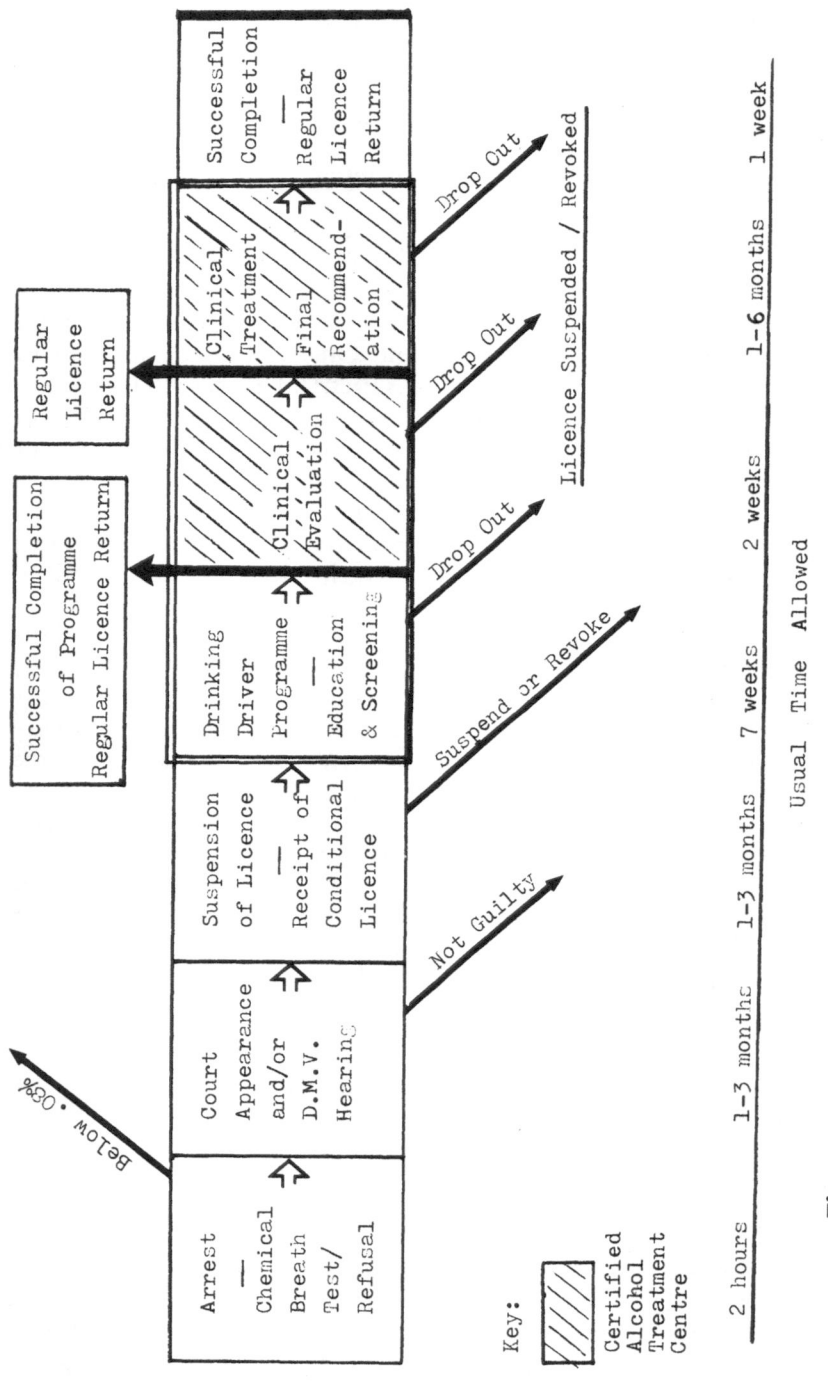

Figure 14.1 Progression of arrested motorist, New York State Drinking Driver Programme

The 16-hour education programme, conducted by agents appointed by the State, works with groups of 20 motorists and is led by two counsellor/instructors. The convicted motorists pay the fee for the programme which is set by the State. The programme teaches self-analysis of drinking behaviour and a curriculum which includes:

(1) an overview of the problem of drinking and driving,
(2) driver responsibilities,
(3) emotional responses affecting driving,
(4) pharmacology of alcohol,
(5) levels of use and abuse,
(6) alcoholism,
(7) effects of alcohol on the driving task,
(8) decision making skills.

Participants are not categorized as problem drinkers by virtue of their conviction of Driving While Intoxicated. During the 7 weeks of the programme, the counsellor/instructor is responsible for screening participants. A determination is made whether or not to send them on to a certified alcohol treatment centre for evaluation and possible treatment at the conclusion of the 7 weeks.

The New York State Drinking Driver Programme was designed with the knowledge that drinking driver schools in other parts of the United States have not significantly affected arrest or crash rates among their participants. The Programme's intervention and 'mandated' treatment of motorists has been a rarely used concept. Although the Programme is voluntary, the motorists often feel coerced and trapped by the narrow choice offered: loss of licence or treatment!

The New York State Programme, with the blending of education, treatment and enforcement, works. A summary of research findings shows that the New York State Alcohol and Drug Rehabilitation Programme drivers:

(1) have a lower rate of conviction for alcohol related violations,

(2) have a lower rate of conviction for all types of traffic violations,

(3) experience a significant reduction in both number and rate of accidents.

Referral criteria for clinical evaluation and possible treatment

Referral is one of the most difficult and challenging parts of the Drinking Driver Programmes for DDP staff, treatment staff and clients. The motorists do not want to believe that:

(1) they are in trouble with alcohol;

(2) someone who observes them for 16 hours in a group setting can know them very well;

(3)   they have time to spend 'talking' to a counsellor,

(4)   it is fair! Motorists believe they have 'paid' their debt to society by attending the educational programme segment.

The referral criteria used in the Drinking Driver Programme are presented in Table 14.2 as an alcohol assessment matrix of events to be considered when referring a client for clinical evaluation and possible treatment. Each of the indicators for referral has been developed to identify persons whose drinking patterns demonstrate possible dependency problems.

Table 14.2   New York State Drinking Driver Programme alcohol assessment matrix for problem drinker drivers

Indicators	Number of indicators required for referral into clinical treatment		
	No referral	2 or more	1 or more
Blood alcohol concentration	0.05%–0.14%	0.15%–0.19%	0.20% or more
Previous DWI/DWAI arrests/Convictions	0	1–2	3+
MAST questionnaire score	0–2	3–5	6 or more
Consistency of verbal responses in class exercises	High	Variable	Low
Willingness to submit to chemical test	Willing	Refusal	Refusal

The staff from the Drinking Driver Programme and the clinical treatment agency each review the client for possible treatment needs. Information gathered on the Drinking Driver Programme level is integrated and enhanced by the clinical agency interview. Areas of concern such as blackouts, rationalization, contradiction and denial can be addressed by the treatment counsellor in the interface evaluation for possible treatment.

Blood alcohol concentration

A blood alcohol concentration (B.A.C.) of more than 0.10% is considered by the National Council on Alcoholism as clearly and definitely associated with alcoholism. As a guideline, a B.A.C. of 0.15% should be considered as a valid criterion for referral unless proven otherwise. Programme staff can become desensitized when the majority of clients seem to have B.A.C. levels over 0.15% and range up to 0.40%. The prevalence of these high levels can begin to seem 'normal'.

DWI convictions

Driving While Intoxicated (DWI) arrests are relatively rare in the United States. Surveys show that the arrest rate per officer in the average jurisdiction is two DWIs per year. This indicator is interpreted to mean that anyone who is apprehended for two or more Driving While Ability Impaired offences (DWAIs) or DWIs has a drinking problem until proven otherwise. Other alcohol related arrest or treatment information may be available. If so, this can be a further sign of alcohol use or abuse and another indicator for help.

MAST questionnaire

The Michigan Alcohol Screening Test (MAST), Table 14.3, is a simple paper and pencil test of 25 subjective questions to be answered by either 'yes' or 'no'. The test is given to the entire group at the start of the Drinking Driver Programme. It is easy and fast to administer, and reliable in that honest answers are considered valid and dishonest answers can lead to defensive and hostile behaviour. The test results also provide a catalyst for personal interview and confrontation.

Classroom behaviour

Classroom responses and behaviour during the 16-hour programme are observed and noted by the counsellor/instructors. Consistency of subject's behaviour in classroom interactions, dialogue and written responses proves to be helpful in the assessment of the problem drinker. These observations, coupled with the other indicators, are often considered positive identification signs.

Breathalyser test

In New York State, refusal to submit to the Breathalyser test is, in itself, an infraction of the law. Motorists who refuse the test will be arrested and lose their licences. Many citizens believe they should have an attorney present before they submit to any questions or tests. The New York State law is quite clear. The implied consent law is in effect when motorists sign for a driving licence. The motorist is bound by the alcohol testing ability of the police officer, much as one is with a radar test for speeding.

Drinking Driver Programme referrals for evaluation and possible treatment

New York State designed the Drinking Driver Programme with the intention that certified alcoholism agency personnel would make the clinical evaluations. The role of the Drinking Driver Programme personnel is to gather information, weigh it against the criteria and decide whether or not

Table 14.3   Michigan Alcohol Survey Test as used by New York State Drinking Driver Programme

1. Do you feel you are a normal drinker?
2. Have you ever awakened the morning after some drinking the night before and found that you could not remember a part of the evening before?
3. Does your wife, husband, a parent or other near relative ever worry or complain about your drinking?
4. Can you stop drinking without a struggle after one or two drinks?
5. Do you ever feel bad about your drinking?
6. Do friends or relatives think you are a normal drinker?
7. Do you ever try to limit your drinking to certain times of the day or to certain places?
8. Are you always able to stop drinking when you want to?
9. Have you ever attended a meeting of Alcoholics Anonymous?
10. Have you gotten into fights when drinking?
11. Has drinking ever created problems between you and your wife, husband, a parent or other near relative?
12. Has your wife, husband, a parent or other near relative ever gone to anyone for help about your drinking?
13. Have you ever lost friends because of drinking?
14. Have you ever gotten into trouble at work because of drinking?
15. Have you ever lost a job because of drinking?
16. Have you ever neglected your obligations, your family, or your work for 2 or more days in a row because you were drinking?
17. Do you drink before noon fairly often?
18. Have you ever been told you have liver trouble? Cirrhosis?
19. After heavy drinking have you ever had delirium tremens (D.T.s) or severe shaking?
20. After heavy drinking have you ever heard voices or seen things that weren't really there?
21. Have you ever gone to anyone for help about your drinking?
22. Have you ever been in a hospital because of drinking?
23. Have you ever been a patient in a psychiatric hospital or in a psychiatric ward of a general hospital?
24. Have you ever been in a hospital to be 'dried out' (detoxified) because of drinking?
25. Have you ever been in jail, even for a few hours, because of drunk behaviour?

treatment may be needed and if a clinical evaluation must be made. The motorist is then directed to the treatment agency.

Clinical evaluation and treatment

Clinical evaluation and treatment may be carried out by any New York State Division of Alcoholism certified alcoholism treatment centre in New York State. These centres include mental health facilities, alcoholism treatment centres and private physicians. Drinking Driver Programme clients who are referred for evaluation are seen, on average, twice by the treatment agency. They are interviewed by a professional clinician, who also has access to the findings of the staff of the Drinking Driver Programme.

The treatment modalities available are intensive inpatient and outpatient treatment programmes, therapeutic groups and individual therapy. The majority of motorists referred are sent to outpatient treatment centres. Eighty per cent of the treatment centres surveyed refer clients to Alcoholics Anonymous as part of treatment planning.

Stages of referral

There are four distinct stages in the referral process for the Drinking Driver Programme referrant:

(1) the referral to the treatment agency by the DDP,

(2) the appointment must be made and kept by the client with the treatment agency,

(3) the evaluation of the client by the treatment agency,

(4) the carrying out of the treatment programme.

This four-stage referral process is critical. The Drinking Driver Programme and the treatment agency must communicate and interface with each other and the motorist in a very clear manner. Motorists who are in strong denial regarding their alcohol consumption level can find many possible ways to drop out of the system. The incentive for the motorists to stay in is the conditional licence and the early return of full driving privileges. A final recommendation from the treatment agency ensures the restoration of the regular licence by the Drinking Driver Programme administrator.

At any of these stages the client could drop out of the Programme, or at some later time appeal to return for further evaluation or treatment. As a result, it is often difficult to keep accurate statistics. The range of referred clients retained for treatment in 1980 was 49%–88%, an average of 73%.

EVALUATION OF NEW YORK STATE OUTPATIENT ALCOHOLISM AND TREATMENT PROGRAMMES

The New York State Division of Alcoholism, in collaboration with the Department of Motor Vehicles, recently completed an evaluation of over 80 outpatient programmes which treat drinking driver referral clients. The evaluation specifically examines demographics, evaluation and treatment processes, staffing patterns, treatment modalities, numbers of clients, linkages with other agencies and costs. Each of these factors is examined as it affects the drinking driver client and is then compared to the treatment of the traditional outpatient receiving alcohol abuse services. The following is a re-examination of the data questioning how these special clients have affected the available treatment systems.

The motorists in this study can be characterized by these common factors:

(1)   They have been arrested and convicted and have chosen, under pressure, to participate in a treatment programme.

(2)   They are generally in an 'early stage' of alcohol dependency, with support systems such as job, family and social contacts still intact.

(3)   They are often hostile and angry and feel victimized by the 'system' for having been referred for treatment.

Profile of Drinking Driver Programme participants

The average Drinking Driver Programme participant who is referred for treatment is male, white, employed and between the ages of 21 to 49, as in Figure 14.2. These factors alone have an impact on the treatment agencies. Most outpatient programme patients are in the 31−50-year age group, unemployed, a higher proportion of women to men, and a greater number of minority patients.

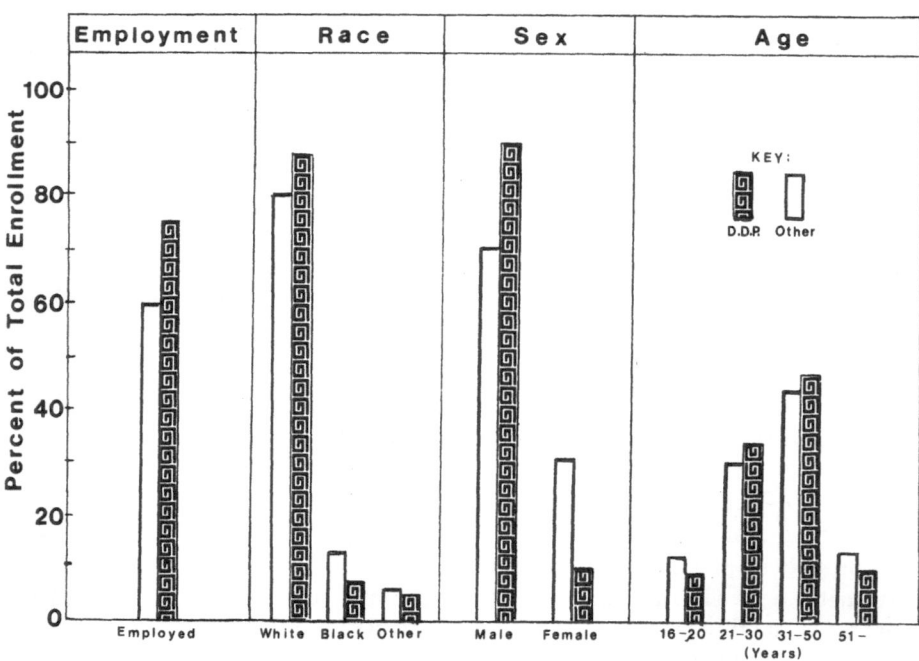

Figure 14.2   Demographic profile of outpatients in treatment

Sex

The fact that the proportion of males to females has been 9 : 1 since the Programme began is significant at the educational level of the Programme as well as at the treatment level. Over the years, several reasons for this have been proposed: women drive less than men, women drink at home more often, the legal/enforcement system tends to 'let women go'. As a result of this trend, Drinking Driver Programmes and some treatment programmes tend to be oriented toward the male client.

Age

The age factor is a complex one. Some of the age trends are not reflected in statistics which are available. A major factor is the Youthful Offender status. No records are kept on clients who are 16 – 19 years of age, in an effort to keep them from developing criminal records. This offers a difficult situation to the referring Drinking Driver Programme as well as to the treatment programme, because the offender's licence is not being withheld. The 'typical' young, white male of middle and lower middle class background falls into a statistically high-risk group in alcohol related crashes. Also, many of these drivers are not eligible for the Drinking Driver Programme and are therefore under-represented in the data.

Most treatment facilities admit they have no treatment programme designed for these young clients. Many of the youth 'drug' programmes do not focus on alcohol or middle class alcohol problems and are not appropriate referrals for these clients. As a result of poor treatment programme feedback from both clients and agency staff, Drinking Driver Programmes do not refer this high-risk group as often as needed. This is because presently there are no suitable treatment facilities.

A similar case can be made for the elderly. However, statistically, they are fewer in number and are involved in less serious accidents.

Employment

Employment must be examined from several aspects. First, the fact that 75 % of Drinking Driver Programme referees are employed must be viewed as a positive factor, because it implies that the intervention into the alchohol abuse has come at an early stage. Yet this has often caused confusion within treatment centres, which are used to working with more unemployed clients. Rates and methods of payment have not been geared to the working client, nor have the hours been set with this group in mind, i.e. evenings and weekends.

According to State legislation, the convicted motorist is to bear the cost of the Drinking Driver Programme. The treatment of referred motorists, which is an integral part of the Programme, has not been as clearly addressed. Treatment agencies have been admitting the convicted motorists as they admit anyone for treatment, using sliding fee scales and deficit financing. Therefore, some of the costs are paid by tax dollars.

Race

The racial balance in the outpatient population figures matches the general population figures for New York State. The Drinking Driver Programme population differs significantly. The over-representation of whites may reflect the theory that more whites drive and are, therefore, subject to arrest.

There are a few Drinking Driver Programmes offered in Spanish in the New York City area. Treatment in Spanish is available in most urban areas, or by minority group counsellors.

Organizational considerations of treatment agencies

Of great concern to the New York State Division of Alcoholism is the effectiveness of alcohol abuse and alcoholism treatment State-wide, in terms of staff, programme and financing.

Costs

The very nature of the Programme, as an alternative to punishment *per se*, creates a critical and delicate public policy issue on financing. On the public taxpayer side is the issue — no free administrative or treatment services' costs for offenders. On the offenders' side — if this is not punishment, why should they have to pay hundreds of dollars for 'treatment' which is unwanted and appears like a punishment in disguise? On the treatment agency side, new fee structures need to be set which will identify entire treatment costs. This would put the agencies into a new business-like treatment mode, 'pay as you go', as opposed to the conventional social service attitude of availability to all regardless of cost.

Treatment staff and programme

Most of the outpatient treatment agencies surveyed have been in operation for at least 8 years. Programme and staffing patterns have been developed to work with the 'traditional alcoholic patient'. In most of these programmes there is a strong link with Alcoholics Anonymous. They also tend to use the same treatment methods for all types of clients.

The motorist who is referred may not be diagnosed as an alcoholic by the agencies' standards. Dependency may be an emerging issue or even a transient one. Treatment agencies, in the first few years of receiving Drinking Driver referrals, were likely to turn away early stage alcoholics as well as alcohol abusers, classifying them as persons not needing treatment. These clients, however, had been identified as problem drinkers from a community safety aspect and in need of some kind of treatment. Some of the agencies have begun to meet this need with special motorists groups, pre-treatment groups and continuing care groups. From these groups, motorists will frequently be re-evaluated and found in need of more traditional alcoholism treatment. Other motorists often need more time and understanding than the basic 7-week programme to make changes in their lives in regard to the use of alcohol and their motor vehicles.

Drinking Driver Programme referral rate changes

Since the first full year, October 1975 to September 1976, the Drinking Driver Programme referral rate has increased markedly. As indicated on Figure 14.3, the Programme population has increased over the 5 years surveyed from 18 736 enrolled in the first year 1975–76, to the 1979–80 enrolment of 22 773 motorists. The referral rate of motorists for evaluation during this time period has risen from 15 % to 32 %. It has more than doubled! This increase has been attributed to the developing skills of the Drinking Driver Programme personnel. Improvement in the interagency communications has led to the acceptance of the mandated client for treatment by the outpatient centres.

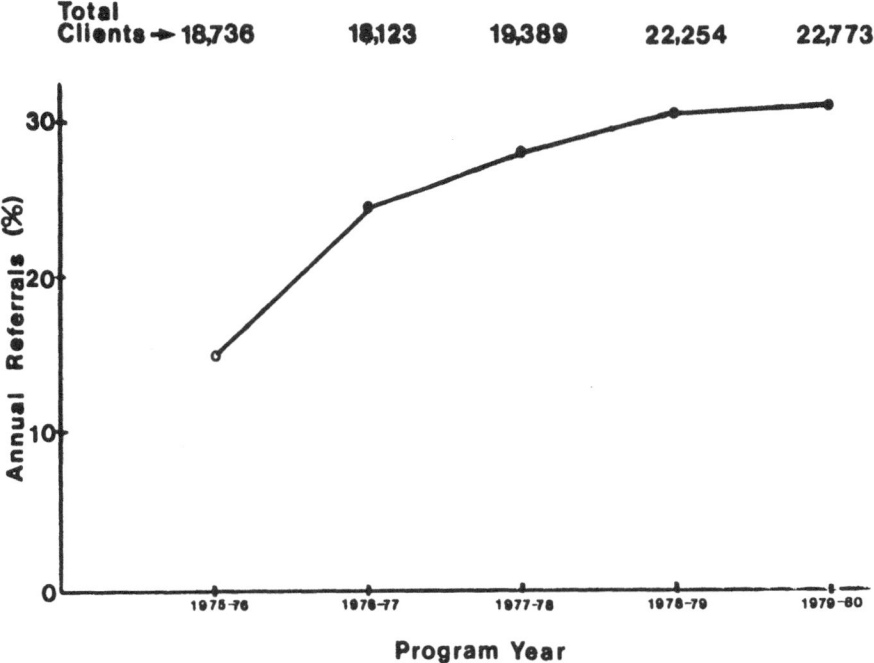

Figure 14.3   Percentage of total DPP clients referred for evaluation

Impact of Drinking Driver Programme patients

There was an influx of 10 000 patients into the outpatient treatment centres for evaluation in 1980 from the Drinking Driver Programme, with 6700 continuing on for treatment. Twenty-seven per cent of agency caseloads were Drinking Driver Programme clients! The average length of treatment was 13 visits, a total of 21 hours.

Also to be noted was the wide difference in referral rates from Programme to Programme across the State. The rates in 1980 ranged from a low of 22 % to a high of 46 %. This may be due to an absence of standardized training in evaluation skills and a lack of referral agencies to treat some types of clients. Often cases are seen as 'borderline' because regionally there has been no awareness of treatment possibilities.

As the level of training and experience increases among the Drinking Driver Programme staff, the number of referrals tends to increase. However, the treatment agencies are not in agreement that the same clients need treatment. The agency staff are accustomed to determining whether their specific programme can help an individual patient. Although the agency could refer clients to other treatment centres, agency staff are not often trained to do so. Also there are not as many specialized treatment facilities as needed for youth and the elderly.

In other states, drinking and driving behaviours were not changed by attendance of short term 'school' programmes. The major difference appears to be the long term education and mandated treatment approach using the loss of driving privileges in New York State as an incentive.

Of growing importance in this comprehensive approach is the need for treatment agencies to work with the identified early stage alcohol abuser or alcoholic. Most treatment centres have worked traditionally with the later stage, self-reporting alcoholic. This is someone to whom it has become apparent through work or lack of it, family trouble, or health breakdown, that something must be done about the problems caused by drinking. The mandated client often does not have the personal history or long term impetus of job, family and health problems to make the need for help implicit. The offender is being sent to an alcoholism treatment centre where in fact, the usual diagnosis of alcoholism may not even be made. Nonetheless, help is needed in order to ensure health and safety for all motorists on the highways.

SUMMARY

Many New York State citizens die or are seriously injured as a result of drinking and driving. The development of the Drinking Driver Programme has demonstrated that, through education and treatment, convicted motorists' drinking and driving behaviour can be changed. The motorists offer great resistance to treatment and require early intervention from traditional treatment agencies and their staff. The Drinking Driver client tends to be at an earlier stage of alcohol abuse than other outpatients in treatment. The treatment of these motorists has increased the number of referrals to outpatient treatment centres. Drinking driving convictions also have increased over the 5 years of the Programme study and the rate of referrals into treatment has increased even more sharply. There is a growing demand to meet the treatment needs of this population for the health and safety of the community at large.

AFTERWORD

The New York State Drinking Driver Programme works as well as it does because of the tremendous cooperation among police, courts, Department of Motor Vehicles, Division of Alcoholism and the treatment centres. However, there are several areas which need attention and improvement. To the credit of all concerned there have been many dialogues, programmes and committees appointed to identify and work out possible solutions to these problems.

Ending needless death and injury on the highway is of paramount concern. The Drinking Driver Programme is helping the already convicted motorists to not drink and drive again. The Drinking Driver Programme has not, however, made an appreciable difference in the incidence of accidents in a preventive way.

Stricter enforcement and sure conviction can make a difference in the death toll. One county in upstate New York used special funds to provide extra police, equipment and additional training and court personnel. Also the District Attorney was unwavering in his stand for prosecutions in Driving While Intoxicated cases. This county, although by no means the largest in population, has more arrests and convictions by half than any other county in the State. In June 1981 there were *no* deaths or injuries due to drinking and driving — the first death-free month since the records have been carefully kept!

Does this mean that treatment is a waste of time and money? Other countries have stricter laws and enforcement which help cut down on death on the highways, yet alcohol abuse seems to be soaring. Drinking and driving have evolved separately, yet together, to impact society powerfully. To counter that, another impact must be made. This one can be a thoughtful, positive, yet powerful movement.

The Governor of New York appointed a Task Force in February 1980 to study the entire drinking driver problem in the State. They set one goal: to reduce dramatically the incidence of drunk driving in New York State. The report of the Task Force has just been submitted to the Governor (1982). They recommend a three-pronged attack:

(1)   A systems approach to educate the public of the increased risk of apprehension

(2)   Swift removal of drivers' licences and certainty of punishment

(3)   Access to appropriate treatment services for all who need them

The Task Force Report goes into detail about how the education and treatment programme could be changed. The major recommendation is a prescreening programme based on blood alcohol concentration, previous driving records and paper-and-pencil testing. Motorists who appear to need treatment based on those points alone will be sent for a clinical evaluation. The others will attend the regular Drinking Driver Programme, which is considered by the Task Force as highly successful for the majority of motorists.

The new treatment plan would call for even further expansion of services than the pressure of the Drinking Driver Programme has already caused. The report calls for:

(1)   more certification of treatment services,
(2)   treatment costs paid by motorists,
(3)   short term, weekly outpatient groups,
(4)   treatment contracting with goals and objectives, timetables and costs,
(5)   strengthened incentives for Programme participation by motorists.

In alcohol and drug treatment it is well known that denial and self-delusion are critical issues to confront with the patient. The difficulty in impacting drinking and driving is that the entire population seems deluded!

Everyone knows they should not drink and drive, but most motorists do, even if it is a relatively small amount of alcohol.

Bibliography

1   Corbin, M. (1981). *Case Studies from New York State Drinking Driver Program.*
2   Department of the Environment Report of the Departmental Committee (1976). *Drinking and Driving.* (London: HMSO)
3   Report from the Secretary of Health, Education and Welfare (1975). *Alcohol and Health.* (New York: Scribners)
4   Report of a Special Committee of the Royal College of Psychiatrists (1979). *Alcohol and Alcoholism.* (London: Tavistock Publications)
5   Sokolo, L., Nathanson, B. and Williford, W. R. (1981). *Evaluation and Treatment of the Drinker Driver: The New York System.* Presented at the *National Council on Alcoholism Forum*, 15 April, New Orleans
6   State of New York Division of Alcoholism and Department of Motor Vehicles, Project Director B. E. Smith (1978). *Workshop and Resource Manual for the Drinking Driver Program Staff Training Project.*
7   State of New York Division of Alcoholism, S. B. Blume, Director, W. R. Williford, Project Director (1979). *Problem Drinker Drivers: Evaluation and Treatment.*
8   State of New York Governor's Alcohol and Highway Safety Task Force, J. P. Melton and S. B. Blume, Chairpersons (1980). *Testimony of Public Hearings.*
9   State of New York Division of Alcoholism, L. Soklow, Project Director, S. B. Blume, Director (1981). *Evaluation of New York State Out-Patient Alcoholism and Treatment Programs.*
10   State of New York Division of Alcoholism. *Report on Survey of Outpatient Alcoholism Treatment Centers and the Drinking Driver.* (In preparation)
11   State of New York Governer's Alcohol and Highway Safety Task Force, L. G. Foschio and S. B. Blume, Co-chairpersons (1982). Final Report, *Driving While Intoxicated.*

15

Can we treat alcoholism?

A study on the interrelationship of treatment and organization in a treatment centre in Geneva

M. A. DAVIES

The Centre Revilliod, the only institution in Geneva specifically created for the treatment of alcoholism, was started in 1927, and attached to the *Centre Psycho-Social Universitaire*, the outpatient sector of the Department of Psychiatry, in 1977. Care for alcoholics in Geneva is divided between the Centre Revilliod, the general hospital and the Psychiatric Clinic, other medicosocial institutions, general practitioners and private psychiatrists, and temperance societies. The Centre deliberately rejected the idea of having its own inpatient clinic as we did not want to give the impression of creating an alcoholic 'ghetto'. Since its inception, the Centre's aim has been to provide medical and psychosocial help for our patients. The multidisciplinary team is made up of psychiatrists, psychiatric nurses, social workers, 'animators' and secretary-hostesses. The Centre itself is divided into three sectors, the outpatient clinic, the day hospital, capable of receiving up to 16 patients from 9 a.m. to 5 p.m., and a club open a few nights a week and occasionally at the weekend.

The philosophy which underlies the treatment offered in the Centre has been developed over many years, as a result of our confronting theoretical considerations with clinical data. There is insufficient space to summarize the different controversies surrounding the concept of alcoholism – after all, even as far back as 1952, a WHO Expert Committee on Mental Health pointed out that a 'serious obstacle to international action in this field lies in the lack of a commonly accepted terminology.'[1] Over the years better nutrition appears to have helped to slow down the negative effects of alcohol abuse, and treatment of many of the physical disabilities resulting from alcoholism has improved.

But, as a recent WHO report[2] states, 'clinical experience suggests that, so far as the natural history of alcohol dependence and its response to treatment are concerned, there are important interactive effects with emotional problems or mental pathologies'.

The treatment of the underlying dependence syndrome has often relied heavily on the use of drugs intended to decrease alcohol consumption. Some of these aversive drugs, such as disulfiram and calcium carbimide, appear to be effective for periods of 3–6 months among a certain category of patients, but are rarely effective over longer periods. A recent article suggests that a decline from initial improvement 'probably reflects both the low potency of the drug and the increased importance of non-pharmacological factors as determinants of long term outcome of treatment'[3].

We have observed that these drugs are unlikely ever to be more than an adjunct to treatment, and should be used in conjunction with behavioural and psychosocial therapies. They have their primary use for those who are seeking abstinence, and should be appropriate to the goals of therapy.

Few medical practitioners or psychiatrists would today dispute the notion that alcoholism should be regarded rather as an illness than as a sin or as a weakness of will – which cannot by definition be treated – but it cannot be considered as an illness in the traditional physical sense defined by symptoms, diagnosis and treatment. Many of the demands from the medical world to alcoholism treatment centres are essentially concerned with the reduction of a medical symptomatology based on a somatic medical model, either 'get rid of the agent alcohol' (causal treatment), or 'suppress the repetitive behaviour pattern' (symptomatic treatment), both of which are based on the supposition that the toxic agent – alcohol – is merely external. 'Alcoholism is a sickness in the sense that there is an encounter between an individual and a toxic substance which will eventually destroy him physically and psychologically: but it is a strange sickness because the patient shows us, through his words and his repetitive, recurrent behaviour that this destructive relationship is essential for him'[4]. Alcoholism is thus neither alcohol nor the alcoholic but the powerful relationship which exists between the patient and 'his alcohol', a relationship that is both deadly and at the same time vitally indispensable to him. Many contemporary therapists have stressed the adaptive function of alcoholism: alcohol or drugs used to alleviate subjective feelings such as loneliness, emptiness, rage, depression, rejection etc.

Before I elaborate further on our practice, I should like to give a few sociological details concerning the patients who are seen in the Centre. The figures given refer to admissions for the year 1981. 78.9 % of patients were male and 21.2 % female. The majority are working class (73.5 % Swiss, 26.5 % foreign), and have no vocational training or qualifications (over 72 % are without occupational qualifications, and 35.9 % are unemployed); their life courses are dramatically marked by premature loss and/or separation (divorce, death, separation, emigration); their occupational histories show multiple difficulties; they have normally passed through the hands of many

institutions, either medical, social or psychiatric (or all), and more than 50%
have been in psychiatric treatment of one form or another.

Only a minority consult us of their own accord: most are either sent or
channelled to us in different ways. In 1981, 51.8% were sent from the medical
world, 32.8% from family and entourage (this figure includes 23.7% who
referred themselves), and 15.2% from social and legal organizations.

When patients come into care, a history of problems associated with
alcohol has already existed for a considerable period. The 'alcohol' problem is
often only the tip of the iceberg, one symptom in a complex psychopathology. Contemporary theoretical orientations[5], plus our own clinical
observations, lead us to consider that the majority of our patients have
troubles of personality development (borderline states) or narcissistic personality disorders. Equally obviously these do not necessarily lead to alcoholism.

Clavreul states[6] that 'the alcoholic never comes by himself: he is preceded
by a letter, a telephone call, even a visit by someone in his family, in order to
put us on our guard against his lies'. As we have seen, few patients come into
treatment on their own account: most are sent, more or less explicitly, or
come in order to please others who are worried about their drinking
problems. Frequently little notice is taken of the fact that the demand for help
is *not* one formulated by the patient. Hartocollis has drawn attention to the
fact that . . . 'the alcoholic patient tries to spare himself the embarrassment of
critical confrontation and the threats of forceful limitation of his freedom'[7].
Over the years we have learned to dissociate the *'predemande'* − that is the
whole constellation of factors underlying the complex that brings the patient
into treatment − from the actual demand posed by the patient himself. His
own demand may either be non-existent, different from the *'predemande'*, or
occasionally the same. We would argue that by not having distinguished the
demand formulated by the patient from that formulated by a third person, we
push him into the position of using one of his favourite and necessary defence
mechanisms, that of denial. In other words could he not be saying 'I am not
just an alcoholic, I am something more'? It is fundamental to differentiate these
two approaches as they refer back to different theoretical models, and can thus
exercise a considerable influence on the therapist's attitude, because, as we
have seen, a *'predemande'* which sees alcoholism as a vice, a fault or a lack
cannot by definition be treated.

On the theoretical level, therefore, we in the Centre have chosen to refer
primarily to psychodynamic and sociological models. The psychodynamic
approach is fundamentally based on three postulates[8]:

(1) Treatment can begin only when there is an explicit demand by the
    patient, and when the therapist feels that a therapeutic alliance has been
    established.

(2) Alcoholic behaviour is not the unique and central problem; the
    underlying suffering experienced by the patient is much more import-

ant, therefore we cannot expect him to renounce his own form of self-medication*[9] immediately. From the respect which we accord to his initial wariness, and our implicit acceptance of his disappearance from treatment and possible relapse, we try to get behind the caricatural image of the staggering alcoholic to the individual with his personal history, capable of entering into a therapeutic relationship.

(3)   It is therefore necessary to create a therapeutic situation which can receive both the demand and the suffering of the patient, and within which he can seek out and understand, with the help of the therapist, the meaning of his drinking behaviour.

In practice our patients show us, in their acts and in their words, that this toxic substance is not merely their enemy: it has become so essential that the patient cannot accept the image of himself as an alcoholic that is fed back to him by those around him. Thus drying-out cannot be the primary or only aim of therapy and a therapeutic relationship can only take place and develop once the therapist understands that alcohol has become a vital solution for his patient. Only when this is recognized can one begin the long and patient search for the significance behind the drinking behaviour. The price the therapist pays lies in his acceptance of the patient's acting-out, in its most dramatic form, relapse, knowing that addiction often represents a defence against intolerable and uncontainable affects.†[10].

Our initial hypothesis is based on the fact that the patient must become the subject of his treatment and *not* the object of our care. If, for example, during an initial interview or series of interviews which have explored the question in depth, the patient still maintains his demand for drying-out only, then we will respect this, in the knowledge that this initial respect frequently leads him to return to treatment when it becomes clear to him that drying out was not the miracle solution that he expected. For each patient the therapist has to create a new therapeutic setting based on careful analysis of the initial demand, the patient's particular personality, and the context within which the symptom alcohol manifests itself and which is related to its genesis and its maintenance. Duncan Stanton[11] maintains that symptoms serve functions within a context, both for the symptom bearer and for those closely involved with him, and that the latter may, in fact, have an investment in

---

*   'If the essential part of treatment is stopping drinking and if the ethylic personality structure demands alcohol, it is difficult to see how the therapist and the alcoholic can meet on the level of prohobition or prescription'[9].

†   'In a classificatory system of character pathology, alcoholics display a severe disturbance in object relationships reflecting inadequate object constancy and identity confusion; a pathological condensation of genital and pre-genital aggression: a primitive, poorly integrated and largely insufficient super-ego; and a developmentally mixed picture of ego defenses, predominantly denial, splitting, projection and omnipotence'[10].

maintaining the symptom. He goes on to state that 'treatment does not take place in a vacuum, and if the external variables which impinge before (*"predemande"*), during and after treatment are not changed, or at least evaluated, both treatment and investigatory efforts operate at a considerable disadvantage'.

There are three aspects of the ethylic personality which seem central to us and which need to be taken into account. These are acting-out, separation and denial. Acting-out, an externalization which takes the form of provocation and hetero-aggressive acts, tends to induce an aggressive response on the part of the therapist, made up of fear, hostility and rejection — which has been the traditional response of society to the alcoholic. To this acting-out by the patient, we try to oppose a therapeutic acting — to perceive and use in therapy the profound significance underlying the patient's acts. This is one of the main reasons for the frequent meetings of the team, who try to elucidate the basic meaning (*signification*) underlying acting-out, and work together over the problems of the countertransference situation. Each therapist also has the possibility of individual case supervision by an outside psychiatrist or psychoanalyst.

An important aspect of the therapeutic setting is that of 'holding' — by which we mean the creation of a structured setting (time, space, rules) capable of receiving the massive, primitive and often uncontrollable affects which invade the patient. Should outpatient therapy prove insufficient at certain critical moments, then a transfer into the day hospital can be negotiated. To this function of holding is related another — that of reception: the therapist's capacity to retain the words, the acts and affects of the patient and ultimately to restore them to him in such a fashion that he can utilize them. The conjunction of these two essential functions, holding and reception, enable crises to be used as instants in time which help both the construction and the consolidation of the therapeutic relationship.

The personal histories of our patients show a predominance of premature loss or separation (divorce, death of one or both parents, institutionalized childhood), and thus the deep fear of attachment, seen as inevitably bringing the threat of loss. This can lead to underinvestment in therapy, which is seen as too full of threat, or overinvestment in the therapist (seeking a maternal care/love relationship). Such patients can awaken primitive affective and relational transference in the therapist. For such patients, the significant other is not recognized in his otherness, but is immediately transformed into a 'good object', capable of repairing their fundamental lacks. The therapist therefore, can be experienced as both frustrating and disappointing. Every demonstration of a lack of total involvement (sickness, holidays, refusal of gratification) can awake feelings of rage and abandon, often marked by temporary disappearance from therapy, and eventual relapse (i.e. 'if I am not everything to you, you are nothing to me'). Often the therapist is led to feel responsible both for the patient and for his acts. Only a careful working through of the countertransference can help avoid the rejection which the patient's acts can arouse.

So the structured therapeutic setting, which is always agreed to first with the patient, defines symbolically the limited help which can be given, and counteracts the illusion of an all-powerful therapy. Perception of, and verbal restitution to the patient of his affects permits them slowly to become accessible to him. Treatment is thus often long, interspersed with relapse and crises, which gradually diminish in severity, as the patient progressively discovers with the therapist the underlying sense of his suffering.

Denial, another important aspect, is, as we have seen, a characteristic defence for the alcoholic: it often shows itself as a refusal to admit any problematic which needs help, even that of alcoholism. What lies behind this is the intense desire for help, which is seen as impossible, and the drawing back before a relationship which could bring intolerable affects to the surface — alcohol appearing when the patient's defence system is weakened.

In the Centre's work, teamwork is the cornerstone whereby the individual skills of the team are drawn out, thus enabling us to provide a structured therapeutic setting, which is subject to constant re-examination in our twice-weekly meetings. Constant elaboration of the different aspects of our work, elucidation of its underlying philosophy, confrontation with the analysis of clinical data, the possibility of introducing other members of the team into casework where necessary, even on a temporary basis, regular presentation of new cases to the entire team, including the secretary-hostesses, so that attitudes will remain clear and coherent, are all seen as essentials. Help for the therapist and through him, for his patients, is always present: even the seeming rejection of certain patients can be situated in a therapeutic context.

Treatment is always adapted to the individual and can range through psychotherapy, individual consultations, couple and family therapy; drying-out at home or in the day hospital; treatment at home etc. The teamwork in various combinations and treatment takes place either in the Centre or outside. Classic medication is used limitedly, physical check-ups and necessary physical treatments are carried out in the general hospital, either during full-time hospitalization or in the outpatient clinic with a gastroenterologist, who is associated with the work carried out in the Centre.

We also act as consultants for other institutions, general practitioners, social workers etc., always trying to avoid the situation of 'you take care of his alcohol, and I'll take care of the rest'. This fragmentation of care, which is only too prevalent in these days of increasing specialization, can only reinforce the fragmentation already existent in the alcoholic. Thus we also try and avoid the transfer of these patients from one therapist to another as it can arouse feelings of rejection, which will lead them to drop out of all therapy.

It is evident that the Centre's organization could be discussed at much greater length. However I would return to one fundamental proposition: in a treatment centre, every decision that is taken, even an organizational or administrative one, will have its effect on the therapeutic setting, and through it on the patient — and can therefore not be dissociated from the goals of therapy.

Acknowledgements

I should like to thank the team of the Centre Revilliod whose work this paper represents, and I would particularly like to acknowledge my debt to Dr V. Bähler, our Head of Clinic, on whose theoretical formulations it is based.

References

1 WHO Expert Committee on Mental Health. Alcoholism Subcommittee (1952). *Second Report.* (*WHO Tech. Rep. Ser.* No. 48.) (Geneva: WHO).

2 WHO (1977). *Alcohol Related Disabilities.* No. 32. (Geneva: WHO)

3 Sellers, E. M., Naranjo, C. A. and Peachey, J. E. Drugs to decrease alcohol consumption. *N. Engl. J. Med.* **305,** 1257

4 Bähler, V. (1979). A propos des patients 'dénommés alcooliques' et d'une pratique dans un centre 'dit spécifique'. *Méd. Hyg.,* **37,** 3025

5 Hartocollis, P. and Hartocollis, P. (1978). Alcoholism, borderline and narcissistic disorders: a psycho-analytic overview. The Menninger Foundation, Topeka, KS. (Not yet published)

6 Clavreul J. (1958). La parole de l'alcoolique. *La Psychanalyse,* **5,** 257

7 Hartocollis, P. (1978). Denial of illness in alcoholism. *Bull. Menninger Clin.,* **32,** 47

8 Bähler, V. (1981). A propos d'un Centre Thérapeutique de Jour pour patients dénommés alcooliques. *Psychol. Méd.* **13,** 70

9 Pellet, J. and Cottraux, J. (1972). Alcoolisme et structure psychotique. *Confrontations psychiatr.* **8,** 21

10 Kernberg, O. (1970). A psychoanalytic classification of character pathology. *J. Am. Psychoanal. Assoc.,* **18**

11 Stanton, D. M. (1980). A family theory of drug abuse. In Sayers, M. and Pearson, H. (eds.) *Theories on Drug Abuse: Selected Contemporary Perspectives.* NIDA Research Monograph Series No 30. (Washington, DC: US Government Printing Office)

12 Bähler, V. and Bourrit, F. (1981). Peut-on traiter les alcooliques? *Méd. Hyg.,* **39**

16
Outreach . . . a spiritual prescription for success

J. PIPER

There exists a misconception that alcoholism 'outreach' and alcoholism 'advertising/public relations' are one and the same. Not so, we say. Were we to accept this advertising/public relations definition, the *real* meaning of outreach would be overlooked. And with it, unlimited opportunity to take decisive action against the disease of alcoholism and drug addiction.

To understand 'outreach', let's examine a viable outreach programme. The following programme was established at Scripps Memorial Hospital, La Jolla, California in June 1979.

First, a general goal was adopted: to provide help for the alco-holic/chemically dependent person and his afflicted family, friends and employer − directly, by referral and through education/awareness.

Objectives are as follows.

(1)   To create an awareness that Scripps Memorial Hospital Alcoholism Treatment Center exists − that we care and are here to help.

(2)   To make 'chemical dependency' a household word.

(3)   To create an awareness that alcoholism/chemical dependency is a treatable disease − one that affects the entire family.

(4)   To create an awareness that Scripps Memorial Hospital has an in-depth inpatient treatment programme for alcoholism/chemical dependency followed by 2 years' supportive aftercare for the patient and his family.

(5)   To make 'intervention' a household word and establish the need for professional intervention services.

(6)   To increase public awareness of alcoholism/chemical dependency through the media in a warm, dignified manner that continues to promote the quality that Scripps Memorial Hospital stands for . . . ensuring that we operate to maximum capacity.

(7)   To promote our vision of expansion on this campus, and to foster a spirit of co-operation among all treatment centres in the area, keeping in mind our ultimate goal . . . the finest treatment for number one . . . our patient.

From the general goal and objectives a general outreach plan was designed to reach all sectors of the population. The breakdown into segments/programmes is dictated by programme implementation rather than socioeconomic groups, demographics or potential marketing segments. This has been done because of Scripps' unique position in the corporate marketplace — meaning that while maximization of services must always be of prime importance, other factors such as education and responsibility to the community at large as a 'source' of information will require input and activity (both financial and in goal achievement). Therefore, breakdown is as shown in Table 16.1 with no weighting of importance.

Table 16.1   Breakdown of segments/programmes

Importance			
25%	(A) *Public*	General	
		Educational establishments (schools, universities etc.)	
25%	(B) *Industry*	General	
		Specific (those requiring an internal programme)	
25%	(C) *Medical*	Physicians	
		Nurses	
		Psychologists	
		Social workers	
		Other hospitals and/or facilities	
25%	(D) *Teaching*	Seminars/symposiums	
		Counsellor training	
		In-house training	
		Special interest groups*	

* Note that special interest groups include peer groups as well as other organizations united for their own specific reasons — i.e. Kiwanis, Rotarians, Junior League, unions, etc.

This plan looks good on paper but two big questions need to be answered. Number one is, 'Does it work?' and two, 'How much does it cost?' I will answer the second question first.

The practicality of an investment (financial) versus return (patient census) is a prime consideration by management. A multi-million dollar television advertising campaign may fill beds simply because of the critical need for treatment beds. Experience shows, however, that institutions that pursue this type of advertising don't thrive over a period of time. True, you have to consider the financial balance sheet, but it must be kept in mind that more is involved.

Outreach is as much a part of the treatment team as is medical care and counselling. Why? Because outreach is the vehicle through which the alcoholic learns about treatment. We need money for outreach but our yardstick for 'how *much*' is based on the institution's acceptance of the *concept of outreach*.

Let's review this concept: outreach shares the successful Alcoholics Anonymous philosophy, 'Our primary purpose is to help the suffering alcoholic' — help the alcoholic no matter *where* he or she may seek treatment. Outreach makes referrals that are in the best interest of the patient. Outreach means going the extra mile to help. It is *love in the purest sense*. Herein lies the difference between 'outreach' and 'public relations'. *Outreach is a spiritual programme* based on giving — giving without expectations. Giving with the hope that the alcoholic will seek treatment wherever best suits his needs.

And now to answer the first big question, 'Does it work when you base an outreach programme on the spiritual concepts of giving and sharing?' Following is a case history of one such treatment facility.

The Alcoholism Treatment Center at Scripps Memorial Hospital opened its doors to patients on 30 July, 1979 with 10 beds. Within 18 months the treatment centre expanded to 40 beds. The occupancy rate has an overall average of 90 %!*

Because of the need in the community for more treatment beds Scripps Memorial Hospital is now building a new 88-bed Chemical Dependency Recovery Hospital. This will include a special 24-bed adolescent treatment centre. This dramatic growth is a direct result of the awareness of the community. In order to build a new Chemical Dependency Recovery Hospital the need and the support must be generated in the community and in order for that to happen one must have a viable outreach programme.

Some hospitals set up alcohol programmes just to fill empty beds. Their primary goal is financial gain. With a similar goal for outreach many fail.

Scripps Memorial Hospital began treating alcoholism and chemical dependency to fill a need in the community. Outreach with a spiritual concept is a vital component of this programme.

Is it outreach that makes the difference? Is it the subtle spiritual aspect of sharing ideas and concepts when the opportunity arises, making referrals to other treatment centres when the occasion presents itself, of providing seminars and workshops free of charge in order to spread the word that alcoholism is a treatable disease? We know that its success can be measured. Outreach . . . our spiritual prescription for success. We offer it to you for consideration. Our cup runneth over.

---

* Average occupancy rate of 12 treatment centres serving the same area: Scripps — 90 %; others — 69 %

Part 3:
ALCOHOLISM – THE NEED FOR SELF-HELP

17

AA and the growing self-help movement

D. ANDERSON

I am reminded that someone said that human beings are constantly amazed at common sense and so am I, and this is the theme of what I should like to discuss. I think that the self-help movement must represent a tremendous social revolution in psychotherapy and how sick people can help themselves by helping each other, and this is all called the 'self-help group movement'. The subject is extensive and I will briefly make some essential comments.

The movement has many different cryptic titles: thus the literature speaks of mutual aid groups, mutual support groups, mutual help systems, a community support system, the fellowship of the afflicted, and expressions like 'banding together is the best way to cope', etc. There are a number of definitions of self-help groups and the one I like best is very simple – people with similar problems get together to share ways to overcome them, to trade experiences to lessen worries and to provide hope for each other.

Briefly I would like to review the explosive growth of this movement, especially in the USA and over the past 10 years. In the past 10 years the self-help movement seems to have spread from coast to coast. It now includes over 500 000 groups. These are not parent groups but separate distinct cells of a lesser number of parent groups. The groups now involve over 15 million people. The US Department of Health and Human Services predicts that by 1990 the number of people reached by such groups will have doubled. In 1974 the alarm was sounded for psychiatry and other professionals, I think. An article in the *American Journal of Psychiatry* said that if psychiatry does not catch up with this new group movement, psychiatry will be left behind. By 1975 a self-help clearing house designed to collect and exchange information just on self-help groups was started. They even have a national newsletter, *The Self-help Recorder*.

To give some idea of the extensiveness of this movement, the various areas of human concern, let me list a few of these self-help groups. You have all heard of AA, Al-Anon, Al-Ateen. You may not have heard yet about the new group, The Adult Children of Alcoholics. You will have also heard of Narcotics Anonymous, Gamblers Anonymous, and Emotions Anonymous, but in addition there are self-help groups for almost all the chronic physical illnesses listed in the World Health Organization classification and I am not going to try to list them here. There are also self-help groups for a wide variety of psychosocial problems. Language like this — Cheques Anonymous for people in chronic debt, Crooks Anonymous, Delinquents Anonymous, Divorcees Anonymous, Fatties Anonymous, Sexual Child-Abusers Anonymous, Parents of Youth in Trouble Anonymous, Psychotics Anonymous, Recovery Incorporated, Recidivists Anonymous and it goes on and on and on — Abused Women, Parents Anonymous, Suicides Anonymous, The Widow to Widow Programme. There are a number of grief groups which handle any and all kinds of forms of grief that human beings become involved in. There are new groups for people doing human service work helping others, care givers, doing something to help them.

With all of these self-help groups, there are bound to be some jokes about them. An old one which comes to mind is about Paranoids Anonymous — I wanted to join the group but they wouldn't tell me where the meetings were being held.

What are some characteristics these groups have in common? Here are some that are suggested in the literature. The groups always serve a perceived, yet unmet, need for many people. Groups seem to be of spontaneous origin — they come from the people up, rather than formal authority. They start from a condition of powerlessness and the members somehow get together and agree on some helpful action. Participation is always personal, always voluntary. There is face to face interaction in small groups, the focus is on mutual aid for common special problems and the goal is simply to improve one's and the group's psychological functioning and their effectiveness in living, but the major source of help is the group members' efforts and skill, their combined mutual experience and their knowledge and concern. Now professionals may be asked to participate to lend their expertise — this occurs especially with chronic illnesses — but their role is always ancillary and they serve at the pleasure of the group. Professionals have even started a number of groups, but wisely they move aside and let the group take over control. I think the most important characteristic of such groups, however, is that they are inexpensive and they are productive. They appear to be directly helpful. When you talk to members of such groups they say that the groups help them. The groups are non-bureaucratic and there is no red tape; they are anti-authoritarian, their activities are based on real life experiences and common sense and it looks like these groups have found that banding together is the best way to cope.

With that taken care of, I should like to say something about self-help groups in historical perspective. Despite this rapid growth of the self-help group movement, self-help activities are not new — depending on how you define them, and that's the rub. Efforts by people to provide mutual aid for common problems are endless and include things like consumer movements, religious groups, various political groups, citizens' leagues, underserved groups, minority groups, and other groups too numerous to mention. I don't believe that such overinclusion really helps us to understand the present movement and its immediate practical origins. Thus I differentiate between political, religious or racial advocacy groups, which are not new, and self-care, self-help groups, which are new. Self-care, self-help groups are groups which tend to focus on helping people with chronic physical problems or chronic psychosocial problems or addictions. Now with that distinction in mind, I believe that the present self-help group movement can best be viewed as a self-care, self-help movement that has grown directly out of, and has been powerfully influenced by, the Alcoholics Anonymous movement.

This movement is primarily concerned, I believe, with helping people with socially stigmatizing shame- and guilt-inducing problems, be they physical or psychological, or both. Thus for me, AA seems to be the model or prototype for most of the new self-help groups representing an almost direct extension or expansion of the practical philosophy and ideology of our largest and most effective self-help group. Someone once said that AA is the single largest unorganized organization in the world. Let me illustrate. Did you notice how many of the groups which I have listed have Anonymous in the title? Somehow AA has become the reference group for most of these new self-help groups. As a matter of fact, General Service Headquarters in New York City report that they are inundated increasingly with requests from different self-help groups asking for advice, information and counselling on how to start a new group and model it after Alcoholics Anonymous.

In an attempt to understand the ropes of this new movement better, we should take another look at AA, at its origins, its philosophy, its perception of the human condition, its practical wisdom. Looking at AA now as the prototype, or model, of these other self-help groups, it is hard to remember that it started in 1935 by a stockbroker and a physician and it is difficult to realize that the movement was initially rejected. It was rejected by practising alcoholics — who wants to admit you have a drinking problem and can't drink any more or hang around with people like that? It was rejected by the general public out of indifference. It was rejected by clergymen who at first thought it was another competing religion and it was rejected by professionals, particularly in medicine and psychiatry, as being much too simplistic ever to come to grips with a disease like alcoholism. But now, 47 years later, we know with the conviction of experience that AA is a powerfully effective organization which is recognized throughout the world as perhaps the most effective planned philosophy ever developed to help alcoholics, and there are over a million members throughout the world. We must also remember that the spirit of AA started before 1935 and its spiritual roots grew out of an organization called the Oxford Group Movement, a movement that started in the 1920s and 1930s and experienced its greatest growth then. This is not the Oxford Movement of Cardinal Newman of the 1830s. This was the movement of moral rearmament — a form of pietism —

and it is still in existence. It was started by a Lutheran minister from the USA who went to Scotland and England and passed through Oxford — somehow the term Oxford Group Movement became attached to the organization called Moral Rearmament. Thus the first alcoholics really sobered up on its six principles:

self-examination of conscience,
acknowledgement of faults in group,
make restitution for wrongs done,
prayer and meditation,
meet in small study groups and share experiences,
carry the message to others and solicit other people.

Only later did AA develop its own spiritual programme independently of the Oxford Group Moral Rearmament, becoming a new group based on 12 steps rather than six principles and also based on attraction rather than active proselytizing.

AA's origins also include certain psychological principles and here I think Bill Wilson's thinking must be credited for his interpretation of what he learned from several people, Dr Carl Jung, the Swiss psychiatrist who was later to be called the spiritual midwife of AA, William James, the philosopher and psychologist from the turn of the century and Dr Harry Tiebout, Bill Wilson's personal psychiatrist and friend. This is grossly oversimplified — the pattern looks something like this. Bill Wilson and the early founders of AA learned really from Dr Jung, who in 1931 treated a man by the name of Rowland Hazad from the USA for his alcoholism, in terms of seeing Dr Jung regularly. Rowland stayed sober for almost a year and then he got drunk and again went back to Dr Jung and said 'help me again'. Dr Jung wisely said, 'I can't help you, you're a hopeless case'. He surrendered him, in other words, and Rowland said, 'What can I do?' Dr Jung said, 'Well, in some cases, perhaps if a person has a real religious or spiritual experience it might help'. Rowland then sought out a spiritual fellowship and found and joined the Oxford Group Movement. It worked for him. He sobered up, sobered up another man and that man in turn sobered up the worst drunk he knew in New York and that was Bill Wilson. Later Bill Wilson learned from William James's book, *The Right to Religious Experience*, his interpretation of the book — that people who have had a spiritual experience have it after having an ego deflation at great depth — after an experience of being broken, a feeling of being crushed and hopeless. Still later, from Dr Harry Tiebout Bill Wilson learned, first as a patient and later as a friend and confidant, about His Majesty the Baby, the concept of infantile omnipotence (that's a Freudian concept, it could just as well come from Adler). This is the concept that the infant's perception of the world is one of being omnipotent and grandiose — 'I am all-powerful, I am in control. Everyone is an extension of me. I cry and I can make people jump'. The infant feels powerful and demands control and yet all at the same time the infant feels completely helpless, completely dependent and demands complete attendance. In some ways what Harry Tiebout said to

Bill Wilson was, the way to help an alcoholic is to help them with their infantile immaturity by deflating this defiant infantile individuality. Remember now, no one is saying that this immaturity is the cause of alcoholism, but somehow it is the condition that accompanies and progresses in chronic alcoholism; it is part of the adaptive impoverishment following from the alcoholism. So in terms of AA thinking: what is the human condition of alcoholic immaturity, the personality of the practising alcoholic, the lifestyle of the practising alcoholic? The AA literature says it many different ways. The alcoholic has two basic drives: one is for absolute control and independence and the other one is for absolute dependence and these drives exist simultaneously all at the same time. The alcoholic says: 'I must have absolute control, we'll do it my way. Limitations are for other people, I demand it, I am in control here, I am completely independent'. And yet all at the same time the practising alcoholic also demands complete dependence: 'When I need you, you be there, there will be no exceptions, I come first'.

I am convinced that AA wisely realizes that domination and dependency go together. It's a reciprocal relationship and this is reasonable. Domination of and dependency upon someone else do go together. Notice the powerful insight into the addictive personality. AA says that addiction is also addiction to power to control. In fact AA says that addiction is an insatiable drive to control everything and yet still always wanting more and more and never getting enough. There's an old joke in the States to illustrate this — the story about a bar in a pub — there's a big sign in the bar, 'All the beer you can drink for a dollar'. An alcoholic walks in, sees the sign and says, 'Give me two dollars' worth'.

In this expanded sense then, all the practising alcoholic really wants is to feel well, to have emotional security, to be happy by controlling everything, by ruling everything. But what does the practising alcoholic get — again these are AA statements — terrible feelings of inadequacy, terrible feelings of insanity, swings of elation and depression, a terrible sense of isolation, a sense of apartness from God and man, and more and more loss of control, and more and more feelings of self-pity and resentment.

Finally the person hits bottom. Now the person is really licked, the terrible sense of hopelessness, helplessness, loneliness and despair and finally ego deflation at great depth can occur — a terrible personal crisis takes place. A personality disintegration, if you will, takes place, but all at the same time, with the despair and the suffering is the growth potential of that very crisis, the possibility of a spiritual awakening, a finding of a new perspective of reality. And somehow AA understands this terrible crisis and its growth potential and how to grow out of it and how to find maturity. The practical steps now seem so terribly simple that they contain, I believe, the basic principles of the whole self-help, self-care group movement: the healing value of facing up to a chronic disabling condition — any terribly frightening condition that won't go away, but that keeps getting worse — an association with other fellow sufferers.

Dr O. Hobart Mowrer, a psychologist from the USA, was, I think, one of the first professionals to recognize the helping potential of AA and its direct influence on the then budding self-help group movement. He called AA, and these extensions, 'the new group therapy' and he wrote a book about it, called *The New Group Therapy*. What he said was that AA and all of these other self-help groups, as well, represented a new form of group therapy, one in which there is no doctor – patient relationship but just a group of fellow sufferers and all of them share a common chronic problem – a problem for which they can get no help from science, it won't go away no matter what you do about it or who you blame it on. Such a group is based on peer relationships, not the authority of formal leaders; there are no experts, everyone is equal. The equality derives from the fact that each person shares a common chronic problem. Then he observed that members of peer groups who have common chronic problems tend to practise what he called honest self-revelation at least in the groups with respect to their common problems. There is a certain freedom to reveal negative aspects about the self. To be transparent, to be open, is an opportunity that few of us have – and to sense that one is understood by someone else, even the dark side of one's self. In such groups self-deception is difficult, one's peers have been there, they know what it's like and they intuitively sense one's genuineness or lack of it. One lady who surveyed the self-help group movement wrote an article and she titled it 'People who know just how you feel', and that describes it pretty well.

Mowrer later observed that in peer groups, in self-help groups where common experiences are shared, where honest self-revelation occurs, where an honest searching for a solution takes place, that under these influences, this kind of searching and probing, gradually leads to a change in attitude, to a change in values and a change to the response to disturbing feelings. Somehow (and this is not his quote) people learn to accept some things that can't be changed, they learn to change some things that can be changed and learn to find the wisdom to know the difference – and that's now called the Serenity Prayer.

For the AA member, this new response to chronic alcoholism, this reconceptualization of this problem, is very simple, practical and straightforward. What the alcoholic does is begin to admit that 'I am powerless over alcohol, my life has become unmanageable.' The person begins to practise the 12 steps, to go to meetings, to identify with the group, get a sponsor, a role model, and not take that first drink and somehow keep it simple.

Finally out of all this emerges, Mowrer says, some degree of mental health, some peace of mind and some serenity. I would briefly like to say something about how AA describes this change of values and attitudes involved in this maturity. Remember the original immaturity was the demand for complete independence, complete dependence. Maturity is reached by the alcoholic only after great pain and suffering, only after multiple assaults on the prideful self, the controlling defiant self. This maturity, AA says, is a gradual realization that to be human is to have absolute control over nothing, absolute dependence upon nothing except absolute dependence upon some Higher

Power. This Higher Power is a spiritual concept, it is not a specific religious denominational concept.

What fascinates me about AA's interpretation of this sickness, is that I think it gives us a new look at other forms of chronic behaviour pathology, not just alcoholism. It gives us another way of thinking about chronic human suffering and our reaction to it, another way of looking at the self-help group movement and what takes place there. Suppose you ask most of us professional behaviour pathologists, psychiatrists, psychologists, social workers, people like that, ask us what are the real origins of neurosis, alcoholism, mental illness and things like that. If we don't find it in physiology, then psychologically we say it will be found in a person with low self-esteem, terrible feelings of inadequacy, inferiority, rejection, anxiety, depression – in other words, a person who is down and too hard on the self. AA says that, for alcoholics at least, the roots are found in human pride and defiance, 'I am an exception to the rules, limitations are for other people' – the roots of alcoholism are found in infantile grandiosity, omnipotence, power seeking, infantile dependence, massive denial of reality – really a person who is too proud of the self, rather than a person feeling too inadequate.

For me, for many years, the problem has been how to resolve this terrible conflict, what's wrong, is it really superiority or inferiority. I think the conceptual breakthrough comes in realizing the reciprocal, dialectical relationship between inferiority feelings and superiority feelings, between feelings of dependence and feelings of independence. Maybe they're just two sides of the same coin. Perhaps the ultimate in infantile immaturity is pride: defiance of accepting human limitations, trying to live up to grandiose expectations which can't be met – trying to make demands that can't be met, on ourselves and on others. If we have grandiose expectations we're bound to fall short of them and if we deny or defy human limitation we will certainly fail, and if we fail we will pay the price in lowered self-esteem and feeling inadequate. Perhaps under the mask of inferiority feelings lies the real problem. Our delusions of grandiosity and omnipotence are dashed down over and over again.

Someone once said to me, isn't the alcoholic's grandiosity just a mask covering up his inferiority feelings? The answer is yes, but his or her inferiority feelings are also a mask just covering that person's grandiose perfectionistic attitudes. It is reciprocal. The relationship is dialectical. Somewhere Jung is supposed to have said that man's whole history consists from the very beginning of a conflict between his feelings of inferiority and his arrogance. Perhaps we all must live with good and evil, being part beast, part angel, must all reconcile the polarities dialectic within us and which perhaps do contain their own opposites. What is the only way out of this inferiority/superiority bind that we all must confront? AA and the other self-help groups say, as do many of the major religions of the world, that you can do something, but not everything. One of the things you need to do is to develop a sense of humility, realism, straight thinking – 'solid honesty' is what AA calls that. Human beings are limited and AA says that one should give up all claims to being special. Somewhere Bill Wilson says, 'It seems absolutely necessary for most of us to get over the idea that man is God, and that we as individual alcoholics have any omnipotence whatever. The minute we make this admission at depth the sky starts to clear'.

Now for me at least, looking at AA and its power over alcoholism and looking at other self-help groups, seeing their basic wisdom, much of it borrowed from AA, what is seen is, I think, a very fundamental recovery process. It is one we don't understand very well but we must acknowledge it and we must value it. I think what we see there is the certain developmental thing. A person develops a chronic physical or psychosocial problem and it won't go away despite multiple attempts at resolution and this is a demoralizing experience. Crises occur over and over again. Stresses occur, but gradually the person is overwhelmed with feelings of hopelessness and helplessness and then in that condition one very reluctantly joins a self-help peer group. A person gets involved in small group meetings, learns the roles whatever the guiding steps happen to be. The person then learns to model his or her behaviour after that of other fellow sufferers. In other words the person learns to surrender to learning from the group, to listening to its experience and its wisdom. And then gradually the person's attitudes and value of behaviour begin to change. I think that the most fundamental attitudinal changes involve going from feelings and attitudes — 'I am in control, my life is completely manageable, I'm running everything' — to a more reasonable feeling of 'there are many things that I am powerless over, my life in many ways is unmanageable'. Other changes seem to be going from either 'I'm a very inferior person,' or 'I am a very superior person' (and remember it all means the same thing) or 'I am a very independent person' or 'I am a very dependent person' to another attitude, 'I'll learn to be realistic. I am going to try to be honest, I'm a pretty ordinary human being, I can do some things but not everything. With the help of this self-help group, with the help of a Higher Power, I can cope with this chronic problem just for today with help. I can help myself by helping another fellow sufferer in need'. The outcome I think, is some kind of growth to maturity, increased honesty, increased responsibility, increased caring about other people and increased hope, some kind of mental health and some kind of courage to live with the chronic condition.

It really seems that this can be done. AA is the living testimony of this, I believe, and so are many of the other self-help groups which are modelled after it. It looks like strength can come from weakness and this is a paradox. Dr Ernest Kurtz[1] who wrote a beautiful book, Not God, a history of AA, has, I think, described not only the root metaphor of Alcoholics Anonymous, but the root metaphor guiding all of the other self-help groups as well. He uses the expression, 'The shared honesty of mutual vulnerability openly acknowledged'. When fellow sufferers can get together and experience this shared honesty of mutual limitation or mutual weakness openly acknowledged, then they can find the strength to overcome, not only alcoholism, but many other human problems as well.

Reference

1 Kurtz, E. (1979). *Not God — A History of Alcoholics Anonymous.* (Center City, MN: Hazelden Educational Materials)

Part 4:
ALCOHOLISM – MEDICAL ASPECTS

18
The medical aspects of alcoholism*

S. E. GITLOW

What are the 'medical aspects' of an illness?

Are they the criteria that justify the term 'disease'? Do they consist of the interface between the clinical physician and the illness? Perhaps they represent its relationship to the use of acute and chronic care medical facilities? Its impact upon morbidity and mortality rates? Or, in the case of an illness associated with the repetitive ingestion of a toxic substance, should we discuss the pathophysiology resulting from the chemical, its pharmacology or toxicology[2]? More likely than not, physicians would expect such a title to direct attention to the metabolic and anatomic derangements resulting from excess ethanol ingestion, the complications of alcoholism rather than the disease itself[3-5]. For completeness, let us examine each of these.

Alcoholism may be defined as a disease[6] characterized by the repetitive ingestion of any sedative drug, ethanol representing but one of these, in such a way as to result in interference with one or more aspects of the patient's life: interpersonal relationships, career, physical health. This definition is broad enough to encompass most of the euphemisms applied currently to patients suffering from it. Obviously such a definition permits variability in the presentation of this illness. But what illness does not have variability? Can typhoid fever or tuberculosis not present in one person with barely detectable stigmata and in another with overwhelming and perhaps fatal consequences? Might one patient respond to therapy and another not? Might one patient acquire complications of an illness and another not? Might the disease not vary in its presentation and course with age, race, or the presence of other adverse medical conditions? For many years, attempts were made to subdivide alcoholism into words or phrases designed to project an aura of moral turpitude or denial of the illness by society: 'alcohol abuse', 'misuse', or 'problem'.

---

* Presented in part at The Conference on Alcoholism and the General Hospital held at the New York Academy of Medicine on 26 May 1982.

The term 'misuse' implies that healthier individuals use ethanol 'properly', and 'abuse' makes the perjorative implication even clearer. Although the message of 'self-abuse' is clear (since abuse of the inanimate object alcohol is obviously ridiculous), some scientists have attempted to legitimatize this term by a pseudoscientific definition: the ethanol 'abuser' using the drug without the production of physical dependency[7]. This becomes a cute trick since evidence of physical dependency and a subtle withdrawal manifestation can be demonstrated when a single dose of ethanol is administered to any mammal[8].

More recently, the terms 'primary' (arising *de novo*) and 'secondary' (representing a complication of a separate and distinct illness) have been applied to alcoholism. This arbitrary terminology overlooks the fact that alcoholism has been observed both with and without any and all psychological patterns and that the latter occur with and without alcoholism[9]. The concept is more specious since it is based upon the temporal sequence of appearance of the illnesses rather than any demonstrated relationship. The rare disclaimer clarifying the anomalous and unusual manner in which the terminology is being used is then rapidly lost in the literature[10].

One even hears of definitions of alcoholism incorporating the term 'progressive'. Now there is little doubt but that this illness, like many other chronic ones, is frequently progressive. Nonetheless, a medical definition must not include such a term. If we were to use it to define neuroblastoma, an illness with substantive tendency to be progressive, would we not be bound to reclassify that occasional instance wherein spontaneous regression occurred? When such a term is shifted from the description of a disease to its definition, it becomes self-fulfilling and arbitrary, restricting our understanding of the illness rather than broadening it.

Obviously, medical science has had little influence over the nomenclature of this illness. Rather social values, morality, personal bias and fear seem to dictate our terminology. Unfortunately, the resultant confusion tends to mislead our highest court[11], our legislative bodies, and eventually ourselves. We lose the very purpose of medical nosology, scientific communication.

Although often attacked from both within and outside of the medical profession[1, 12, 13] the disease concept of alcoholism persists. Why? If we examine the derivation of the term disease, *lack of ease* (old French), there is little doubt but that our patients suffering from alcoholism possess it. Our real problem turns about our assumption of self-induction. We seem to have less difficulty with the overweight diabetic or hypertensive subjects. Their diseases, resulting in gangrene or myocardial infarction, might have diminished or disappeared without self-induction. Although we have less difficulty applying the term 'disease' to these conditions, there is still a detectable level of disapproval regarding circumstances commonly viewed as resulting from lack of control. Such a view suffers from (1) a total absence of scientific substantiation, and (2) a failure to achieve clinical corroboration. In clinical practice, one rarely observes a subject whose entire life is weighted down with greater efforts at control than that of the alcoholic. To be honest, the rest of us do not control our alcohol intake; we don't have to. In fact, the need to exercise such control is pathognomonic of the illness alcoholism.

Rather than failure to control oneself, let us turn to the reverse side of this coin: level of need for relief (i.e. appetite). It is unbelievable that this biological mechanism, upon which our very survival as a species rests, would replicate without variation. Indeed, patients with alcoholism commonly claim, 'When I had my first drink, I finally discovered what it was like to feel normal like everyone else'. Such a concept was substantiated with the observation that alcoholism is associated with stimulus augmentation and that this circumstance could be relieved by alcohol[14]. Of potentially greater significance is the recent finding of Hennecke that children of subjects with alcoholism have not only an increased likelihood of developing this illness but are more apt to reveal stimulus augmentation than children of normal parents[15]. This is believed to be the first pre-morbid (prior to drinking) finding associated with this disease.*

Let us put aside the very questionable issue of self-induction (lack of control) and examine the applicability of the term disease in its more sophisticated or modern definition: *a dysfunctional state with characteristic form*. Ultimately, the fulfilment of this definition separates 'symptom' from 'disease'. Does alcoholism possess a recognizable pattern when examined from such aspects as aetiology, history, physical findings, complications, course, prognosis and therapy? If one is experienced with the variation of expression common to all illnesses and the problems inherent in classifying all disease for which a known, singular, and specific aetiology is lacking, the answer of clinicians who have laboured in this field is a clear 'yes'. One need go no further than the local AA meeting to hear the recurrent and common histories. The physical findings are frequent enough to permit their expression in cartoon form. What medical student cannot recite readily the list of complications of this illness? Its untreated course and prognosis are so well known as to influence some physicians to avoid involvement with these patients. Effective treatment techniques, on the surface so dissimilar, all share the singular element of a caring person (or better yet, group) with whom the patient can establish a successful interpersonal relationship. It matters little whether you electrocute, Rolfe, or hug your patients, as long as you care, share and support them in their abstemious lifestyle[6, 17].

Is the pattern not as clear as it is for most diseases? Certainly we cannot persist in the belief that only gross anatomic derangements and infections are entitled to the label 'disease'. If a biochemical disorder of the liver or pancreas can represent a disease, why not one involving the brain? If we must separate psyche from soma, how do we deal with the intellectual impairment

---

* Along with a failure to identify with the parent of the same sex and a culture in which exposure to alcohol is common, it represents one of a triad of aetiologic circumstances which has been referred to as the mosaic theory of the aetiology of alcoholism[16].

associated with the biochemical disorder of brain metabolism, phenylpyruvi-coligophrenia? A disease?

Let us turn to the more pragmatic issue: medicine has an interface with alcoholism because, like it or not, the patient eventually feels sick, isolated, and confused. He* rarely seeks initially the advice of the teacher, social worker, alcoholism counsellor or cleric; rather, he sees his doctor.

Alcoholic patients do this with such frequency that they account for a disproportionate share of health expenditures in the USA[18]. Although physicians are often the earliest resource to whom the alcoholic turns for help, we fail to identify the nature of the problem, often diagnosing only the complications. And why not? We spend hundreds of hours teaching medical students how to recognize the complications of alcoholism but rarely more than 2 or 3 hours during a 4-year curriculum on the subject of recognition of alcoholism itself. The patients may present with vague complaints reflecting in a general way their dysfunctional state, or the troubles may be more somatic in nature, including headache, pyrosis, flatulence, asthenia, palpitations or abdominal pain. From an objective standpoint, one may observe labile hypertension, tremulousness, diaphoresis, tachyarrhythmias or recurrent tracheobronchial infections. Repeated injuries, often complicated by fractures or pulmonary infections, are common. One may see evidence of poor compliance with therapeutic suggestions for other illness — hypertension, peptic disease, tuberculosis and radiculopathies proving especially nettlesome. The patient may note symptoms of depression, especially insomnia, or more simply lament the fact that he is cursed with family members or career associates who are impossible to satisfy. More often than not, modest problems are perceived by the patients as overwhelming and unresolvable.

Not only does the generalist see the stigmata of alcoholism in the family (that autocracy governed by its sickest member), the work place, and the community, but every medical specialist is in contact with some aspect of alcoholism as well. The obstetrician delivers the child suffering from an alcohol related birth defect (ARBD) or, worse, fetal alcohol syndrome (FAS). The pediatrician treats not only this group with the most common of all preventable birth defects, but the abused children growing up with alcoholic parents or surrogates. The surgeon and/or orthopod treats the injuries resulting from an auto accident or fire, until the delirium tremens demands the assistance of a psychiatrist or internist. The ENT surgeon attempts to resect the laryngeal or pharyngeal carcinomas that are relatively uncommon except in the heavy drinker. The subspecialists have their own contacts with these patients, whether through primary myocardial disease, cirrhosis, myopathies, gout or pancreatitis. One may wonder which patients would require our efforts, should the alcoholics no longer need them.

But it is not only our offices that patients with alcoholism fill but our

---

* Although almost half of such patients are female, the male pronoun will be used for convenience.

hospitals as well. On numerous occasions, it has been apparent that some 30 % of the service medical beds in my own institution are filled with patients whose illnesses or admissions are somehow related to alcoholism. This, despite the fact that admissions to this unit for 'alcoholism', 'detoxification', or 'withdrawal syndrome' are extremely uncommon. More formal studies of other institutions yield similar results — 30–50% of medical beds being occupied for alcoholism or some illness related to or resulting from it[19].

This interface between medicine and alcoholism is perhaps one of our sorriest. Rarely does the diagnosis of alcoholism appear on the charts of these patients and even more rarely are they referred for appropriate care of their alcoholism[20]. Resident physicians who would never confess to ignorance about a liver function test express readily their lack of information concerning local Alcoholics Anonymous (AA) meetings, their whereabouts or techniques of referral. Is it not an anachronism that AA meetings fill more church basements than hospitals? It is extremely rare to find any house staff or attending physician who knows whether his own institution houses AA meetings, or if so, when and where. This, despite the fact that each physician is in some manner treating the alcoholic. Most hospitalized alcoholics are discharged eventually without inpatient or outpatient treatment for their primary illness.

Another interface between medicine and alcoholism relates to the mortality resulting from this disease. When asked to examine my unsuccessful efforts a few decades ago, I was shocked to learn that many such patients had died suddenly and violently. Certainly this observation should have evoked no surprise since 50% of all vehicular deaths are somehow associated with ethanol use and in like manner the figures for drownings and fire are 60% and 75% respectively. Sudden unexplained deaths (dysrhythmias?), the mixing of solid and liquid sedatives, occasional intentional suicides, and falls within the home resulting in head trauma completed the list. One need not even add the 85% of the over 11 000 yearly liver deaths ascribed to alcohol in order to realize that alcoholism is related to more deaths between 15 and 45 years of age than any other single factor.

Our biggest killer of young adults — yet largely unlabelled. We hardly needed the text by Haberman and Baden[21] to remind us of the frequency with which alcoholism is omitted from the death certificates that we fill out. When the son of a reputable townsperson suffers a fatal vehicular injury while his blood alcohol concentration is 0.3%, is 'alcohol' entered on his death certificate? If this represented his third such accident and not the first related injury, is 'alcoholism' entered? Not likely.

Perhaps the 'medical aspects' of this disease should encompass the pharmacology of ethanol, the withdrawal syndrome, tolerance and the nature of the addictive (physical dependency) state[22]. One can lecture for many hours about this unique sedative, its absorption, the caloric and metabolic load it presents to the body and its enormous toxicity for the gastrointestinal tract, liver, pancreas, heart, skeletal muscles, neurons (central and peripheral), bone marrow and endocrine organs. Its ability to disorder the metabolism of neurohumoral transmitters, alter fat and carbohydrate metabolism, and modify the redox of NAD can only intrigue the toxicologist. The treatment of the disordered bodily metabolism resulting from alcohol ingestion, especially the abnormal c.n.s. function requiring detoxification, may result in yet another interface between alcoholism and medicine.

Maybe the genetic studies, by supporting the biologic nature of the transmission of this illness, represent the interface which should really concern us?

No, in the final analysis most planning committees would agree that the 'medical aspects' of alcoholism are simply the complications of alcoholism. Many of us in medicine continue to doubt the medical aspect of addiction itself, favouring its perception as a social, moral or political problem. Our prestigious acute care facilities reflect our attitudes, few possessing even rudimentary detox units. And when it comes to long term rehabilitation units, we have largely quit the field. Classically, these entities have had minimal input from the medical sciences and schools.

It would appear that we are long overdue in changing our perceptions as to what the medical aspects of alcoholism might be. Today, we will not err again in mistaking the disease complications for the disease. But will we persist in the maladaptation of medicine to this illness? There is an ancient Talmudic quip that relates 'for the man who does not know where he is going, any road will take him there'. Let us choose our road more carefully than those who embraced the illusion of 'controlled drinking' therapy for the alcoholic just a few years ago[23]. In the final analysis, the patient has chosen the physician to meet the onslaught of alcoholism. Our path and our aim with this disease as with any other, should meet that need.

References

1 Gitlow, S. E. (1973). In Bourne, P. and Fox, R. (eds.) *Alcoholism: a Disease. Progress in Research and Treatment.* (New York: Academic Press)

2 Sellers, E. M. and Kalant, H. (1976). Alcohol intoxication and withdrawal. *N. Engl. J. Med.*, **294**, 757

3 Sherlock, S. (ed.) (1982). *Alcohol and Disease.* (London: Churchill Livingstone)

4 Kaelber, C. T. and Barboriak, J. (eds.) (1981). Symposiums on alcohol and cardiovascular disease. *Circulation*, Part II, **64**

5 Eckardt, M. J., Harford, T. C., Kaelber, C. T., Parker, E. S., Rosenthal, L. S., Ryback, R. S., Salmoiragbi, G. C., Vanderveen, E. and Warren, K. R. (1981). Health hazards associated with alcohol consumption. *J. Am. Med. Assoc.*, **246**, 648.

6 Gitlow, S. E. and Peyser, H. S. (eds.) (1980). *Alcoholism: A Practical Treatment Guide.* (New York: Grune & Stratton)

7 American Psychiatric Association, Task Force on Nomenclature and Statistics (1980). *DSM III. Diagnostic and Statistical Manual of Mental Disorders*, 3rd Edn. (Washington, DC: American Psychiatric Association)

8 McQuarrie, D. G. and Fingle, E. (1958). Effects of single doses and chronic administration of ethanol on experimental seizures in mice. *J. Pharmacol. Exp. Ther.* **124**, 264

9 Feighner, J. P., Robins, E., Guze, S. B., Woodruff, R. A., Winokur, G. and Munoz, R. (1972). Diagnostic criteria for use in psychiatric research. *Arch. Gen. Psychiatry*, **26**, 57

10 Schukit, M. A. (1973). Alcoholism and sociopathy − diagnostic confusion. *Q. J. Stud. Alc.*, **34**, 157

11 *Powell vs. Texas*, (1968) 392 U.S. 514.

12 Emory, M. L. (1969). Medical management of the effects of alcohol and alcoholism. *J. Louisiana State Med. Soc.*, **121,** 279

13 Kendell, R. E. (1979). Alcoholism: a medical or political problem. *Br. Med. J.*, **1,** 367

14 Petrie, A. (1978). *Individuality in Pain and Suffering*, 2nd Edn. (Chicago: University of Chicago Press)

15 Hennecke, L. (1982). Stimulus augmenting and field dependence in children of alcoholics. *Doctoral Dissertation*, Teachers College, Columbia University. (University Microfilms)

16 Gitlow, S. E. and Hennecke, L. (1982). The mosaic theory of alcoholism. (In preparation)

17 Marlatt, G. A. and Nathan, P. E. (eds.) (1978). *Behavioural Approaches to Alcoholism*. (New Brunswick, NJ: Rutgers Center of Alcohol Studies)

18 Califano, J. A., Jr. (1982). *The 1982 Report on Drug Abuse and Alcoholism*. A report to H. L. Carey, Governor, State of New York, June 1982

19 Mc Cusker, J., Cherubin, C. E. and Zimberg, S. (1971). Prevalance of alcoholism in general municipal hospital population. *NY State J. Med.*, **71,** 751

20 Zimberg, S. (1978). Alcoholism: prevalance in general hospital emergency room and walk-in clinic. *NY State J. Med.*, **79,** 1533

21 Haberman, P. W. and Baden, M. M. (1978). *Alcohol, Other Drugs and Violent Death*. (New York: Oxford UP)

22 Gitlow, S. E. (1966). Treatment of the reversible acute complications of alcoholism. *Mod. Treatment*, **3,** 472

23 Pendery, M. L., Maltzman, I. M. and West, L. J. (1982). Controlled drinking by alcoholics? New findings and a reevaluation of a major affirmative study. *Science*, **217,** 169

19
Mortality and alcoholism – the need for urgent detoxification

D. H. MARJOT

First and last it is the physician's task to prevent death. Yet many doctors subscribe to the aphorism, 'You should not kill nor need you strive officiously to keep alive'. When death is inevitable and expected and when the patient's position is helpless then heroic, distressing or degrading treatments should not be attempted.

But this view is capable of subtle distortion. Handicapped babies may be thought unfit for survival. A modest shift can provoke the frequently expressed view that putative deviants such as alcoholics are better off dead – both for their own sakes and those of family and society.

Such views lead to the rejection of the alcoholic as a patient in spite of alcoholism being a disease, and the alcoholic the victim of the disease complications of his dependence. The intellectual dissonance provoked by the rejection of the alcoholic forces the compassionate subscriber to that view to deny that his patients are alcoholics. Thus an advanced and advancing cirrhotic will be advised to cut down or cut out his drinking but never formally diagnosed as alcohol dependent and offered appropriate treatment.

Inevitably many alcoholic lives are punctuated with crises. When these threaten life or the impairment of health, medical intervention is essential and an obligation on the attending doctor and any other individual involved. But some crises, such as homelessness or delinquency, are not the primary responsibility of the physician; nonetheless, if alcoholism is the cause, prompt advice, support and appropriate treatment of the dependant is the physician's duty.

Interventions in the alcoholic's career are justified by the adage, 'prevention is better than cure'.

Detoxification is outside the scope of primary intervention. In most cases secondary prevention – the detection of asymptomatic or early cases – is again not concerned with detoxification. However, tertiary prevention – the prompt intervention in established disease so that the illness may be arrested, improved or induced to remit — is the very proper place for detoxification.

MORTALITY STUDIES

The causes of death in alcoholism and the natural history of such disorders should constitute rationale for acute intervention in such cases. Published papers highlight the causes of and relative importance of deaths in alcoholics[1-5].

Adelstein and White[1] showed that out of a sample of 2070 alcoholic inpatients in psychiatric hospitals between 1953 and 1974, 794 deaths had occurred. This was for males 2.1 times the number expected for an average population of men and 2.7 that for females.

They found that the ratio was very much higher for both sexes in the younger age groups. Of course, this is in part a statistical artifact, as the older you are the more likely you are to die of causes other than those related to alcohol. This makes the express mortality equally startling for *all* ages. (The graph, Figure 19.1, shows these findings to good advantage.)

Table 19.1 shows the Adelstein and White figures[1] in tabulated form.

Table 19.1   Deaths of alcoholics by age and sex, 1953−74, England and Wales

Observed	Male/female		Expected	Ratio
15−30	M	35	3.04	11.7
	F	4	0.23	17.4
30−39	M	339	101.7	3.3
	F	90	18.4	4.9
60 +	M	231	185.0	1.2
	F	95	50.0	1.9
All ages	M	605	290.0	2.1
	F	189	68.0	2.7

Adelstein and White[1] found an obvious excess of deaths among alcoholics in diseases of the circulatory, respiratory and digestive systems as well as among accidents, poisonings and violent deaths.

Polich[2], analysing the 'Rand' reports, described the mortality in 758 male alcoholics followed-up for 4.33 years, as shown in Table 19.2.

The analysis showed that 56% of the deaths in this sample could be directly or indirectly attributed to alcohol.

De Lint[5] surveyed excess mortality from a number of studies (Table 19.3).

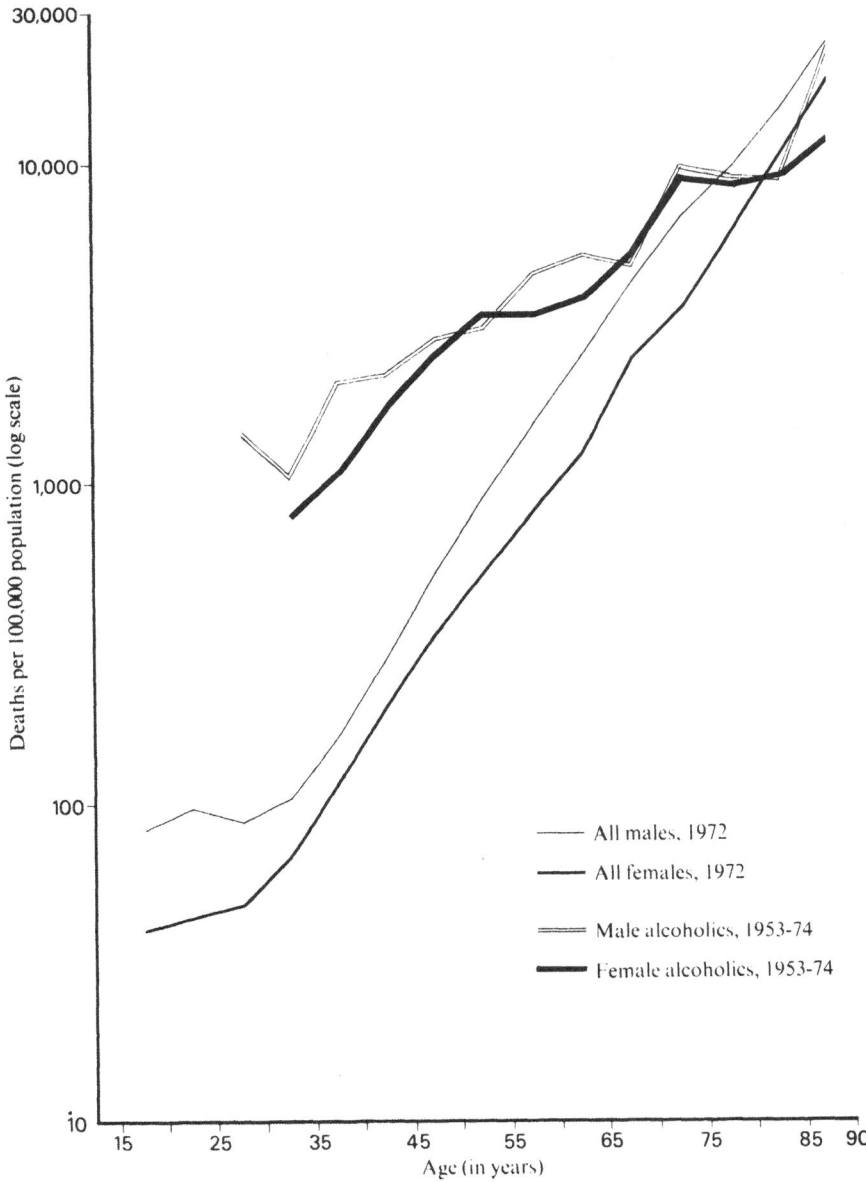

Figure 19.1 Death rates of alcoholics: age and sex, England and Wales

Table 19.2   Analysis of mortality in 758 alcoholics[2]

Causes of death	Actual mortality %	Expected mortality %	Ratio
All causes	14.5	5.9	2.5
Alcoholism	0.6	0.03	21.0
Suicide	2.3	0.1	23.0
Cirrhosis	1.6	0.2	8.0
Accident	2.0	0.4	5.0
All others	8.0	5.2	1.5

The mean age of the contact was 45 years

Table 19.3 Results of survey of excess mortality

Investigator	Sample	Number of Deaths Observed	Number of Deaths Expected	Observed / Expected
*Gillis (1969)	802 patients treated for alcoholism, S. Africa	90	22.9	3.9
*Pell and D'Alonzo (1973)	899 "alcoholic" employees, USA	102	31.7	3.2
*Brenner (1967)	1343 patients treated for alcoholism, USA	217	72.6	3.0
*Nicholls et al. (1973)	935 patients treated for alcoholism, England	309	112.7	2.7
*Sundby (1967)	1722 male patients with diagnosis of alcoholism, Norway	1061	496.9	2.1
*Giffin and Oki (1971)	343 male drunkenness offenders, Canada	191	89.7	2.1
*Schmidt and de Lint (1969)[4]	6514 patients treated for alcoholism, Canada	738	346.2	2.0

* Studies listed, as cited by de Lint[5]

In a large sample (5395 male and 1119 female) of alcoholics Schmidt and de Lint[4] found the mortalities shown in Table 19.4.

Thorarinsson's findings[3] on mortality among male alcoholics in Iceland, 1951–1974, are detailed in Tables 19.5 and 19.6.

Table 19.4 Mortalities in sample of 5395 male and 1119 female alcoholics

| | Number of Deaths | | | | | |
| | Men | | | Women | | |
	Observed	Expected	fo/fe	Observed	Expected	fo/fe
All causes	639	315.24	2.03	99	30.98	3.20
Malignant neoplasm of upper digestive and respiratory organs	49	17.55	2.79	1	0.53	1.88
Other malignant neoplasms	28	40.56	0.69	9	9.48	0.95
Alcoholism	29	1.03	28.16	3	0.06	50.00
Vascular lesion of central nervous system	27	23.67	1.14	9	3.69	2.44
Heart disease	247	142.10	1.74	30	8.99	3.34
Pneumonia	22	7.15	3.08	5	0.71	7.04
Cirrhosis of the liver	56	4.87	11.50	12	0.48	25.00
All violent causes	114	34.21	3.33	22	1.92	11.46
Other	67			8		

Table 19.5 Observed and expected causes of death male alcoholics in Iceland

Cause	No. Observed	No. Expected	Ratio O/E
Accident	146	36.84	3.96
Heart disease	143	79.14	1.81
Suicide	45	10.20	4.41
Cancer	29	8.68	3.34
Cirrhosis of the liver and faulty liver	14	1.24	11.29
Alcoholism	13	1.16	11.21
Vascular lesions of the c.n.s.	26	22.93	1.13
Other	72	39.58	1.82

Table 19.6   Observed and accidental deaths of Icelandic male alcoholics for four types of fatal accident

Cause	No. Observed	No. Expected	Ratio O/E
Drowning by water transport accident	36	11.09	3.25
Drowning	14	4.03	3.47
Falls	23	4.65	4.95
Poisoning	30	1.91	15.71
Other accidents	43	15.16	2.84

Four causes accounted for 70 % of the excess mortality: (1) accidents, 35 %, (2) arteriosclerotic heart disease, 19 %, (3) suicide, 11 % and (4) lung cancer, 6 %.

CAUSES OF MOST EXCESS DEATHS

Looking at such studies we can see that

(1)   suicide, violence, poisoning and accidents
(2)   cirrhosis and other digestive disorders
(3)   respiratory disorders
(4)   circulatory disorders

are responsible for most excess deaths.

Suicide, violence, poisoning and accidents

There is clearcut clinical evidence that very heavy drinking, particularly if it occurs on consecutive days (i.e. in binges or bouts), can produce a stereotyped emotional shift.

Unfortunately terms such as 'depression' are used indiscriminately for a trait (with a presumptive normal gaussian distribution), an explicable reaction to adverse circumstances, even if severe and distressing, the distress of loss including bereavement, a symptom, a syndrome and a disease. Often when patients describe depression they usually mean anxiety, anger or that state of impotence called frustration.

In my experience, such heavy drinking produces a stereotyped emotional shift whereby

anxiety
depression
aggression
suspiciousness and
sexual disorganization

are subsyndromes[6, 7].

Mayfield and Montgomery[8] called the depressive subsyndrome the 'depressive syndrome of chronic intoxication'. In my experience this is a melancholic picture with abnormal moods of sadness, guilt and despair. As intoxication increases recklessness, impulsiveness and impaired control of all modalities of emotion, it is not surprising that violent acts – whether they be self-injury, accidents, assaults or other violence – are much more frequent than in sober life.

Suspiciousness and aggression can involve the alcoholic in violence towards others and to property. If a motor vehicle is involved then a complex of aggression, impulsiveness, recklessness and depression can lead to accidents or deliberate harm. (Ritson[9], Proudfoot and Park[10] and Havard[11] have well reviewed alcoholism and suicide, self-poisoning and accidents).

Cirrhosis of the liver

Nicholson[12] reviewed alcoholic liver disease. He pointed out that alcoholic hepatitis itself caused a real mortality and leads to cirrhosis. Those with established cirrhosis have a 50 % survival rate after 5 years and this increases to 80 % with abstinence. Improvement includes those with ascites and jaundice but not haematemesis.

Detoxification and subsequent measures to establish abstinence should improve mortality and morbidity in such patients.

Respiratory disorders

Many alcoholics are very heavy smokers and this may be responsible for part of the excess deaths. But there is considerable evidence that alcohol alters the defences of the body against infections and this assists the development of respiratory disease[13].

(The one death on our own Unit (at St Bernard's Hospital, London) in 1981 (from 670 admissions) was of a man with a respiratory infection who collapsed and died suddenly and at postmortem was found to have had bronchopneumonia.)

Cardiovascular disorders

Alterations in blood cognability, thiamin deficiency, alcoholic myocardial disease and alcohol induced hypertension may all contribute to increased mortality and will respond to treatment and abstinence.

(The only death other than that cited above on our own Unit in the past 5 years (in 1979) was a sudden death due to pulmonary embolism.)

DETOXIFICATION – ITS NATURE AND ROLE

Redmond[14] cited Pittman and Gordon[15] as saying 'A treatment centre should be created for the reception of the chronic drunkenness offender. This means that such offenders should be removed from gaols and penal institutions, as the mentally ill were removed from gaols in the last century. . . . Given the present state of knowledge concerning alcoholism the time is right now for such a change'.

In 1971 a Home Office Report on the Habitual Drunken Offender accepted such a principle and recommended the establishment of detoxification centres in the larger cities where there would be the demand. The Report suggested that in London 150–450 places would be needed. Those arrested for public drunkenness would have the choice of arrest or going to such a centre.

Two pilot centres for such offenders were set up in England. One was under the aegis of social services with a strong nursing and medical input and the other was hospital based. Both were open by 1977.

Already, however, other units were moving into the field of detoxification. The Oxford Regional Alcoholism Unit provided urgent detoxification on a very significant scale in 1965[16]. An *ad-hoc* arrangement came about in Edinburgh in 1976 at the Regional Poisoning Treatment Centre. These units did not cater primarily for the drunken offender but had a much wider remit. They saw such crisis intervention as an integral part of the treatment offered by regional units and it was an effective way of drawing a different group of alcoholics into treatment.

Ritson[17] has written of his experiences in Edinburgh with helping the habitual drunken offender as part of a wider scheme for detoxification of the alcoholic.

For the drunken offender, the peak hours of admission were at or after the closing times of the bars in that city. Peak admissions were on Friday and Saturday — the traditional days for heavy drinking.

Those drunken offenders who were admitted to a positive programme of help rather than just sobering-up and detoxification spent more time with caring agencies and their quality of life had improved.

In 1979 The Regional Alcoholic Unit at St Bernard's Hospital, London, was unable to admit patients for nearly 8 weeks. We accumulated 80 patients on our waiting list which took over 3 months to clear. Five patients died while on the waiting list. While we were aware that our patients seemed to die too readily, we were nonetheless shocked.

In the next year we allocated 13 beds to urgent detoxification; another 7 beds were regularly in use detoxifying patients admitted for our treatment programme. The stay was expected to average 7 days and the patient was counselled and assessed for further treatment. A total admission rate of over 800 per annum is now established.

It now seems that the centres established to cater for the drunken offender and those which were developed as part of a regional alcoholism service are moving closer together.

A detoxification centre will carry out some or all of the following functions:

(1)   Sobering-up service: in the case of the drunken offender the majority of the people admitted discharge themselves with 24 hours of admission,

(2)   safe management of withdrawal from alcohol,

(3)   diagnosis and arrangement for treatment of the disease complications of alcoholism,

(4)   assessment of the alcoholic patients and their introduction to treatment services and caring agencies,

(5)   a clearing house or referral sink (an ugly expression!) for alcoholics and those involved in their care,

(6)   providing a brief stay in an alcohol-free environment.

The incidence of the serious disease complications has been studied by Redmond[14] (1980) at the detoxification centre at Manchester. Of 50 consecutive admissions to that centre, one third had serious medical complications and 10 % needed immediate medical attention.

In our Unit nearly half have serious medical disorders and 15 % need immediate care, quite apart from withdrawal from alcohol.

Of 194 consecutive patients admitted in 1982 to the Regional Alcoholism Unit at St Bernard's Hospital, 74 % had evidence of liver damage; in 38 % this was severe and in five cases there was liver failure. Of those with liver damage, 24 % had other serious problems including peripheral neuritis, hypertension, heart disease etc. A further 8 % of these 104 admissions were ill but had no liver damage, but cardiovascular disorders predominated.

At present, however, there is no hard evidence that such urgent detoxification does reduce mortality and morbidity, but *a priori* it should do so.

References

1 Adelstein, A. and White, G. (1976). An examination of deaths in the period 1953−76 in a sample of alcoholics. *Population Trends*, 7−13. (London: HMSO)
2 Polich, J. M. (1980). Patterns of remission in alcoholics. In Edwards, G. and Grant, M. (eds.) *Alcoholism Treatment and Transitions*, pp. 95−112. (London: Croom Helm)
3 Thorarinsson, A. A. (1979). Mortality among men alcoholics in Iceland, 1957−74. *J. Stud. Alc.*, **40**, 704
4 Schmidt, W. and de Lint, J. (1969). Mortality experiences of male and female alcoholic patients. *Q. J. Stud. Alc.*, **30**, 112
5 de Lint, J. (1975). Current trends in the prevalence of excessive alcohol use and alcohol related health damage. *Br. J. Addict.*, **70**, 3
6 Marjot, D. H. (1982). Alcohol, aggression and violence. *Practitioner*, **226**, 287
7 Marjot, D. H. (1982). The disease concept of alcoholism redefined. In Golding, P. (ed.) *Alcoholism: A Modern Perspective*. (Lancaster: MTP)
8 Mayfield, D. and Montgomery, D. (1972). Alcoholism, alcohol intoxication and suicide attempts. *Arch. Gen. Psychiatry*, **27**, 349
9 Ritson, B. (1977). Alcoholism and Suicides. In Edwards, G. and Grant, M. (eds.) *Alcoholism − New Knowledge and New Responses*, pp. 271−278. (London: Croom Helm)

10 Prondfoot, and Park, (1977). Alcohol and self-poisoning. In Edwards, G. and Grant, M. (eds.) *Alcoholism — New Knowledge and New Responses*. (London: Croom Helm)

11 Havard, (1977). Alcohol and road accidents. In Edwards, G. and Grant, M. (eds.) *Alcoholism — New Knowledge and New Responses*. (London: Croom Helm)

12 Nicholson, G. (1980). Alcoholic liver disease. In Clark, P. M. S. and Kricka, L. J. (eds.) *Medical Consequences of Alcohol Abuse*, pp. 51 − 86. (Chichester: Ellis Horwood)

13 Smith, F. E. and Palmer, D. L. (1976). Alcoholism; infection and altered host defences. A review. *J. Chron. Dis.*, **29,** 35

14 Redmond, A. D. (1980). The medical morbidity of 50 individuals admitted to a detoxification centre − a preliminary study. In Madden, J. S., Walker, R. and Kenyon, W. H. (eds.) *Aspects of Alcohol and Drug Dependence*, pp. 361 − 367. (Tunbridge Wells: Pitman Medical)

15 Pittman, D. and Gordon, G. W. (1958). *Revolving Door. A Study of the Chronic Police Inebriate*. (New Brunswick, NJ: Rutgers Center for Alcohol Studies)

16 Arroyave, F., McKeowan, S. and Cooper, S. E. (1980). Detoxification − an approach to developing a comprehensive alcoholism service. *Br. J. Addict.*, **75,** 187

17 Ritson, B. (1975). Detoxification − an evaluation. *Br. J. Addict.*, **70,** Suppl. 65 − 73

20

The family doctor as a scientist and friend of his alcohol-diseased patients

H. BRAMMER

INTRODUCTION

The profession of local general practitioner is not limited to the prescription of medicaments. It also cannot be described in the way an experienced practitioner did with the following ironical remark: 'In the morning I talk to the people and in the afternoon I drive my car around'.

The entire spectrum of human life with its manifold phenomena is characterized by anxiety and by the hope of finding relief during the consultation hours of the doctor who has the unique potential to accompany suffering humans during a part of their lives. This does not necessitate his forgetting science. A science, not conceiving itself as an example of '*l'art pour l'art*', should aim at directing the human's way back to the original divine harmony. However, for achieving this aim, the investigator should question his own personality and be aware of his subjectiveness. Only the one who is aware of his own limits and thus his susceptibility to mistakes also knows and recognizes subjectiveness and human incompleteness in the other person. The physician examines the damaged liver and with a considerable technical effort he tries to readjust the 'derailed' metabolism — the doctor shows compassion for human suffering and wants to participate in the sorrows and anxieties of the other human being. Medicine is a suitable means to reach this aim.

The diseased human is in a situation of exception which in our standardized world of postulated health and performance induces anxiety. Fear as a factor in our development cannot be denied. Each domination of fear is a victory which makes us stronger, each flight from it is a defeat which weakens us. Therefore the doctor also must dominate his own anxiety and penetrate into a profound discussion with the patient. But frequently enough the doctor —

appearing to be the teacher — for reasons of defence against his own anxieties remains 'on the stage of inaccessibility'. We deem ourselves free and liberal, but we fear the responsibility involved. However, if humans no longer want to take on responsibility, their freedom is endangered and this can mean that complete groups tend to aggressions induced by unreal anxieties. This aggression frequently originates from the fear of being in some way hampered in personal development[1].

In spite of excess adaptation and 'substitute mentality' the doctor must endeavour to look behind aggression and 'impressing attitude' and recognize the anxious and helpless human being, a grown-up person needing help.

The recognition of my own subjective susceptibility to mistakes as well as the intensive experience of my own addiction may have caused a greater tolerance towards the alcoholic. The fact that I myself have been an alcoholic since my twelfth year of age, which I do not try to hide at all, can surely explain the circumstance that the proportion of alcoholics in my practice increased from 2 % in the beginning to about 4 %[2, 3].

Evaluation of the last quarter of the year even showed that the proportion of addicts in my total number of patients was 8.5 %[4].

As long as we cannot accurately diagnose with relevant statistical significance whether a person may become an alcoholic, and as long as alcohol is produced and is sold without limitation in our pluralistic society, we must live with the fact that everybody who drinks alcohol — without exception — can become an alcoholic, but this does not justify the reproach that he is a person of inferior character. Yes, I am even convinced that those who do not become alcoholics in spite of consuming alcohol have been lucky. But this does not give them the right to deduce therefrom some personal merit — many other human beings did not have such luck!

It should be remembered, however, that we often entrust our lives to alcoholics in anaesthesia or during a taxi ride; bridges and high-tension transmission lines are erected by alcoholics; alcoholics regulate traffic and teach our children; they preach in the churches and teach in universities. Alcoholism is not a privilege of masons and beer truck drivers, it is a disease — and not one which stops before reaching a certain social class, but one which penetrates into the whole structure of the population.

The alcohol addict lives a miserable life on the margin of society, like a wolf turned out of his pack. He no longer drinks alcohol because of the taste, but because he needs it to hide the shakes, to overcome stomachache, to relieve nausea and the tendency to vomit, to 'polish up' his feeling of self-esteem which has been almost destroyed and to be able to carry out the simplest daily work. The alcohol addict in the chronic phase is no longer the centre of a happy circle in his favourite pub, he sits in a remote corner and gloomily broods upon himself and complains of his fate. He develops almost autistic traits and is unable to perceive anything beyond the bottle. For escaping the fate of being 'the odd man out' or being considered an unsteady asocial creature, but primarily so as not lose his almost vanished self-esteem entirely, he has developed whole systems of explanation, however transparent these may be. The alcohol addict is a deeply disturbed person in extraordinary psychic distress who has reached the lowest point of his existence, is often aware of his miserable state and thinks frequently of ending this unworthy existence by committing suicide.

But if a relationship can be achieved in which physician and patient no longer avoid each other[5] and the helper speaks with the alcoholic about the consequences of his state, i.e. about the disease itself and not about ethics and morals, then the addict will have found in his family doctor a therapist who works with him and accepts him as a suffering person, and therefore the addict can finally give up running from one doctor to another hoping to find one whom he can still deceive with his 'explanations'.

In a multi-morbidity study in 1977[2] the following items were investigated:

(1) the number of alcoholics related to the overall number of patients
(2) age distribution and male:female ratio
(3) frequency of all diseases
(4) period of observation of the patient
(5) mortality.

Out of 3159 patients investigated within the period of observation the proportion of alcoholics was 2.22%. The male:female ratio was 5:1 and the average age of males 45 and of females 37. The number of diagnoses of alcoholics was in the median 3.47 and of the other patients 2, so that the morbidity of the alcoholics was 62% above the entire sample. In detail, the higher sensitivity to infections of the alcoholics could be proved, as well as the higher participation in accidents and the greater frequency of heart disease and disturbances of the stomach and intestine organ. Especially pronounced was the fivefold increase in involvement of the vegetativum, such as headache, perspiration, sleeplessness, states of anxiety and tremor. These were, however, syndromes of an alcohol disease. By contrast, other risk factors such as diabetes, hyperlipidaemia and hypertonia were not more frequent in alcoholics, and illnesses of the urogenital region were five times less frequent in these patients. The frequency of treatment of non-alcoholics is in the median 2.5, whereas the alcoholics frequent the practitioner about three times more often, i.e. the median was about 6.

In 1977 we performed an extensive epidemiological investigation for which 5000 questionnaires were sent out, of which 881 could be evaluated[6]. In this investigation the male:female ratio shifted to 2.5:1 — unfavourable for the women — and the start of drinking in women was on average 3 years later than for men.[7]

In an investigation in 1981 about 'iatrogenic addiction'[3], the male:female ratio even reached 2.2:1. The question was investigated as to whether the age at the beginning of drinking has an influence on the frequency of relapses and it has been established that the group of those persons who drank alcohol for the first time prior to their eighteenth year was clearly over-represented for numerous relapses, indicating that development of personality and steady social position prior to the beginning of the disease are of prognostic significance for rehabilitation[8].

In the epidemiological investigation in 1977 as well as in the subsequent investigation in 1981, the average duration of addictive drinking was 11 years for males and females. The high portion of 74% of the persons questioned who reported having undergone inpatient treatment was astonishing, but no indication was given as to whether this inpatient treatment related exclusively to alcoholism or also to other somatic causes, so that a more precise diagnosis is required. Of the persons questioned, 43% abstained from addiction as a result of outpatient treatment, 39% of them without any inpatient treatment; 61% were subjected to inpatient treatment, but were rehabilitated and readapted to society only by the self-help groups[6]. Only 13% of the persons questioned had been informed about the disease and self-help organizations by their practitioner – an observation which has also been confirmed in the later investigation, which showed a 17% participation by the family doctor in the recovery from addiction.

As in the epidemiological investigation, 72% of the patients indicated that – contrary to correct practice – they were treated with hypnotics and sedatives; this question was to be further investigated by a study on iatrogenic addiction and an attempt made to find some causes for the aversion of alcoholics against the physician[9]. In this evaluation 185 alcoholics were involved; 59% of them asked a doctor for help during their drinking phase to recover from addiction. Out of these 107 persons, 86% were treated with hypnotics and sedatives, and even out of the 82 persons who asked for help after recovery from addiction, 66% were treated with these drugs[3]. In 15% of the patients treated with hypnotics and sedatives – in spite of the known alcohol addiction – an iatrogenic addiction was developing[10] necessitating, for one half of the patients, additional therapy[11]. This also explains why the clinical physician – deemed in some way anonymous – is reported as being helpful for recovery from addiction by 35% of the patients, and the general practitioner by only 13% in the investigation of 1977 and 17% in the study of 1981. This coincides with the method of prescription[9] and the fact that for 19% the practitioner even became the 'feared adversary'.

It is completely inconceivable that 69% of the physicians show no understanding at all for their patients, of whom respectively 21% react by feelings of offence and 5% by going as far as rejecting further treatment because the alcoholic does not want to take the medicaments which endanger his life. Obviously the risk does not need any further discussion, if a so-called primary addiction exists in patients genetically disposed for addiction[9]. It could also be proved that inpatient treatment was, to a significant extent, more frequently necessary for alcoholics who – apart from the addictive medium, alcohol – also took hypnotics and sedatives, a situation finally resulting in a severe socioeconomic problem. Under such circumstances, addicts' fear of consulting the family doctor is understandable.

Further causes for the addict to avoid the practitioner can be found in the following answers:

'I fear the lack of understanding and knowledge of the doctor.'
'I feel I am being rejected as a creature of inferior character and fear this rejection and the reproaches.'
'The psychic pressure is treated merely with medicaments.'
'The doctor has neither time nor understanding for my actual situation.'
'I longed for a talk, but instead I received a piece of paper and was called a faker and psychopath.'

There are certainly many physicians who endeavour to help their alcoholic patients in a suitable way. This is also evidenced by statements that the participation of the family doctor in recovery from addiction is increasing due to a better level of information[12]. There are certainly also many alcoholics who try to deceive their doctors because they are not able to judge their situation correctly, are ashamed and do not want to recognize the truth. The investigations available should, however, give rise to deep thought and review of one's own therapeutic efforts for the alcohol-diseased.

As hypnotics and sedatives carry in themselves a danger of converting the prescribing physician into an inhuman technician[13] and the prescription of medicaments with an addiction potential can be considered almost malpractice[14], I searched for possible ways of helping the addict in his withdrawal syndromes without facing the danger of an iatrogenic addiction.

For 2 years now, addicts have been treated with this new therapy[4]. Each voluntary patient receives within 2 weeks, ten treatments with own blood[15] with 1000 y of ozone, 15 ml piracetame (Normabrain, Nootrop) and 5 ml of protein-free hydrolysate from pig's brain (Cerebrolysine). Furthermore, after about three ozone treatments each patient receives a cure with fresh cells[16] of an average of 13.7 injections.

An evaluation of 30 histories and catamnesis investigations has shown the following: 4 weeks after the treatment, the overall state of the patient was clearly improved in 93 % of the cases, performance and capability of concentration was in each case improved to 100 %. 73 % joined a self-help group. A rehabilitation could be predicted for 58 %, as against 33 % of a control group investigated within the same period of time, not treated with ozone and fresh cells. 13 % indicated that their relationship to the environment and family worsened. This can be due to improved critical thinking and increase of the frustration tolerance. The alcohol addict is no longer 'placed under tutorship' as previously and tends now to re-establish his lost position in the family. This can eventually lead to difficulties.

However, it must be emphasized that this therapy does not guarantee the recovery of the alcoholic, it serves merely to overcome withdrawal syndromes, to stop the physical decay and to improve the capacity of performance and concentration. The addict is placed in the position of thinking over his situation for the first time in a sober condition and has the potential to stabilize his personality during the following years, eventually with the aid of a self-help group.

A further problem of increasing urgency is that of alcohol-addict physicians. Although exact figures are lacking in the Federal Republic of Germany, we have no reason to assume that the rate of physicians becoming alcohol and drug addicts is essentially lower in Germany than in the USA and Canada, presuming a rate of 6—10 %[17]. I myself have been more helpless than all my patients. At the same time, however, I was in the pretended position of a 'model', expected to give advice, where I had no advice for myself, to give help, where I myself was helpless, to incite courage, where I myself was desperate. My picture of the alcoholic in no way differed from the imagination of so many people who see in the alcoholic merely the weak character and the misfit. I see also the suffering of many of my colleagues who have an ideal image of the high responsibility and the position of the physician as the model for their patients and this image aggravates the recognition of their own disease, preventing them from accepting help for themselves. They are ashamed of the apparent failure and the presumed weakness of character and therefore many physicians do not join a self-help group. For this reason we have founded the association AÄD — Alcohol-Addict Physicians of Germany. Similar groups are already in existence in Switzerland, England and the USA as 'international doctors in AA'. In journals for physicians throughout the country, medical periodicals as well as radio interviews, I have drawn attention to this discussion circle which meets at regular intervals to talk about different items, such as:

    physician and anonymity
    physician and approbation
    physician and personnel
    the employed physician
    physician and alcohol-addict patients
    dentist and withdrawal — where the tremor can be considered a risk for economic existence.

The friendly discussions, showing also a group-dynamic process, have proved to be very helpful, both for the colleagues already living in the programme of AA and also for those who did not yet dare to join the self-help group because of the high threshold of scruples.

A further way to offer help to alcohol addicts was the foundation of a special group in the form of a registered association. Owing to the differences in human beings, different self-help groups developed — and this is judged positive — but all of them follow the same aim, to make a satisfactory and happy life in the community possible for the alcoholic. However, this necessitates an accompanying group treatment for a lifetime and this can be done only on a voluntary basis. This work is naturally focussing on the inside, as alcoholics remain among themselves and want exclusively to help themselves. Moreover, the self-help group can start to work only when the constant alcohol abuse has induced alcohol disease, and only when the pressure of suffering is so severe for the alcoholic himself and for the family that he finally is willing to accept the help of this organization.

This circumstance was taken into account by the foundation members of

SORRAL, when on 9 September 1979, they created the Social Rehabilitation and Resocialization Centre for Alcoholics. They recognized that the idea of the self-help groups has its limits which the groups cannot exceed without giving up their status of independence. Our aim was to realize a forum for the alcoholic as a starting-point for him to act in public and to use his re-established performance for the benefit of the community.

SORRAL is a humanitarian association of alcoholics and their friends joining in the effort to release addicts from isolation and give them the opportunity to live a normal life. The purpose of the association is help for persons endangered by potential addiction, manifest addicts and their families. The aim of the association is the readaptation of the addicts to society by a behavioural training related to practice and moreover by prevention of the danger of developing addiction, through making consultation available and giving information. The measures for help range from prevention, advice, therapy and subsequent assistance and intervention for help, to self-help.

In the meantime we have two fully professional consultation offices and three consultation hours with the respective offices in our locality, and by numerous publications in newspapers and through radio broadcasts we have been able to carry the idea to other cities, so that SORRAL also has local offices in Bonn, Cologne, Hameln and Osnabrück. In all these places citizens, both in public and private life, are coming together to combat with shared responsibility the abuse of alcohol and medicaments, for the benefit of their diseased co-citizens.

But among all these ways and methods I keep in my mind the words of Max Glatt, when he said that it is not the method which is the decisive factor, but the therapist as a human being who stands behind those methods[18]. The alcoholic in his experienced anxiety and deficiency of contacts often cannot join a group at the first impulse, but rather tries to find an individual. For this reason I ask that the following be considered.

The human being is body and soul — an entity in mind — he always seeks for a personal help in its entity, in other words, he does not search for help, but for a helper, a person of superior healing power who does not only cure his stomachache or his damaged liver or treat his states of anxiety, but who strengthens him as an individual entity, as a living creature. Only when he is accepted in his entity does he feel safe, and this is the only premise for a recovery process. Therefore the doctor must find a contact of confidence with the patient being in a state of anxiety, must show compassion for severe human suffering, must accept the patient in his entity and accompany him on his way to a better life.

References:

1 Battegay, R. (1976). *Anxiety and Being*. (Stuttgart: Edition Hippokrates).
2 Brammer, H. (1980). Multi-morbidity study in a general practice with special regard to alcoholism. *Therapiewoche*, **30**, 3268
3 Brammer, H. and Fritz, W. (1981). The iatrogenic addiction. Presented at the *27th Congress of ICAA*, Vienna

4 Brammer, H. (1981). Treatment of the alcoholic with cells. Presented at the *Deutscher Zelltherapietag*, Hamburg

5 Schulte, W. (1966). The treatment of addiction and abuse by the general practitioner. *Suchtgefahren (Hamburg)*, **12**, (1)

6 Brammer, H. and Fritz, W. (1979). Epidemiological investigation of some aspects of alcoholism. *Z. Allgemeinmed.* **55**, 2017

7 Jasinsky, M. (1975). Alcoholism in school age. *Fortschritte Med.*

8 Schröder, U. (1976). Alcoholism in children and adolescents. *Z. Allgemeinmed.* **52**

9 Hebenstreit, G. (1977). Psychopharmaca in the general practice. *Wiener Med. Wochenschr.* **27**, 561

10 Sattes, H. (1979). Distraneurin and alcohol abuse. *Med. Klin.*, **74**, 3

11 Twerski, A. (1978). Iatrogenic addiction no less devastating because it's legal. *Pa. Med.*, **81**, 21

12 Lohse, (1975). Aspects of treatment of alcoholics by general practitioners. (Hamburg: Neuland-Verlagsgesellschaft)

13 Beckmann, H. (1976). Use and abuse of psychopharmaca. *Med. Welt*, **27**, (11)

14 Huhn, A. (1978). Actual tendencies of alcohol- and medicament dependence and its treatment. *Psycho*, **4**, 132

15 Wolff, H. H. (1979). The medicinal ozone. (Heidelberg: E. Fischer)

16 Schmidt, F. and Stein, J. (1963). *Cell research and cellular therapy.* (Berne: H. Huber)

17 Bissell, L. C. (1975). The treatment of alcoholism: What do we do about long-term sedatives. *Ann. NY Acad. Sci.*, **252**, 396

18 Glatt, M. M. (1971). Attitude and influence of the public to the rehabilitation of the alcohol addict. *Rehabilitation*, **24**, 49

19 Hartenfels, H. (1964). Necessity and possibilities of abstinent organizations in the aid for alcoholics. Presented at the *27th International Congress on Alcoholism*, 6–12 September, Frankfurt/Main

20 Hohelüchter, K. L. (1978). The significance of medical prescription in case of addiction and abuse. *Psycho*, **4**, 137

Part 5:
ALCOHOLISM – SPIRITUAL ASPECTS

21
Spiritual recovery: from addiction to freedom

K. CAMPBELL

In my ordination paper, I used the following illustration from Henri Nowen's book *The Wounded Healer*. A fugitive enters a small village, and begs the members of the village to protect him from the army that is following him. He explains to the villagers that he fears for his life, and that he needs their protection. The villagers agree to hide him, and when the army arrives they are informed that they will all be killed if they do not give up the fugitive. The villagers don't know what to do, feeling both concern for the fugitive and fear for their own lives. After considerable debate, the villagers send a delegation to the local pastor, explaining the situation to him, and asking him to make the final decision. The pastor retreats to his study, where he spends a tormented night praying and reading his Bible. In the light of dawn, he explains to the villagers that he has decided that the best course of action would be to surrender the fugitive to the army, reasoning that the lives of the villagers would be spared. The fugitive is given to the army, and he is killed. That night an angel visits the pastor, and informs him that he has given up the messiah. The pastor is horrified, and exclaims, 'But how was I to know'? The angel responds, 'If you would have looked into his eyes but once, you would have known'.

This story has stayed with me throughout my ministry, because I have come to believe that much of our experience of the holy, the mystical, the spiritual and the sacred happens when we look into the eyes of creation, when we become sacredly profane, and when we enter the lives of those around us with the intention of equality, sharing, vulnerability and a sense of common humanity. The majority of my ordained ministry has been in treatment centres for people who are recovering from an addiction to a chemical. What I have to share with you today is not academic knowledge or research statistics, but the story of one life, one ministry, and some of what I have learned from the people who have participated with me in my life and in my ministry. I hope that during the course of this conference some of you will do the same with me.

I am a pastor, and my approach to recovery is largely pastoral. I am sure that many of you come from other disciplines, and I hope that some of you are also pastors, because I believe that the ministry as profession plays an important role in the interdisciplinary team approach to recovery. I further hope that as a result of this conference, we will come to see the significant impact of harmonizing different skills into an interdisciplinary approach to providing wholistic treatment for addiction.

The definition of addiction that I am most comfortable with is as follows: if a chemical is interfering in your life in any way, you are in need of recovery. There are two distinctly different approaches to addiction. One approach is to focus on the pathology of the situation, identifying the patient according to his or her disease, systematically outlining the symptoms of the illness. In the treatment of alcoholism, drug addiction, and co-addiction, this plays the important role of breaking through the denial that is intrinsic to all of these diseases. The other distinct approach to addiction is to focus on the person in treatment as being in a state of recovery, and having multidimensional aspects of being. In the years that I have been working in the field, I have experienced that the treatment emphasis is often focussed on the pathological, rather than on the process of recovery, which is in essence a return to wholeness. I have become more and more interested in shifting the focus of treatment to the recovery process, and believe that the 12 Step programmes of Alcoholics Anonymous, Narcotics Anonymous, Al-Anon, and many other programmes based on the steps were the forerunners in what we now refer to as a wholistic approach to healing. When the focus is on pathology, we hear such terms as patient, sickness, disease, dysfunction, neurotic, obsessive, and a series of other adjectives. When the focus is on recovery, we move into a vocabulary that includes such words as hope, reconciliation, balance, faith, serendipity, trust, serenity. These words describe states of being and movement, movement from a state of dis-ease to an experience of being at ease.

Addiction is characterized by distinct sets of symptoms, and the most apparent and observable aspect of addiction is bizarre, self-destructive, and unpredictable behaviour, such as lying, car crashes, radical mood swings, verbal and physical violence, suicide attempts, illegal transactions and poor physical appearance. Because these outward characteristics are so shocking, it is tempting to focus on the observable, and to believe that when these behaviours change, the disease has been arrested. This assumption is far from the truth, and represents a carryover of treating a disease by removing the symptoms, rather than striving for the goal of wholeness. It is my belief that beneath the behaviours of any human being is a complex belief system that has the power of healing and restoration. In the twelve steps of Alcoholics Anonymous, it is only the first step that mentions the word alcohol, and all of the other steps speak of taking action, and are spiritual in nature. The recovery programme is based on a spiritual awakening, and it is this spiritual awakening that is the very essence of recovery.

One of my most basic beliefs about healing is that it happens only in the context of community. We do not become whole in isolation, but only in relationship with others. As I mentioned before, addiction carries with it a set of bizarre behaviour patterns, and many professionals and lay people point to these patterns as descriptive of the toll of addiction on human life. In my own opinion, the greatest tragedy of addiction is that the addicted person and the co-addict lose the ability to love and to enter into intimate relationships. I believe love to be the epitome of the spiritual, and further believe that we would benefit from adjusting our concept of the term 'lover' to encompass the many aspects of love, rather than just the sexual component. We are capable of emotional, social, intellectual, sexual, affectionate, recreational, aesthetic and spiritual intimacy. Life pours out to us the opportunity to love life, children, animals, ourselves, skiing, laughing, people and daffodils. One of my main goals as a therapist and as a pastor is to encourage people to be lovers and to be a lover to others. When I took my training at Hazelden Foundation, I met a man named Ben Williams. When he saw me becoming afraid, stressed or overwhelmed, he would say, 'Tina, I love you'. When he thought I was really in trouble, he would say, 'Tina, *we* love you'. Because I knew that he meant it, I was often able to find the stamina to carry on. Another of my mentors, Gordy Grimm, taught me that people grow more from encouragement than from criticism. My friend the Velvateen Rabbit lives in the nursery with the Skin Horse. The Skin Horse is in rag-tag shape, having had most of his hair loved off by generations of children. The Skin Horse and the Velvateen Rabbit have a discussion about what it means to be real. The Skin Horse points out that it is only love that makes us real, and the Velvateen Rabbit then asks, 'Does it hurt to become real?' The Skin Horse responds, 'Sometimes', because he always tells the truth. (*The Velvateen Rabbit* by Margery Williams). In treatment, people are in the process of becoming real, and sometimes it hurts. People become real through the process of a kind of tough love that tells the truth, but the truth is less frightening, less painful, and more easily received when it is told in the context of a community of love. The two most important qualities offered by community are the feeling of being accepted by a group and the responsibility of being accountable to the other members of that group. I believe that both of these qualities greatly enhance recovery, and can be offered in any treatment setting.

Christopher Jones speaks of the love of one professional when he says[1]:

Little girl grown old too soon,
embittered by so many who want so much —
missionary, crying out against man's self-centeredness,
standing in the snow waiting —
shiver girl,
alone.
Little prostitute, I love you.
Joe in black leather
with licenses hands,
tough, hard, yet so very soft,

afraid,
Joe, with your girl and her baby,
homeless and alone,
drinking coffee after coffee in the all-night cafe,
I love you.
Lonely drifter, lovely drifter, crying drifter,
long-haired, tight-legged, hungry prophet,
I love you.
You, beaten in an alley, cursing, drunk, murdered
for the five hundred dollars you flashed to impress
a whore at the bar,
you, silly, absurd, loud mouthed, loud tied, murdered
brother,
I love you.
You violent youth, now on the run,
soon to be caught,
soon to feel the tight, smothering walls of prison,
you, crying somewhere now that it is too late,
I love you.
You, mother of six,
you, prostitute,
you, policeman,
you, addict,
you, pervert,
you, grandpa,
you, black brother,
you, Mister IBM,
you, soldier,
you, Mr President,
You, Reverend Sir,
you, Very Important Person,
you, Monsignor,
you, Bishop,
you, monk,
you, rich executive,
you butcher,
you, candlestick maker,
you, eleven-year old burglar,
you, you, whoever you are,
you are my brothers and my sisters,
you are my God, and I love you.

Our world has become the size of a fifty cent piece, and much of my ministry has been with people from different cultures. I have attempted to develop a global perspective when speaking of a return to wholeness, and have tried to find means of communication that are universally understood. In this attempt, I have come to depend on tools such as music, poetry, humour, story telling, and speaking of matters of the heart. One of the most exciting aspects of moving into the realm of the spiritual is that it is a universal and all encompassing experience. I attempt at all times to elicit from others their own versions of what it means to be real, what it means to believe and what it means to be a lover, and I find that most people have a deep yearning to share this part of themselves.

When people walk into a treatment centre, they bring with them a lifetime of history, experience and background, and the therapist is presented with the task of taking diversified backgrounds, and guiding individuals into a cohesive healing community. All people come with their own sets of values, limits and beliefs. One woman let me know this loud and clear when in her third day of treatment she announced to me, 'I've been shot up, I've been shacked up, and I've been knocked up, but I never let the son-of-a-bitch beat me up.'

The one common denominator of all people who are addicted to chemicals is that they are in a state of broken-heartedness. When I ask groups of addicts to tell me what it feels like to have a broken heart, it takes less than 3 minutes to fill a blackboard full of responses such as: alienation, fear, loneliness, hopelessness, despair, depression, helplessness, rage, desperation, grief, ugliness, unloveliness, separateness, sadness, weariness, homesickness, longing, self-loathing. All of these words describe a terrible sense of being apart from community, apart from love, and all of these words describe the spiritual illness that is a part of addiction. The creation of wholeness within self and within community is the task of spiritual recovery. Spiritual recovery is about mending broken hearts.

The foundation of the 12 Step recovery programme is the concept of spiritual awakening. Most people who are new to the programme are confused about the word 'spiritual', and need help in clarifying what this term means. People entering treatment bring with them considerable baggage from past religious experience and this can create a barrier in the recovery process. I find that people are able to define their own terms when given the opportunity to express themselves. I would like to stress as strongly as possible the importance of offering a non-judgemental forum for the expression of feelings and ideas, fears and reservations, hopes and dreams about the spiritual, about matters of the heart. As soon as we censor or evaluate this free expression, I believe that we lose the opportunity for movement. Those of us who are professionals may have to do some work on our own language, moving from a vocabulary of religiosity into a discourse of the spiritual. I find a tremendous reawakening in myself when I listen to others describe their own pilgrimage and wonderment.

I would like to take you through the process that my clients and I share together. The first question I raise is: What words do you associate with the word religion? Some of the responses I have received are: money, Sunday, hypocrisy, Jamestown, self-righteous, phoney, Sunday School, hellfire, organized, confession, ten commandments, offering, rigid, oratory, evangelism, heaven, brainwashing, conflict, churches, music, bingo, war, mandatory, sin, manmade, hell, rules, Jesus, communion, faith, holy, Moral

Majority, charity, Bible, prayer, punishment, million dollar churches in poor neighbourhoods. It becomes quickly evident that many of these responses have connotations of dissatisfaction, judgement, superficiality and pain. Bear in mind that the spiritual symptoms of the disease of addiction are alienation and separateness, and many addicts have felt these symptoms in terms of their religious experience.

The next question I raise is: What are your resentments about organized religion? In response to this question, I hear: Sunday morning Christians, guilt trips, taking the Bible out of context, moralizing, intolerance, unbelievable dogma, immoral clergy, holier than thou, attempts at conversion, tax free, control life, greed, manmade laws, monetary gains, gossip, judging, politics, condemnation, bigotry, rituals, self-deceit, mandatory, institutionalized, threat of damnation, lies, narrow-mindedness, in groups, humourless, door to door soliciting, apathy, fundamentalism, sexism, instilling fear, lack of true understanding. I have learned that the open expression of resentment dissipates the power of the feeling, and allows movement. After listing resentments, I point out to the group that it is their individual decision whether or not they are going to allow these resentments to stand in the way of recovery, or if they are willing to move on to the concept of the spiritual.

I then ask the group to tell me the words that they associate with the term spiritual, and the responses have included: healing, helping, open-mindedness, peace, sharing, self-esteem, awareness, sincerity, Higher Power, choice, conscience, reason for life, values, self-respect, true love, do unto others, compassion, life, faith, understanding, serenity, wonderment, caring, direction, love, forgiveness, hope, beauty, strength, inner peace, contentment, group therapy, how to treat others, joy, tranquillity, rebirth, God, belief, sincerity, divineness, personal commitment. I point out to the group that all of them, alone and together have some or all of these qualities, and that all of these qualities are available to each person. Note that many of these qualities connote wholeness, community, hospitality, love and restoration. I have seen the atmosphere of an entire room change when people begin to share their own heartfelt beliefs: voices lower in tone, the room becomes quiet and there is a sense of listening and open-mindedness.

Much of this process has to do with demythologizing the concept of the spiritual, and bringing it to a level of human understanding. My own notion of the spiritual is that it is inclusive of all of the experiences that we find most difficult to describe in words. For example, it is difficult to describe in words the process of falling in love, imagining a poem, listening to the wind or experiencing trust. I encourage people to reawaken their senses in their search for spiritual recovery. In an addicted state, people are out of touch with the pleasures of sight, smell, touch and hearing.

When we describe the spiritual in terms of the sensual, we come to see that while most of us will not travel the road to Damascus, we are ever encountering the spiritual in our midst. When I invite people to share with me the spiritual in terms of the sensual, I find that there is an immediate outpouring of the very essence and ecstasy of life, and these experiences might include: the swooshing of water along the side of a sail boat, the feel of sweat dripping during exercise, birthing a child, birthing a poem, the feel and smell of bread dough, the contact of hammer to nail or axe to wood, the cut of a skate blade against the ice, a child's touch or a dog's fur, making love, making music, making laughter, the sight of the sunrise or an eagle flying high, sharing coffee at a kitchen table, the touch of a lover, pastor, parent or friend, the breath of life, the breath of love. These experiences represent the movement of being in a lobotomized addicted state into the dance and rhythm of life.

In *Our Town*, Thornton Wilder expresses this experience[2]. Emily has been allowed to return to Grover's Corners from her grave for one last visit, and she says: 'I can't. I can't go on. Oh! Oh. It goes so fast. We don't have time to look at one another. I didn't realize. And all that was going on and we never noticed. Take me back — up the hill — to my grave. But first: Wait! One more look. Good-by, Good-by, world. Good-by, Grovers Corners . . . Mama and Papa. Good-by to clocks ticking . . . and Mama's sunflowers. And food and coffee. And new-ironed dresses and hot baths . . . and sleeping and waking up. Oh, earth, you're too wonderful for anybody to realize you. Do any human beings ever realize life while they live it? — every, every minute?' And the stage manager responds, 'No. The saints and poets, maybe — they do some.'[2] And I would add, so do many many recovering addicts, who come to believe that they have been given a second chance at life.

It is important to acknowledge that the 12 Step programme speaks of a Power Greater Than Ourselves, rather than presenting dogma about a God figure. Many of our clients do not believe in God, and we need to be respectful of the fact that people are at different points on different pilgrimages. I like to point out to my clients that the healing community is in itself a power greater than any one of us, and I encourage other interpretations, such as AA and nature, to be discussed. Self-centredness is one of the prisons of addiction, and any concept beyond self represents movement into the spiritual, movement toward the Holy Other.

Another area where people express fear is in the expression of prayer. In the eleventh step, we learn about prayer and meditation. My clients often tell me that they do not know how to pray, and this is one area where I draw heavily on music as a tool. I would like for you to listen to this song as a form of conversational prayer:

Hello again — hello!
Just called to say hello.
I couldn't sleep at all last night, and I know it's late, but I couldn't wait . . .
Hello again, my friend, hello!
Just called to let you know
I think about you every night,
and I'm here alone,
and you're there at home —
hello.
Maybe it's been crazy and maybe I'm to blame,

But I put my heart above my head.
We've been through it all, and you love me just the same.
And when you're not there, I just need to hear —
Hello, my friend, hello!
It's good to need you so!
It's good to love you like I do,
and to feel this way when I hear you say . . .
hello!
Hello, my friend, hello!
Just called to let you know,
I think about you every night,
and I know it's late, but I couldn't wait . . .
hello.
('Hello Again', sung by Neil Diamond.)

I am very grateful for the opportunities that I have had to talk about faith and hope and belief with a diversity of people. I have received countless gifts. I believe very much that it is important for people to acknowledge that they are experiencing the spiritual during their treatment. When I walk into group therapy, I often think of the Biblical phrase, 'Take off your shoes, for this is holy ground'. One of the things that we know about addiction is that it does not happen unless we go against our internal belief systems, and therefore, recovery is the process of discovering what we believe and acting accordingly. I would like to close my remarks by sharing with you a song that we have used to describe our concept of a Higher Power, and I would like to thank the countless addicts who have allowed me to look into their eyes, and who have been so willing to share their hearts with me. They have taught me that we have tremendous, magnificent and powerful abilities to heal and to love. We appreciate this opportunity to share our journey with you. Thank you.

I cried a tear, you wiped it dry.
I was confused, you cleared my mind.
I sold my soul, you bought it back for me,
and held me up and gave me dignity;
somehow you needed me.
You gave me strength to stand alone again,
to face the world out on my own again.
You put me high upon a pedestal,
so high that I could almost see eternity,
you needed me, you needed me.
And I can't believe it's you,
I can't believe it's true,
I needed you, and you were there.
And I'll never leave, why should I leave?
I'd been a fool, cuz I finally found someone who really cares.
You held my hand when it was cold.
When I was lost, you took me home.
You gave me hope when I was at the end,

and turned my life back into truth again.
You even called me friend.
You gave me strength to stand alone again,
to face the world out on my own again.
You put me high upon a pedestal —
so high that I could almost see eternity.
You needed me,
You needed me,
You needed me,
You needed me.
('You Needed Me', sung by Anne Murray.)

References

1 Jones, C. (1968). *William*, pp. 9—11. (Milwaukee: Bruce Publishing)
2 Wilder, T. (1938). *Our Town*, Act Three

22
The spiritual dynamics of recovery

J. R. DOLLARD

Those involved with people who are recovering from alcoholism or other addictions through 12 Step programmes will have heard references to 'the spiritual part of the programme' or such phrases as 'this is a spiritual programme'. 12 Step programmes clearly distinguish themselves from religions and by putting the emphasis on 'God as we understood him' avoid doctrinal and moral issues. The question for many a recovering person is 'Can I be spiritual without being religious?'; 'What does it mean for me to enter a recovery process which leads to and depends upon a spiritual awakening?' Many alcoholics have had negative experiences of religion and view anything having to do with it with suspicion. Others have sought through religion for answers and feel religion has failed them. Some will view religion as a naive and childish attempt to explain reality that has been superseded by other explanations in our modern culture. Some will have very positive attitudes toward their religious backgrounds and will find religion a great aid in recovery. Many will discover that as they progress in recovery they will become more interested in religious aids and practices. In this chapter I want to affirm that the insight that the 12 Step programme is spiritual rather than religious is a valid one and that recovery depends upon the development of a new spiritual lifestyle.

In a very real sense the addicted person has been living AWOL, an Addicted Way of Life, which is a negative spirituality that is self-destructive. The 12 Step programme is intended to provide the person a foundation for a new way of life, one which is characterized by a positive spirituality. Spirituality and religion are related to each other as infrastructure to superstructure. Spirituality is concerned with inner core of a person's capacity to relate through attitude and action to others, one's self and God. All of us, addicted or not, have a way of relating to our own lives, other people and God which tends either to be positive, healthy, fulfilling and lifegiving or tends toward

271

the negative, self-defeating and destructive. We cannot help but be spiritual. The question is what kind of spirituality will we live. Religion, I believe, is not a matter of indifference. It is not simply a question of 'all religions being the same' underneath. It makes a difference whether one takes refuge in Amida or Jesus, accepts the Koran or the Gita as telling the truth about life, views history from a Marxist point of view or human behaviour from a Freudian perspective. Religion, understood as a world view which confers ultimate meaning to life, is not a matter of interchangeable superstructures. Religion and spirituality may be distinguished as content to form. Frequently what the recovering person requires is attention to spiritual needs, i.e., development of his or her atrophied spiritual capacities and too often perhaps the well-meaning greet them with religion. They are offered a religious superstructure which their personal spiritual infrastructure is unable to bear because addiction has not nourished the infrastructure but has caused a deterioration of the capacity to be spiritual. The 12 Step programme is intended to renew the personal infrastructure of the recovering alcoholic and encourage growth from a negative spirituality to a positive spirituality. In this way the AA programme is spiritual rather than religious.

It seems there are four major characteristics of a negative spirituality which constitute an addicted way of life. The first of these is fear. Fear is not in itself evil. For the alcoholic fear has become the foundation of a way of life. Many people are unaware of the negative role fear has played in their lives. Fear of rejection, of being hurt emotionally by others, can lead a person to an isolated life, or to try to develop a series of defences which make one invulnerable to attack. Either through aggressive bravado or withdrawal such fear leads to the isolation which was originally dreaded. Fear of failure, of not measuring up to others' expectations, can lead to a life of anxiety about what others think and the constant question, 'Am I good enough'. Particularly for one addicted to alcohol or other chemicals the fear of being found out, of 'running out of my supply', of being challenged about performance can lead to the 'sense of impending doom'. Fear is at the foundation of the exaggerated mood swings characteristic of addiction.

Fear of not getting what we think we need is, perhaps, characteristic of being human. But as fear becomes a dominant fact of life and foundation for action for the addicted person it ceases to be a healthy motive for self-preservation and ends by destroying the self. Fear as a characteristic of addiction is not always easy for others to detect and many people, whether addicts or not, have repressed their fears to the point of being consciously unaware of them. The more one lives out of fear the more a foundation is being laid for a negative spirituality. The opposite of fear is trust. Our capacity to trust others, self and God is vitiated by fear. As we develop our capacity for trust fear exercises less control over our lives. Trust is not simply intellectual assent to propositions nor is faith believing 10 000 impossible things before breakfast. To trust is to risk placing one's confidence in another, to hope for the eventual well-being of that over which we do not have total control, whether it be our lives or the lives of those close to us. To trust is not to be irresponsible but to recognize and act on the fact that I am not and cannot be totally in control. The first act of trust is to stop drinking or using. Many alcoholics while actively drinking will say they cannot imagine life without alcohol. Again, this is true of any addictive attitude or behaviour. The addicted person's capacity for trust has been severely limited and it may take time to develop this vital spiritual capacity. As a general observation it seems fair to say that we will not trust a God whom we do not see if we fail to trust others whom we do. The sharing of experience, strength and hope among alcoholics and their families has been a hallmark of recovery. For many it is only in the context of AA or a similar group that this dimension of our infrastructure can be awakened and developed. The sense of relief that there are others like me, who have done what I have done, felt what I have felt, who can and will help is the awakening of trust which will be the foundation of recovery.

It seems others are trusted first and then there is a gradual expansion of this to God and self. If we recall that we are concerned with the spiritual, i.e., the personal, infrastructure of the recovering person we can grasp that one of the first important issues in recovery is the development of the capacity for trust.

A second characteristic of a negative spirituality, and one that flows from fear, is self-pity. The tendency to view one's life as unrelieved tragedy and failure, or the inability to respond to real injury or failure in a realistic way, can become part of a consistent pattern of attitudes. Self-pity as an attitude is seen in the tendency to catastrophize a situation. Sadness is a normal part of life. Sadness is not incompatible with serenity and is an appropriate response to some events in life. Self-pity is an egocentric misuse of sadness for other purposes, e.g., to drink (poor me, pour me a drink); to get attention (the pity party); to provide an excuse for other attitudes and actions (anger, buying sprees etc.). As self-pity is more and more frequently chosen as a response to life it can lead to severe depression. But short of clinical depression it can still be part of a person's basic relationship to others, self and God. In self-pity a person begins to view life as a series of 'if onlys' (if only I had a better job, had married someone else, lived elsewhere, had better clothes, more education, less education – the list is inexhaustible). Fear and self-pity reinforce each other. It may seem curious but they both result in lower self-esteem but tend to inflate the ego. Fear and self-pity as attitudes and the actions that flow from them usually leave people feeling worse about themselves. For example, they can lead to a person taking less care of their appearance, health, because 'what difference does it make'. Yet this increasing inability to 'take care of oneself' which results in lower self-esteem is also very egocentric in that the person and their troubles and fears are on centre stage all the time.

Developing our capacity for gratitude is a way of overcoming the negative effects of self-pity. Gratitude and sadness may coexist, but not gratitude and self-pity. The capacity to give thanks/be thankful is destroyed by the addictive process. The regaining of the capacity takes time and is a good indication of the progress of recovery. At the start it may be impossible for a person to be thankful for the whole of their life, including their disease. The very structure of gratitude is relational and positive, for it is a recognition of something good that has happened to or for me. Even when I am grateful for doing something positive for myself it is a building of a new self-image and understanding that is the opposite of self-pity. The maintenance of an attitude of gratitude rather than occasional spontaneous feelings (which are not to be discounted) is hard work. But a daily listing of good events, or the momentary stopping to admire and give thanks for a beautiful sunset, or the cultivation of the practice of saying 'thank you', may, on a daily basis, go a long way towards developing the personal capacity to be grateful. As aspects of a developing positive and healthy spirituality, trust and gratitude are correlative.

An addicted way of life is marked by resentments. The word resentment comes from the Latin *re-sentire*, to 're-feel'. A resentment is not simply a thinking about a past situation but is a re-feeling of it. The continual replaying and going back over a situation, event, old hurt or anger usually distorts it. A resentment may begin with being hurt or threatened in some way. However, in resentment the anger which comes up as part of our defence against such things is not dissipated after the event is over. It is as though we have videotape cassette inside of us and a whole library of resent tapes we can play. There can be quite elaborate internal wars a resentful person can carry on with people, institutions, values. We can even resent ourselves and direct the anger toward ourselves. Resentment is not always a blunt and obvious anger. It is the repetitive, circular, non-resolvable quality of the anger that is most damaging. A person caught up in resentments is living a very tense and anxious life even though outwardly it may seem calm. Resentment has been called the alcoholic's number one enemy. It is the chief block to spiritual growth not because it involves anger but because more than any other attitude it involves a judgemental spirit. As a resentful attitude becomes a way of life, it can develop in any number of directions. A person may begin to take revenge on others for real or imagined hurts. A bitter and carping spirit may develop which manifests itself in every conversation. A person may make greater efforts at control of others or events. It frequently happens that a person new in recovery is unaware of resentment in their life and such people do not see they are devouring themselves when they feast on old hurts, wrongs done to them and harsh judgement of others. As we judge others either we make ourselves superior to them or we make them superior to us. In either case it is the resentful person whose isolation is increased and self-worth is attacked or whose ego is inflated. It renders identification with the other and acceptance of the other or a situation impossible.

To move away from resentment is to develop a capacity for acceptance (forgiveness). Acceptance is not being pusillanimous. Acceptance is the acknowledgement of the limitations on our capacity to control people, events, institutions. Acceptance is not indifference. It happens, however, in the process of recovery a person frequently discovers that many things they at one time considered to be vitally important are in fact of secondary concern or of no moment at all to them. Even where there has been real hurt and anger an authentic acceptance of the givenness of a situation can replace a resentful attitude. The spiritual capacity for acceptance seems to derive from the development of our potential for trust and gratitude. The 'Serenity Prayer' may provide a clue here to what the process of acceptance is. The prayer asks for the gift of 'serenity to accept'. It does not read 'grant me acceptance that I might have serenity'. If we understand serenity as a combination of the basic trust that 'all will be well' and gratitude for the good already present, there is a foundation for acceptance. One can begin to let go of the need to control and the judging and comparing that have fueled the repetitive anger of resentments. Resentment flows directly from fear and self-pity; acceptance proceeds from trust and gratitude.

A fourth characteristic of the negative spirituality of the addictive way of life is dishonesty. The tendency of the alcoholic to deny or minimize the extent, power and effects of addiction is well-known. This is not only true for alcoholism but is also true for any addiction, whether it be to a mood-altering chemical, food, cigarettes, a person, work or goal. It is dishonesty which allows the person to see but not to see that they have chosen (are caught in) a negative spirituality, to pretend that the discomfort they feel with themselves and others is an occasional minor annoyance rather than having become a lifestyle. The deception practised by the addicted person is so often effective because they believe their own lies. When the addicted person says next time will be different or 'if I get that bad I'll stop', he or she frequently believes it and means it. The very depth of sincerity is what makes it possible to convince others. One can be sincere without being honest.

The dishonesty of the alcoholic as it relates to a negative spirituality is compulsive and unfree. Dishonesty is not simply an intentional lie now and then. It becomes a characteristic of a person's lifestyle. One of the chief effects of dishonesty is the growing fragmentation in a person's life. It might seem that the single-minded pursuit of an addiction would lead to a kind of unity but the negative spirituality we have been describing here is one which leads to disintegration. Dishonesty begins to relate not only to a person's addiction but infiltrates other areas of life as well. Recovery begins when there is a capacity for honesty at least *vis-à-vis* the addiction. The admission that 'it' is out of control, that I need help, is the foundation for recovery. Without this honesty there can be no openness to place trust in others. Trust, gratitude, acceptance lead to a greater sense of personal integrity. For the recovering person honesty is both foundation and process. Honesty is in a sense a starting point and a goal of recovery. It implies a sense of wholeness in which a person is able to acknowledge both strengths and limitations, joys and sadnesses of life, a need for giving and receiving with others without absolute dependency on them. There is growth from dishonesty to personal integrity as one becomes more free from addiction.

Review. We can distinguish religion and spirituality as superstructure and infrastructure. Alcoholism is a threefold illness which attacks not only the physical, the mental—emotional, but also the spiritual dimensions of a person. It attacks a person's capacity to lead a positive spiritual life, for as a disease it works to destroy the infrastructure. Viewed from a spiritual perspective the person is in a vicious, ever-tightening downward spiral of: fear leading to self-pity leads to resentment leads to dishonesty leads to drinking (using, or other addiction) which in turn leads back to fear. It is not simply a linear process but a circular one and can begin at any point. This is why recovery is not simply removing the addictive substance. If fear, self-pity, resentment and dishonesty continue to characterize a person's life there is a good chance the person will drink or use again. As a spiritual programme of recovery the 12 Step programmes provide a means of developing a new positive way of life based on human spiritual capacities of trust, gratitude, acceptance and integrity. The concern is with rebuilding the personal spiritual infrastructure, which will permit and empower a person to live a life free of addiction. The movement looks like this:

Fear	Trust
Self-pity	Gratitude
Resentment	Acceptance
Dishonesty	Integrity
Drinking	Sobriety

Recovery involves the restoration of the personal infrastructure that is an individual's capacity for a positive spiritual life. This involves a willingness to change, and there are three observations I would like to put forward regarding the spiritual growth.

The first observation is to note the perfectionistic tendency in many alcoholics which can block any kind of spiritual development and recovery. The 12 Step programme emphasizes that the goal is progress not perfection, to be sober not saints. Perfectionism as a block to recovery takes many guises, e.g., setting impossible standards and ideals for oneself and others, or the reverse of this by taking the attitude 'if I can't be the best of the best I'll be the worst of the worst'. As a self-directed tendency, perfectionism feeds the sense of failure and frustration characteristic of alcoholics. Directed towards others the tendency encourages a resentful attitude because others don't live up to my expectations.

Perfectionism is one manifestation of the 'big ego/low self-worth' phenomenon that is so prevalent among addicted people. It can be seen in the tendency to compare onself to others rather than identify with them. As a factor in recovery the chief reason perfectionism is an enemy of progress and the development of a positive spirituality is that it paralyses a person and keeps them from action by convincing them action is either unnecessary or will end in failure.

A second tendency which can severely retard progress in recovery is impatience. Impatience is characteristic of recovering people, perhaps of our modern culture. Impatience as a block to recovery frequently appears in the 'flurry of activity' in which a person engages in order to force a situation, person or themselves. The result of impulsive activity is frustration. The attempt to do too much too soon, to resolve all problems within the family or at work within the first months of sobriety, can result in disaster. The development of our vital spiritual capacities is not entirely under our control. There are things we can do and need to do to develop a positive way of life — to start trusting, being grateful, accepting and becoming honest — but there is not always a direct and measurable correlation between perceived effort and results.

In regard to perfectionism and impatience it may be helpful to encourage people toward small changes, e.g. to aim for the 2 % change you can make (rather than the 98 % you cannot make). An obvious kind of example would be to realize that a person may not be able to be grateful that they are alcoholic but may be able to be grateful that they are sober today. The small change in developing our capacity to trust by talking with others, expressing gratitude or letting go of a resentment can have enormous benefits.

A third block to the development of the personal infrastructure is the tendency toward intellectualization. Many recovering people seem to think if they can talk about it they've done it. Understanding what acceptance is, why it is important in recovery, and fully grasping that it would be a good thing if I were to let go of my resentment against John or Mary, is not the same thing as actually taking the necessary steps to let go of the resentment and begin accepting a person. Another dimension of problem of intellectualizing spiritual growth is the tendency to cut off feelings from thinking. More than most the addicted person has separated mind and heart. The tendency to act inconsistently solely from one or the other has caused problems. Recovery demands a willingness to allow the intellect and feelings to grow together so that the recovering person can in fact learn 'to stand before' God, self and others with the mind in the heart.

I hope the suggestions I have made in this chapter are helpful in understanding that 'this is a spiritual programme' which has a limited goal, i.e., total abstinence from alcohol or drugs or whatever dependency a person needs to be free of to live a more full life. I have attempted to show that the negative spirituality of addiction works to destroy the human potential for growth, to develop a positive spirituality is to become open to the possibility of transcendence. The life of negative spirituality leads to isolation, fragmentation and a disintegration of personality. It is an egocentric life in one sense but the ego is centred on the addiction which has on a practical level become a person's God. The spiritual dynamics of addiction point to the disintegration of the personality in terms of infrastructure, and to idolatry as the addiction becomes the person's religion. (The spiritual dynamics of recovery lead to continuing freedom from dependency.) The abiding and valid insight of the AA 12 Step programme is that it is concerned with the spiritual, i.e. the infrastructure, and as a person develops capacities for trust, gratitude, acceptance and integrity there do emerge new relationships to others, oneself and to a power greater than oneself.

23

A pastoral approach to the use of the 12 steps

R. R. LESLIE

THE PERSONAL–PROFESSIONAL JOURNEY

A reality – some personal illustration

Ever since the first thoughts of becoming a minister or pastor crossed my mind, somewhere around the age of 14 years, my life has been what I call a personal and professional journey. My belief is that most of us who have entered a religious vocation have experienced this reality and have had a similar journey. So in this presentation I want to share my thoughts from the context and experience of both the personal and the professional. The major and primary concept I want to share and encourage for your consideration could be called the 'personal–professional journey'. I don't believe my life process, both personal and professional, has been unusual or abnormal. Thus, I believe that as persons (men or women) and as theologians, we find ourselves involved in a search, a struggle, a journey that motivates us to integrate the personal–professional in ourselves as ministers and pastors.

I would like to share with you some of the story of my own personal–professional journey, and I think the elements in my story reveal this combined search and journey. I will list them in brief descriptive terms, and I ask that you use them to reflect upon your own similar journey experience and the meaning that it has had for you.

My initial vocational thoughts and feelings about the ministry during my high school education years . . . the encouragement I received from my own pastor . . .

My vocational struggle and decision-making during college and seminary years . . . should I become a doctor, minister, businessman? . . . going to

279

my campus pastor and seminary pastoral counsellor for counselling and guidance . . .

My involvement, enthusiasm and liking for Clinical Pastoral Education . . . my seminary internship in a 1 year CPE Residency Program . . .

My parish ministry years . . . hoping to demonstrate that pastors were fellow human beings . . .

My decision to enter chaplaincy and to become a CPE Supervisor . . .

My anxiety, depression, stress, and contact ulcer of the larynx leading to some brief individual psychotherapy, speech therapy, and vocational decision-making again . . .

My exposure to and training in alcoholism and chemical dependency . . . attending AA and Al-Anon meetings to learn about the programme . . . my envy of recovering alcoholics who seemed to have something spiritually that I longed for . . .

My discovery of and personal entry into the Emotions Anonymous (EA) programme . . .

My new position as a Chaplain at Hazelden in an alcoholism treatment centre . . .

My continued involvement in EA . . .

My recent family and life crises – grieving . . . feeling helpless . . .

My attempting to use daily the 12 Step programme . . . its tools . . .

The above have been some of the personal points along the road that has been my personal–professional journey. All along I can see that my profession as a pastor has influenced my person, and that my person has influenced my profession as a pastor, and that integration of the person–pastor has been most important for me.

A necessity – in giving pastoral care

I believe that a pastoral approach to using the 12 Steps necessitates a personal–professional journey in the Steps. If I'm going to work with alcoholics and recovering chemically dependent people, I need to have journeyed in the 12 Step programme personally and professionally. Other ways of saying this are: we can't *give* unless we have *received* . . . we can't *help* unless we've *been helped* . . . we can't *influence* unless we have *been influenced* . . . we can't *journey with another* unless we have *journeyed with another* . . . we can't *spiritually guide* another unless we have been *spiritually guided* . . . we can't *give* what we don't *have* . . . we can't *use* the 12 Steps unless we have *used* the 12 Steps!

So I am suggesting that for you and me to be effective pastors and helpers with alcoholics and chemically dependent people, we need to have accomplished some personal–professional integration of the 12 Step programme for ourselves.

USING THE 12 STEPS IN AN ALCOHOLISM TREATMENT PROGRAMME

The foundation of programme structure

At Hazelden the treatment programme focusses on the 12 Steps of Alcoholics Anonymous and on the overall philosophy of AA. The major focus of the treatment programme is on Steps 1–5. Chronological structure of the programme is built around these Steps. Treatment is divided into three phases, with the first phase centring on Step 1; the second phase centring on Steps 2 and 3; and the third phase centring on Steps 4 and 5. We talk about the first phase as focussing on recognizing the problem, recognizing the need for help, recognizing 'powerlessness and unmanageability'. We talk about phase two as recognizing that change is possible and making a decision to change. We talk about phase three as engaging in further self-assessment and honest admission.

Patients are assigned readings in the AA 'Big Book', *Alcoholics Anonymous* and in the *Twelve Steps and Twelve Traditions*. They are asked to memorize the Steps, to do written self-assessment assignments focussing on personal application of Steps 1, 2 and 3. They attend lectures on the Steps and other elements of AA and attend 'Step Groups' on their unit.

The Chaplain or 'clergy' on the treatment unit do a spiritual assessment interview, facilitate a Second and Third Step Group, conduct Fourth Step interviews, listen to Fifth Steps, facilitate a Grief Group.

The philosophy, language, treatment goals and methods are rooted in and structured around these Steps of AA.

Integration and practice in pastoral care

The 12 Step programme is a spiritual programme of recovery. It places emphasis on the need for 'a power greater than ourselves', a higher power, 'God as we understood him' in order to recover. Step 12 refers to the 'spiritual awakening' that occurs in the individual 'as the result of these Steps'. There are many different concepts and realities in alcoholism and in the 12 Steps that have spiritual–theological meaning and background. Acquaintance with alcoholism and the 12 Step programme has helped me 'put some meat on the bones' of my theology. There are many deep and rich spiritual and theological concepts involved — such as the concept of loss of control; surrender; powerlessness; the Big Ego; pride and grandiosity; hopelessness; loneliness; low self-worth; guilt and shame; anger and resentment; and grief. Most of these are referring to and describing aspects of the spiritual experience the alcoholic has in his active disease. In his recovery equally rich and deep realities, concepts and spiritual experiences are seen, such as increasing peace and serenity; hope; trust; honesty; willingness; letting go; coming to believe; humility; a sense of self-worth and self-acceptance.

All of these above terms, concepts and realities integrate easily for me into some of my theological and pastoral foundations, concepts and beliefs. It's enjoyable to work with patients around these issues and realities.

Some of the elements emphasized in the 12 Steps are also seen as extremely significant and critical in terms of relationship with a patient as chaplain or clergy, such elements as describing and communicating acceptance, warmth, caring, compassion and honesty.

For me the 12 Steps have personally and professionally seemed to give me the opportunity to integrate spiritual – theological beliefs and realities with real daily living behaviour, problems and issues.

USING THE 12 STEPS IN PASTORAL COUNSELLING – SOME CASE ILLUSTRATION

All of us as pastors or pastoral care givers have done pastoral counselling in our parish setting, hospital setting, or perhaps treatment programme setting. Some of my pastoral counselling has been with people who were not patients in an alcoholism treatment programme. In this section I want to share briefly some counselling experiences with those kinds of people in whose cases I believe the 12 Step programme has influenced my counselling and was used by me in different ways in the counselling process. Following are three such illustrations.

Pat K. – 'From EA to Al-Anon'

Pat and I met in 1976 as members of the same Lutheran congregation which I began to attend after moving to Minnesota. I remember her attending an adult education class presentation that I did in the congregation. My presentation was on alcoholism and chemical dependency. I also remember within the first 2 years of our acquaintance that she attended a series of adult catechism classes that I taught in the congregation, again in which I attempted in my teaching to incorporate some of the concepts of the 12 Step programme into my teaching of Luther's Catechism. During our first couple of years of being acquainted, I learned that Pat had had some emotional difficulties in the past and at one point was hospitalized for some kind of anxiety problems. She learned that I attended EA meetings and was a member of EA, and around 1978 she began to attend EA meetings also. We would usually drive together to go to a meeting which was about 15 miles from our home. Going to and from the meetings we would do a lot of discussing in the car. Pat began to share with me about her husband's drinking and the effects that she felt upon herself and family members. I began to encourage Pat to consider attending Al-Anon. After several months, she made contact with Al-Anon and began to attend some Al-Anon meetings while attending EA at the same time. This went on for a period of many months, and finally Pat stopped attending EA meetings and only attended Al-Anon. In 1981 her husband entered a treatment programme for alcoholism. Pat and other family members attended a treatment family programme and aftercare sessions. I think what I did in all of this was I helped Pat get into the right 12 Step programme eventually! It was a joy to watch her develop in awareness and also in personal growth and change as she moved along her journey. This whole process occurred over a period of approximately 5 years. At this point she's a solid Al-Anon member and we are good friends.

Karen A. – 'Taking a Look'

Karen is a woman around 40 years old, married, lives in my community, who one day in June 1977, called and asked if she could come to see me and talk about her drinking. At our first meeting we talked for about 1½ hours about her and her use of alcohol. I perceived what I believed to be symptoms of alcoholism: loss of control, use of alibis, rationalizing, preoccupation with alcohol, self-pity, alcohol-related sexual behavior, effects in family relationships.

I met with Karen for pastoral counselling sessions four times between June and December 1977. My main approach with her in counselling was, 'If you are an alcoholic, then . . .'. I tried to help her begin looking at her drinking and looking at herself as possibly having alcoholism. After our first meeting I gave her some reading material on alcoholism as a treatable illness, suggested she attend an AA meeting, and suggested that she try a 30-day test of controlling her drinking, and made an appointment with her for approximately 1 month later.

At our next meeting, Karen brought her husband along. At that meeting she told me she felt she did have 'a slight problem' with drinking and that she would be willing to investigate her problem further. As I recall she had not attended any AA meetings at that point. At the end of our second meeting I scheduled another appointment for 1 month later; asked Karen to contact the county chemical dependency centre and arrange for an alcoholism evaluation; and gave her a copy of my book by Keller, *Drinking Problem?* I also encouraged her to keep on considering whether she felt AA and/or treatment would be most helpful to her. At our third session, Karen reported that she had gone for an alcoholism evaluation, and that she had been diagnosed as alcoholic. The evaluator had recommended she consider inpatient treatment or outpatient treatment for her alcoholism. She was not willing at this point to make a decision about entering treatment. At the end of this session I encouraged her to continue considering treatment for herself; encouraged her to keep reading and gave her my own copy of the *Twelve Steps and Twelve Traditions*. I made an appointment with her for 3 months later. (Part of my approach in letting her use my own personal books was that she would feel obliged to return them to me!)

Karen did return for our fourth session. She reported that she was having no further problems, that everything was under control, that she was drinking but minimally, and that she wasn't worrying any more about her drinking. I stated to her, 'If you are alcoholic, you may still be hoping and controlling for right now'. The outcome of our session was that we agreed to meet again in 6 months. Karen didn't show for our appointment 6 months later. I called her on the telephone and she stated she had forgotten to mark it on the calendar. She also reported that she was having no problem, but did describe a few times of heavy drinking to me over the phone. My response to her was, 'If you are alcoholic, then some of the things you are talking about with me sound like reasons for drinking'. I again simply encouraged Karen to keep looking at the possibility of having alcoholism, and to give me a call if she felt it was necessary in the future. I have not seen her since.

Kris C. – 'Al-Anon to EA and back again'

Kris is a 27-year-old married woman who came to see me in October 1981. She wanted to counsel with a pastor who also had knowledge of the Emotions Anonymous 12 Step programme and someone had referrred her to me. She came to me as an EA member. She shared and we discussed her history of emotional problems. We met for pastoral counselling sessions five or six times at 2-week intervals. During the course of counselling she also described a family and marital history that included alcoholism and chemical dependency, as well as her own prior involvement in the Al-Anon 12 Step programme. In counselling with her I gave her support in her EA 12 Step programme. However, I also suggested and encouraged that she consider returning to Al-Anon. She shared and we discussed her negative attitudes toward her previous Al-Anon experience and some of her resentment toward Al-Anon. One of the goals that emerged in counselling was for Kris to do a Fourth and Fifth Step again as part of her personal EA programme. She agreed to this, and in January 1982 we met for three sessions that were designated as her Fifth Step sessions. Currently we are meeting monthly in terms of ongoing counselling and support. Kris did return to Al-Anon and has been attending Al-Anon meetings and EA meetings for the past 3–4 months. She expresses positive attitudes, feelings and thoughts and also some amazement as to how meaningful and helpful her return to Al-Anon has been for her. It looks like she is someone for whom the return to Al-Anon has been very significant and important, and for whom the combination of Al-Anon and EA will be helpful.

SUMMARY

Theology, pastoral care, and the 12 Steps

As a person, theologian and pastor I have not experienced conflict between the 12 Step programme and my own theology and pastoral care concepts. In fact, as I alluded to before, the 12 Step programme has given me a deeper, richer, more alive grasp of my own spirituality. My spiritual−religious life has become more alive for me. My theology has taken on the realities of daily life. God as I understand him and my relationship to him have become more real and practical for me. I do feel a sense of indebtedness and gratitude to the alcoholism field and to Alcoholics Anonymous for nurturing my own spiritual personal−professional growth.

Being involved in the personal−professional journey

As I've stated above, it is my belief that in order to best learn, prepare, serve, and sustain, I believe that we need to be involved in our own personal−professional journey with the 12 Steps. Thus personal involvement in AA, Al-Anon, EA, Overeaters Anonymous (OA) or other 12 Step programmes that are appropriate for us is the best way for us to learn about using the 12 Steps with alcoholic and chemically dependent people. I encourage you to consider this kind of journey for yourself.

Bibliography

1 Jourard, S. M. (1971). *The Transparent Self.* (New York: Van Nostrand)
2 Keller, J. E. (1969). *Ministering to Alcoholics.* (Minneapolis: Augsburg Publishing House)
3 Keller, J. E. (1971). *Drinking Problem?* (Philadelphia: Fortress Press)
4 Kurtz, E. (1979). *Not God: A History of Alcoholics Anonymous.* (Center City, MN: Hazelden Educational Services)
5 Sellner, E. C. (1980). *The Event of Self-Revelation in the Reconciliation Process: A Pastoral Theological Comparison of A.A.'s Fifth Step and the Sacrament of Penance.* PhD Dissertation, University of Notre Dame
6 Sellner, E. C. (1981). *Christian Ministry and the Fifth Step.* Professional Education Series, Booklet No. 8. (Center City, MN: Hazelden Educational Services)
7 Tiebout, H. M. *The Act of Surrender in the Therapeutic Process. Surrender Versus Compliance in Therapy. The Ego Factors in Surrender in Alcoholism.* (And other pamphlets distributed by the National Council on Alcoholism, Inc., 733 Third Avenue, Suite 1405, New York, NY 10017)
8 (Anonymous) (1976). *Alcoholics Anonymous.* 3rd Edn. (New York: Alcoholics Anonymous World Services, Inc.)
9 (Anonymous) (1953). *Twelve Steps and Twelve Traditions.* (New York: Alcoholics Anonymous World Services, Inc.)
10 (Anonymous) (1973). *Came to Believe.* (New York: Alcoholics Anonymous World Services, Inc.)

24
A spiritual foundation

W. F. COX

I am a parson, retired from full-time parish work and therefore trying to find the most worthwhile things to do. I find my weekly visit to Broadway Lodge, an alcoholism treatment centre in Weston-super-Mare, very worthwhile indeed. I feel privileged to take part in what is disciplined teamwork by a dedicated staff interpreting the first five steps of Alcoholics Anonymous as the road to recovery for alcoholics, and as a parson, to have personal contact with individual patients taking their Fifth Step.

Gradually, the general public is beginning to recognize that alcoholism is a disease and that just to help an alcoholic to 'dry out' doesn't tackle the disease at all. Healing is a question of wholeness and that means wholeness in the complete human personality. So this statement in *Not God* by Ernest Kurtz[1], which is a history of AA, is, I think, very important. He says ' "alcoholism is a three-fold disease — physical, mental and spiritual". The clear message is that there is a unity in human life, ill or healthy. The parts of the human experience are so interconnected that to suffer disturbance in one is to suffer dislocation in all; and in recovery, all must be attended to if any is to be healed.'

It is encouraging, indeed exciting, to see this kind of recovery happening; to see alcoholics being changed, discovering a new philosophy of life, finding and keeping sobriety and thus regaining hope, becoming honest and human once again. And this is achieved by acknowledging their powerlessness over alcohol and their need of outside help and that they can't run their own lives by themselves. It is achieved by acknowledging and feeling the damage they have done so that, having been brought low, having reached the bottom as it were, they are willing to hand over their lives to a Higher Power as each person understands that term — in fact to make a daily act of surrender to God. 'Out of the deep have I called unto thee O Lord', and the *cri de coeur* is answered.

The philosophy of AA contains overtones from the Oxford Group of the 1930s with its emphasis on personal conversion and its four 'absolute' standards of conduct — honest, purity, unselfishness and love. It also owes a debt to the writings of William James in his book *The Varieties of Religious Experience*[2] in which he summed up the characteristics of the religious life in all religions:

(1)   That our visible world is part of a more spiritual universe from which it draws its chief significance.

(2)   That union or harmonious relation with that higher universe is our true end.

(3)   That prayer or inner communion is a process by which spiritual energy flows into peoples' lives and produces effects.

(4)   That the effects include a new zest for life, an assurance of safety and a temper of peace, and in relation to other people a preponderance of loving affection.

AA was also influenced by psychologists like C. G. Jung* who openly stated 'among all my patients over thirty-five years of age, there has not been one whose problem in the last resort was not that of finding a religious outlook on life'. This endorses the well known saying of St Augustine that God has made us for himself and that our hearts are restless till they rest in Him.

It seems to me that the realization of the spiritual reality of life can come to a person in three different ways. It can come through intellectual conviction and this may have been the Church's traditional way of approach. It may come from a subjective feeling that God cares, that 'underneath are the everlasting arms'. It may come from doing things for other people, from unselfish action, from love being put into practice. It is in the second and third ways, rather than the first, that I have seen faith coming to alcoholics.

The whole programme at Broadway Lodge helps towards this — as it were, softens the ground. Before treatment and when an alcoholic first arrives, he would much perfer to keep himself to himself. He dislikes company, but in treatment he is placed alongside fellow alcoholics. He helps in the kitchen and in looking after the house, he gets into conversation and shares his experiences, and thus by giving and receiving, he finds himself a member of a caring community. All this, I believe, helps to awaken faith in a spiritual dimension.

I have learned that besides our subconscious mind there is another part of ourselves we cannot see. That is the part which everybody else sees — hence the power of group therapy to enable us to see ourselves as others see us. In this context the Sunday visit of relatives sharing in this group therapy, no longer protecting the patient but honestly pointing out how the patient's past behaviour has caused pain and damage, helps the patient to face reality. It hits home. Again, after listening to a life story — and each patient has to read his or her life story — the power of the group comes out in the 'confrontation' letters

---

* C. G. Jung — one of the greatest medical and psychiatric specialists practised in Zurich, Switzerland and was the friend and adviser of the founding members of AA. Questioned by a despairing alcoholic who had tried every kind of treatment with no success and who asked him whether there might be any *other* hope, Jung spoke of 'a spiritual or religious experience — in short a genuine conversion'. (See *Not God*[1] p. 9.)

that follow. There is no collusion between the writers but it is amazing how each fastens on the things that need putting right. The good letters have a sting in them, but they also give the recipient hope and that is a spiritual virtue none of us can do without.

Every day counts and what happens at the beginning of the day sets the tone for what follows. I am sure that a very important part of the programme is the Quiet Time in the morning, reading the *Day by Day* Book[3], looking up and saying "Good Morning" to God. That is a habit which bears fruit. In the same way, the frequent saying of the Serenity Prayer, 'God grant me the serenity to accept the things I cannot change, the courage to change the things I can — and the wisdom to know the difference', is a salutary reminder of God's presence; and the holding of hands while it is being said brings home the comradeship of seeking, that we are all in this together.

Many who are patients have been out of touch with the spiritual life perhaps since childhood, but the seeds are still there deep down and they begin to grow again. As feeling comes back, it includes a spiritual consciousness that God cares for them individually.

The third step in the programme, the daily handing over of life to a Higher Power, is the foundation of recovery. I am sure that for most people this has to be a daily surrender and the reality of its meaning can only happen gradually. On the other hand some people undoubtedly receive an immediate sense of God's presence. The atheist or the agnostic finds his Higher Power in the group, in each meeting of AA, but if they begin there with an open mind, as a seeker after truth, I believe they are on the way to a deeper experience. 'Seek and ye shall find', as Christ said. 'Knock and it shall be opened unto you.' Expose yourself to the truth and the experience will come. I find the majority acknowledge that they are sure they were meant to come for treatment — it wasn't just their idea. The idea of God's providence in bringing them to recovery begins to dawn. God cares.

The spiritual awakening isn't in any sense 'churchy', though very often patients taking their Fifth Step plan to be in touch with their Church when they go home. It is the feeling of being helped up the stairway of life with a new zest, a new joy in living. It is a feeling that whatever happens, there are banisters there which will hold.

AA literature has many examples of this experience. Let me quote from the book, *Came to Believe*[4]. 'I had four good sponsors. One was my spiritual adviser with whom I felt little empathy. I often listened against my will but one day he struck a responding chord. He said "when you have used up all resources of family, friends, doctors, and ministers, there is still one source of help. It is one that never fails and never gives up and is always available and willing." These words returned to me one morning at the end of a three week binge in a hotel room. I was acutely aware of the shambles my life had become. Now my second marriage was on the rocks, and the children were being hurt. That morning, I was able to be honest. I knew I had failed as a father, husband and son. I had failed at school and in the service and had lost every job or business I had tried. Neither religion, the medical profession or

AA had succeeded with me. I felt completely defeated. Then I remembered some of the words of my sponsor — "When all else had failed, grab a rope and hang on. Ask God for strength to stay sober for one day."

'I went into the filthy bathroom and got down on my knees. "God, teach me to pray" I begged. I remained there a long time, and when I arose and left the room, I knew I never had to drink again. I came to believe that day that God would help me maintain my sobriety. Since then I've come to believe that He will help me with any problem. During the years since my last drink, I haven't encountered as many problems as before. As I grow more capable of understanding the things that have happened to me, I don't think it was on that morning in the hotel that I found God. I think He had been with me at all times, just as He is in all people, and I uncovered Him by clearing away the wreckage of my past.'

'The wreckage of our past' — whoever wrote the *Fourth Step Inventory*[5] was a very wise man. The negative part consisting of examining one's character defects and measuring oneself up against the cardinal sins and the Ten Commandments is a necessary emptying of the dustbin, and a conscious facing up to damage, a confession to God which, when sincere, brings His healing forgiveness. It has to be pointed out that character defects are not all due to alcohol and will always need to be watched and worked at — for we all make habits and it is very hard to change one's habits. But it is the positive side of facing the future with secure foundation which gives balance to the Fifth Step which follows. And the foundation is clearly based on the virtues of faith and hope and love, on working out a plan for daily living, on finding the right attitudes to life, and on acknowledging our responsibility to God, to ourselves, to our family, to our work and, for the alcoholic, the essential responsibility to Alcoholics Anonymous.

There is great encouragement to those in treatment to meet ex-patients who come back for aftercare who have been putting these principles into practice and can share their experience of going out into the world. Life isn't easy for those who go home. It takes a long time to regain the trust of relations and friends. In a sense a centre like Broadway Lodge resembles a greenhouse, and just as new plants must be planted out and face cold winds and storms, so it is for those who leave treatment. They have to discover that they must keep taking in to be able to keep sober and give out to others and this means frequent contact with their sponsor, regular attendance at AA meetings, daily prayer and surrender of one's life to God and asking for help for each day, one day at a time. These are the first things first — the things that really matter. The first five steps lead on to the other seven and to the ability to help other alcoholics, to give as well as to receive, to keep sobriety and to find fulfilment — fulfilment on a spiritual foundation.

What I have been trying to say is, I think, summed up in this little poem:

Upon the wreckage of thy yesterday
Design the structure of tomorrow;
Lay strong corner stones with strength and purpose;

Great blocks of wisdom from past despair;
Strong mighty pillars resolve to set
Deep in tear-wet mortar of regret;
Work well with patience, tho' thy toil be slow,
Yet day by day thy edifice shall grow.
Believe in God and in thine own self believe,
Then all thou hast desired, thou shalt achieve.

Bibliography

1 Kurtz, E. (1979). *Not God: A History of Alcoholics Anonymous.* (Center City, MN: Hazelden Education Services)
2 James, W. *The Varieties of Religious Experience*, p. 464. (London: Collins Fount Paperbacks edition)
3 *Day by Day* (1974). (Center City, MN: Hazelden Foundation)
4 (Anonymous) (1973). *Came to Believe*, pp. 35, 36. (New York: Alcoholics Anonymous World Services Inc.)
5 *A Guide to the Fourth Step Inventory*. (1978). (Center City: Hazelden Foundation)

25
My involvement in an alcoholic treatment unit

L. VIRGO

The title is an opening to describe an effect and a first cause: to describe some current work with the spiritual development of alcoholics, and a first cause in that the basis of my approach today is rooted in my experience in the alcoholic treatment unit of Pinel House at Warlingham Park Hospital between 1965 and 1974. I owe a debt to alcoholics. I believe that anyone who really works with people who suffer in this way will owe them a debt. Those who face up to their addiction and begin the struggle through to sobriety can only do so if they fight for their lives. There is no room for niceness or cover-up, there has to be the exposing of the real person. My debt is due to all those people who trusted me enough to share with me their suffering and themselves. Such suffering experienced, faced and lived through has led me to a completely new view of the theology of suffering – and of health; as well as to a new understanding of revelation. There is a tendency in religious consciousness to turn everything to sweetness and light: to cover up the harsh and hard. The Alcoholic must discover God through the experience of the harsh and hard: thus through the experience of the Cross.

Nasrudin is a sort of prophet or holy man who spreads his gospel by telling stories about himself. One such story tells of the occasion when Nasrudin is looking around in the gutter under the lamp post outside his house. A friendly neighbour comes along and discovers that Nasrudin is looking for his front door key and helps him look. Soon a half-dozen neighbours are all searching under the lamp post for the key. Eventually the first neighbour stands back and asks 'by the way, Nasrudin, where exactly did you lose your key?' 'Inside the house!' 'Why on earth are we looking out here then?' 'But this', says Nasrudin pointing to the lamp post, 'this is where the light is!'[1]

The real problems of life are not resolved by looking where the light is, but by taking the risk of going into the dark. Letting go of alcohol, taking the first step, is always a step into the dark. Most alcoholics will have made all sorts of attempts to solve the problem 'where the light is' by geographical escapes, by going from spirits to beer, from beer to wine, from alcohol to pills. In the end the beginning of recovery comes with that step into the darkness which is saying, 'I don't drink – for the next 24 hours'. That step into the dark can be a discovery of a new light, a new life. The backbone of AA meetings is the 'Chair' in which a person will contrast the darkness of the drinking days with the light of sobriety.

However there will always be those for whom the discovery of the supporting fellowship and family of AA will not be enough – those who may achieve sobriety but will remain flattened or stressed in unfulfilled dryness. For such people a fourth and fifth step will lead them back into the darkness of their interior house to discover the key. In *Paradise Lost* Milton says, 'Long is the way and hard that out of Hell leads up to light'. There are those for whom there is no other way to the discovery of true light in life than through the harrowing of their own personal hell. Milton is paraphrasing Virgil, who even more adequately describes the journey: 'So he prayed with his hands on the altar and while he still prayed the prophetess began to answer: Seed of the blood divine, man of Troy, Archis' son, the descent to Avernus is not hard, throughout every night and every day black Pluto's door stands open wide but to retrace the steps and escape back to upper airs that is the task and that is the toil'.

'To retrace the steps and escape back to upper airs', that is the task and that is the toil that we became involved in in Pinel House. I would like to describe something of our approach to treatment there, and then say how I use this similar approach in work with people on their fourth and fifth step today: the recovery of faith and the deepening of the spiritual life.

In the first 3 weeks of involvement at Pinel House people came to Group 1, in which there was an introduction to the group process. They were encouraged to see that they could only get from a group to the extent that they were willing to put into it. The main focus of the groups was an exploration and release of feelings. The aim was described as a revaluing by each individual of themselves. Sometimes the computer analogy would be used: each person is like a computer – when we are born we are unprogrammed but we are open to programming. The first thing that happens to the child is that she or he begins to be programmed. When your mother picked you up for the first time, how did she hold you? With anxiety and nervousness? With a non-caring rejection, pushing you away? With a feeling that you were dirty and messy? Or was it with a sensuousness and warmth which responded to you as a baby? Whatever way we were responded to began the programming of the sort of person that we feel we are today. The sort of person I am and my response to life goes on having a relationship to that bedrock of early experiences.

To some extent all of us have had wrong answers fed into us. Feelings of valuelessness, basic anxiety; unwantedness may be our bedrock, axiomatic self-evaluation. However people may try and reassure us we still go on giving the basic answers and need to reassess them. This was part of the basis of our approach at Pinel, and has continued to be my approach since in working with people in the community.

To live with established ideas and patterns and then to question and change them leads to confusion. Yet the fact is that those of us who break down in any way are discovering that our way of coping is inadequate. One of the clearest indications that a person is beginning to change is a sense of confusion.

That a baby should be made to feel she or he is worthless, dirty, rejected, is to make the child relate to a lie. It is in the countering of these lies that the group will be engaged: helping each person to come to a new assessment of themselves through joining in a group. The group becomes our echo of the original family. Feelings from childhood are recapitulated, and can be reassessed. This process was made possible by encouraging each person to write a life story and present it to the group after about 6 weeks in the unit. The emphasis of the life story was the emotional biography, focussing as much as possible on feelings remembered during the whole process of life. The life story produces points of identification with others, breaking the common feeling of isolation. The patterns of repeating behaviour in the life experience gave clues to the way the person experienced their world: we tend to reproduce elements of our childhood world in our adult life, since this is the familiar way the world is. However painful that early world may have been, it was 'the world' and goes on providing boundaries in the view of the world today.

Through these Pinel groups I came to my practical understanding of Object Relations Theory which is now a primary tool. This practical use of object relations maintains that we only get to know ourselves in relationship to our surroundings and to the persons who are reacting to us. As infants we are not aware of others as persons but as objects which affect us and which we can affect.

We can imagine the infant in the centre of a circle: the circle of the family environment – primarily, at first, of mother, but also of the atmosphere of 'home'.

The way mother responds to us will begin the process of our learning about life and about ourselves, about femininity, mothering, sexuality, safety, trust and complexity, of learning in relation to Mother as object.

Add to this circle father – what sort of father do you add? The caring, strong, responsive, nurturing and controlling ideal Dad – or the brutal, punishing, threatening dictator? Or maybe something in between? Brothers, sisters, grandmothers and grandfathers – all the significant persons of childhood – take their place in the circle, each having a different attitude to the child in the centre. From each the child is discovering its measurements – measurements of itself, and its world.

That which is modelled in childhood becomes the person's norms. This is what masculinity, femininity, love, life is all about. How we receive life and react to it depends on how we receive communications from these primary objects which surround us in our growth process – not only of family life but of the thought and experience of God.

A frequent question for alcoholics is 'What does "love" mean?' So often the experiences of childhood have been harsh, deprived, often quite demonic. Berger in his *Rumour of Angels* points out that the ordering gestures of mother as she puts her arms round a disturbed baby will have a transcendent significance for the infant. Dis-ordering gestures are also transcendent. God comes with many faces. For most people suffering the deprivations of life that have led to alcoholism, the face of God is distorted. The transcendent is understood and measured by the ordering of early life experience.

The application of Object Relations Theory enables a reconstruction of ideas and attitudes towards God as well as towards others and the self. The model can be invaluable in fourth and fifth step work generally and particularly in helping people to discover and rediscover faith. Many people who go through a recovery process, whether it is with AA or with a treatment unit, are left very unsure of their faith – not knowing where to turn to find somebody who will really understand them and their doubts and fears. Through the object relations process it is possible to build up a personal experience of all that is meant by the injunction to love God with all the heart, soul, mind and strength and to love your neighbour as yourself. This time to begin with loving yourself. To love the self, to accept the self, a person must know himself or herself. A lot of the alcoholic pattern is a defence against self-knowledge. In order not to know the self – drink! The dark and dangerous journey, the journey out of hell, means first of all going back into the hell in order to discover the self. That can be very painful, very hard.

Let us look at an example, Tony.

Tony certainly found the journey hard. But there could be nothing harder than living in the hell of alcoholic addiction for 15 years.

Brought up by a totally non-caring, self-centred mother, and a father concerned only with intellectual success and social mobility, Tony suffered. Rickets in infancy indicate the deprivation he suffered. Hiding under the table was a way to escape parental battles. More often, window shopping through the street was the escape route. The Roman Catholic Church offered a nirvana of security and peace – so long as you kept the rules.

Tony found more rules to keep than even the Church had invented. With guts and determination he made his way to professional excellence. Before his colleagues he appeared assured and confident. To himself he was a terrified child. Marriage and fatherhood produced the final strains: how to be a husband/father? Drinking gave a two-edged solution – a greater feeling of confidence, and an ability to let go and be a tearaway.

Of course the drinking slowly destroyed: ate further into confidence, ability, credibility. Tony crashed. AA rescued and began to restore. Feelings of inadequacy and yet the need to excel remained. Failing God, guilt and remorse waxed large. From this background Tony came into his fourth step experience. He began to look painfully and hesitantly at his feelings today as related to the patterning of yesterday. He began to be aware of his battered child not, as before, as one who deserved all he got, but as a victim. Having felt that the verdict of his parents on the child as spineless, incompetent, useless, were justified, he began to reverse these judgements and to accept the child in all its need and hunger for love.

At the moment he recalled the terrified 3-year-old screwed up in a pool of his own urine trying to disappear, at that moment, seeing the child before him, he could reach out in desire to take, hold, comfort his own child. Becoming a good parent to his own child, Tony begins to ascend the steps that lead up from darkness into light. No easy, quick path; each step worked for, slipped from, regained. With each step sobriety becomes celebrated rather than endured, God becomes the Lover rather than the Judge.

Now whenever he gets into points of tension and stress Tony remembers the little child. He holds the little child's hands and remembers that it was Jesus who said, 'unless you become as a little child you cannot enter into the Kingdom'. It was Jesus who took the little child and sat him on His knee. So Tony acts for Christ, Christ can act for him taking up, nurturing, loving his little child. He can be not only the nurturing parent but also the controlling parent. Finding the boundaries of 'ought' and 'should' for himself, Tony no longer has to be ruled and structured by his parents who themselves were warped and distorted by their past.

Through the process of these object relations exercises, people can come to discover a love for themselves and so for their neighbour. By learning to love the brother they can see to really discover the love of the God they cannot see. No one can really love the neighbour before he has learnt to love himself. I believe that spiritual work, not only with alcoholics but for all of us, must lie in the discovery of the ability to know and love ourselves. If we do not do this all our operations are self-defensive. We are defending against self-knowledge. I think that Christians like to go round saying, 'we are Christians, we must be like cornflakes, crisp and ready to serve', and instead of that they are really all very soggy underneath. We are soggy underneath because we spend our time defending against self-knowledge. We serve other people in order not to look at ourselves. We are running away from the honest admission of who we are. I believe that until and unless we do that we cannot really be of service to our fellow men and we cannot really say that we know and love God. I think that the way back to the upper airs is the task and the toil, it is dark and it is difficult but it is the way that Christ opens up for us because he harrowed hell. One other aspect that I find invaluable in working in the spiritual programme with the alcoholic is to recognize the shepherding element of the atonement − the fact that the shepherd does not come to the edge of the precipice and say 'come along, little lamb, climb up to me', he actually goes down into the darkness to bring the lamb up, carries it back on his shoulders. In the darkness of despair, in the disease of alcoholism, the person has perhaps been closer to Christ than ever before. If you can be with Christ in the darkness then you can be with him in the light of the resurrection. It is the empathetic Christ who from the cross says 'I thirst'. It is for me the Christ who enters into the estrangement, the alienation to which the human soul is heir, who becomes the atoning shepherd. It is he who carries us back and brings us into the fold of our own family, the family of AA, the family of the Church, above all brings us back into the family of humanity. One of the greatest elements of forgiveness that happens in fourth and fifth step work is the forgiveness that comes when the person accepts himself or herself because they find themselves accepted by the one they are working with. The movement outwards in understanding and acceptance to parents, siblings, family and friends is the one proper movement of restoration, for it is restoring to others the genuine self I had denied them, and in denying made them suffer. With such restoration comes release from self-concern and freedom for responsible living.

'I am come that they might have life and have it more abundantly.'

Reference

1   Idries Shah (1966). *Nasrudin*. (London: Picador)

Part 6:
ALCOHOLISM – PSYCHOLOGICAL ASPECTS

26

Behaviour therapy training for social workers, psychologists and physicians working in the addiction field

H. VOLLMER and R. SCHNEIDER

INTRODUCTION

Current situation

In the Federal Republic of Germany, psychotherapeutic care in the field of alcoholism is primarily performed by social workers, psychologists, and physicians. This applies both to inpatient and outpatient institutions. During the training of these professional groups, both at universities and at professional colleges, the use of therapy in dealing with alcoholism is rarely included in the syllabus.

The psychologist, social worker or physician will become familiar with addiction work only when he begins to work in a clinic or in a counselling service for addicts. Normally he will be introduced into this area by his colleagues. The relevant therapeutic skills are acquired through supervision by colleagues, in case discussions and by reading pertinent literature. Depending on the work load in the institution, these forms of training may be utilized to different degrees. Even under favourable conditions, however (personal assignment, working atmosphere, accessibility of literature etc.), it is apparent that attendance at weekend seminars and the availability of other possibilities will not normally suffice for the acquisition of psychotherapeutic abilities and that in fact, extensive postgraduate training will be required.

Training during professional practice

In view of the present organizational framework it will only rarely be possible to have the practical training carried out by the universities and professional colleges, for instance in addiction therapy or therapy for other disturbances. These institutions are occupied to a large degree with the teaching of psychological, medical, and social-pedagogical knowledge. With regard to the university education of psychologists, the 'permanent conference of the representatives of clinical psychology and psychotherapy' (*ständige Konferenz der Vertreter für Klinische Psychologie und Psychotherapie*) has come to the conclusion that 'upon the completion of his studies, the graduate psychologist specializing in clinical psychology and psychotherapy will be in a position to work diagnostically, consultatively, therapeutically, and preventatively, subject to supervision and guidance. In order to reach a level of full responsibility and independence in the practice of psychotherapy he will require inservice training of 2−3 years' duration following the diploma in psychology.' (reference 1, p. 159).

This statement concerning training in clinical psychology may also be applied to the group of physicians and social workers involved in the care of addicts, even though this is a different therapeutical field.

Training during professional practice subsequent to university or college education has the following advantages.

(1)   Social workers, psychologists, and physicians do not have to specialize during the period of their studies. This would be necessary as it is not possible during the short period of university or college education to give equal coverage to all disturbances and relevant practical therapies. Furthermore, such early specialization does not appear to be purposeful.

(2)   Social workers, psychologists, and physicians already have practical experience and professional competence in dealing with alcoholics, which they may contribute in the postgraduate training, and which will enable them to take an active part in compiling seminar subjects within the framework of the training concepts.

(3)   The professional experience of the participants will enable them to suggest various subjects which are important for the practice of therapy. In the case of professional beginners, such subjects could be treated on a theoretical level only, such as the analysis of patient−therapist interaction, the analysis of feelings, thoughts and behaviour of the therapist towards various patients or the effects of organizational conditions on therapeutical action.

(4)   The training programme is tested directly in professional practice. Thus the participants may test what has been dealt with in the training immediately in their practical work, thereby experiencing direct feedback from their behaviour. In accordance with the principle of operant conditioning, learning effectiveness will be improved. In

addition, the instructors will obtain feedback on the feasibility of their instructions and suggestions while training is still in progress and the subjects will thereby be adapted to the needs of the participants in the best possible manner.

(5) The participation of various professional groups in a postgraduate training group will be facilitated by the fact that the participants have similar background experience and this will promote the inter-disciplinary co-operation which is necessary in the field of addiction work.

The necessity for postgraduate training programmes

The need for postgraduate training programmes is supported by the results of interviews, carried out with staff members of outpatient and inpatient institutions. Repeated surveys of counselling services and rehabilitation institutions for drug addicts made between 1973 and 1977 show that there is a considerable discrepancy between the number of staff members who are involved in therapeutical work and the number of staff members who have had an appropriate training in psychotherapy[2]. Based on these surveys, Bühringer[2] recommends that at least half of the case workers involved in the care of addicts should have a completed training in therapy; in this he is taking into consideration the organizational and financial limitations of the institutions.

Interviews with staff members of counselling services which mainly deal with young alcoholics have shown that the most frequently used methods in therapy for addicts are: client-centred therapy, behaviour therapy, gestalt therapy and therapies which are psychoanalytically oriented. Only a small proportion, however, of the persons interviewed had a completed training in these methods. A large number of the case workers (46–64 %) therefore also felt insecure in the application of these procedures (exception: client-centred therapy)[3].

Confidence in the use of therapeutic methods may be increased in various ways. One possibility could be participation in a postgraduate training course[4]. Another factor which appears to increase confidence in the practice of therapy is frequency in the application of a method. Therapists believe that they are more secure in methods which they use more frequently[3]. Especially when one considers the variety of skills required for the individual therapies, this may be seen as an indication that the case worker should limit himself in practice to one line of therapy instead of using several different procedures. He should, however, have a full command of that line of therapy[4].

This principle is realized in two different postgraduate training programmes which differ in their theories without being mutually conflicting. One of these, the behaviour therapy programme, will be presented here (see section on Description of the Training, below). The psychoanalytic postgraduate training programme is discussed by Lindner[5]. Preliminary results have been described by Triebel[6].

DEVELOPMENT AND MODIFICATION OF THE TRAINING

The behaviour therapy training programme was developed and introduced in successive phases. Although the programme development cannot be considered as having been finally completed – despite positive experience in the training achieved so far – the various development phases will be described in detail and the present situation regarding the testing of the training will be described.

(1)   *Determination of the existing situation.*
       The determination of the existing situation may be divided into the situation regarding (a) the therapy institutions and (b) postgraduate training programmes.
       Therapy institutions: A research project, commencing in 1973 and covering the planning, control and evaluation of therapy institutions drew the conclusions, described above, concerning the necessity of supplementary training in psychotherapy[2]. The staff members of the institutes involved in postgraduate training reached the same conclusions on the basis of random personal interviews and observations.
       Postgraduate training programmes: In her article surveying psychotherapeutic training programmes, Matarazzo[7] writes, 'Research on the teaching of psychotherapy skills is still in its early stages, necessarily moving no faster than our knowledge of some of the important dimensions of psychotherapeutic behaviour, as well as our ability to measure them and some of the significant dimensions of patient improvement' (p. 919).
       It is true that at that time various training programmes were in existence[8, 9]. Psychotherapeutic training during professional practice in the field of behaviour therapy for addictions was unknown at that time, when the initial results of experience with behaviour therapy for addictions were only just becoming available in the Federal Republic of Germany. An original training programme in behaviour therapy therefore had to be developed, making use of experience gained in other general training programmes.

(2)   *Interviews with experts.*
       In addition to the analysis of existing literature, experts were personally interviewed (Brengelmann, Kanfer, and others) concerning the structure (subjects and form) of the training. The combination of psychotherapeutic methods and skills to be trained was based on the experiences of a study group which was engaged in the development and testing of behaviour-therapeutical treatment programmes in the addiction field[10-15].

(3)   *Testing of the curriculum.*
       This study group also conducted the first three training courses, based on the curriculum[16] drawn up on the basis of the interviews with

experts and the analysis of the existing situation, thereby establishing a basis of experience for future training courses.

(4) *Modification of the training programme.*

The experience with the first training groups was successful and the feedback from the participants and the instructors made only insignificant modifications of the programme necessary with regard to subjects and didactical and organizational components (for instance: extension of the training by two seminars and microteaching of skills required for behaviour analysis or assertiveness training). Furthermore, the therapeutical methods and skills to be trained were adjusted according to knowledge acquired as a result of more recent therapy investigations (for instance: cognitive therapies, analysis of patient–therapist interaction).

At present, the structure of the postgraduate training as described in its four successive phases is being maintained. The constant improvement of behaviour therapy procedures and the limited knowledge available concerning the teaching of psychotherapeutical skills prevent a final completion of the curriculum. In addition to the continuation of the analysis of the existing situation, the interviewing of experts, the testing of the curriculum and the amendment of the training programme (Figure 26.1), efforts are being made to improve the evaluation of the training step by step. Since this does not primarily represent a research project, but a field study, the scientific evaluation of the training is limited. In accordance with the principle of behaviour therapy to examine empirically the effectiveness of the therapy procedure applied, an attempt is made here to give a rough indication of the effectiveness of the programme by empirical standards (see section on Results, below)

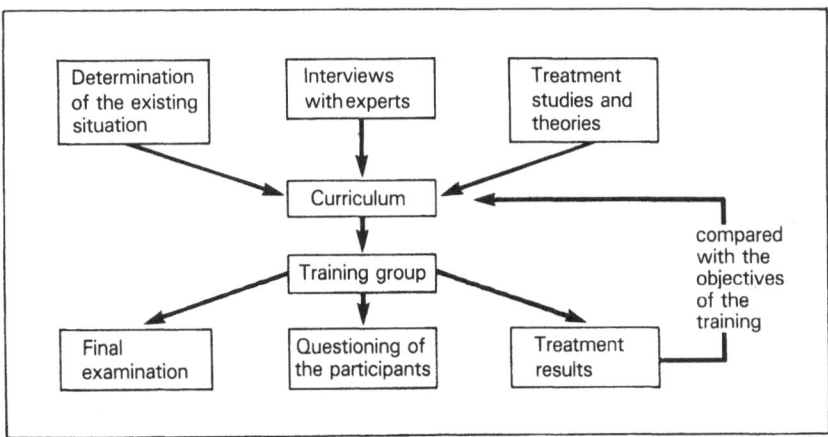

Figure 26.1 Development and modification of the training programme

DESCRIPTION OF THE TRAINING

Participation requirements

Persons interested in being admitted to the training courses must fulfill the following requirements:

(1) A completed university or college education as a social worker, psychologist or physician,

(2) at least 2 years' practical experience in a profession,

(3) at least 1 year's experience in a service for helping addicts,

(4) availability of supervision by a colleague: i.e. the possibility of seeing a colleague experienced in behaviour therapy or another participant in the training on a weekly basis,

(5) no participation in another training course at the same time,

(6) proof of personal qualification and the organizational requirements for the training in behaviour therapy, to be obtained in an admittance interview, as follows:

    The applicant's qualification is evaluated on the basis of his understanding of behaviour therapy theories and on his general abilities in dealing with addicts. With regard to the organizational requirements for the training, it must be clarified whether or not the participant will be able to put into practice the contents of the training course within the framework of his institution. It would not, for instance, be useful to accept onto the training course an applicant who worked mainly in the management of his institution and who had hardly any contact with the patients

It may be possible to make exceptions in individual cases with regard to the conditions for participation.

Training objectives

The objective of training is to enable the participants to work independently using behaviour therapy in the field of addiction.

(1) To *work independently* means to be solely responsible in the performance of therapy, which ranges from diagnosis (primarily by means of behaviour analysis) through interventive action to the examination and analysis by the therapist of his own actions.

    However, independence also means the recognition of personal limitations, which may be due to the level of professional competence (for instance: no experience with certain methods, no professional competence to treat certain psychic diseases) and which may be due to the level of personal competence (for instance: limitation of the therapist's competence due to personal crises). Depending on the limiting conditions, the recognition of personal limitations may lead to a transfer of the patient to another colleague or to personal and professional advanced training for the therapist. To sum up: independence does not only mean to act alone, but it also implies timely consultation with other colleagues − in other fields of specialization also − in order to obtain their advice, to include them in the therapy or to transfer the case to them.

(2) To *work using behaviour therapy* means to proceed according to the theories and models on which behaviour therapy is based, for example learning theories from Pavlov to Skinner and Bandura; the disease model of sociology and the principles of experimental psychology. The discussion concerning definitions of behaviour therapy will not be dealt with here; for further details of this see references 17, 18.

(3) In this training programme, *work in the field of addiction* does not only mean taking care of persons who are suffering from addiction but also taking care of those persons who are in the preliminary stages of addiction, such as juvenile problem drinkers or consumers of soft drugs, who believe their consumption of drugs to be a problem and who wish to change their behaviour.

The general objective of 'working independently using therapy in the field of addiction' can be broken down into several component objectives.

(1) Basic knowledge of clinical psychology, for example: social-psychological errors of observation, test theory, conditions leading to the formation of addiction habits, criteria for experimental psychology.

(2) Knowledge of the theoretical basis of behaviour therapy, for example: learning theories, differences between behaviour therapy and psycho-analysis, possible theoretical explanations for the effectiveness of various behaviour therapeutical methods.

(3) Practical skills in the application of behaviour therapeutical methods, for example: interview methods in behaviour analysis, planning and application of assertiveness training, explanation of the methods in the language of the patient.

(4) Personal qualifications as a therapist. The specification of criteria for qualification as a therapist is difficult and controversial, unless one is willing to limit oneself to obvious criteria for exclusion. Leaving aside concrete criteria, in this training self-experience is expected to have a postive influence on personal qualification, for instance by improving the self-observation and self-evaluation of the participants, so that they can develop self-regulating processes for their own future behaviour.

(5) Organizational requirements for the practice of behaviour therapy, for example: possibility of supervision by colleagues, integration of

behaviour therapeutic methods into an existing clinic conception.

(6)   Development of personal focal points depending on professional training, according to theoretical and practical abilities and interests and according to the general organizational conditions under which the therapist is working. Thus even though the various professional groups attend the same course, they can select particular study topics during the training. For instance, a social worker will give priority amongst other subjects during the training to social competence in dealing with the authorities; a physician will concentrate amongst other things on appropriate methods during the detoxification period; a psychologist might, however, consider therapy planning and evaluation to be his most important field of responsibility.

Within the general objectives of the training, every participant thus sets himself individual goals. The interdisciplinary nature of the training programme is thereby facilitated so that social workers, physicians, psychologists and other professional groups are able to co-operate in a training group and benefit from each other by exchanging knowledge in their specific fields.

Subjects covered in the training

A detailed list of all the subjects covered in the training will not be given here, but rather an overview of the most important subjects.

Clinical psychology

Methods of behaviour observation, structure of an experiment, test theory, origin, diagnostic counselling and treatment disturbances which frequently occur in the case of addicts (for example: partner conflicts, personal insecurity, depression, learning disturbances).

Theoretical basis of behaviour therapy

Classical conditioning, operant conditioning, learning models, self-efficacy theory, social science disease model, reciprocal inhibition, self-control.

Methods

Diagnostic methods such as behaviour analysis and tests which are more frequently used in behaviour therapy and behaviour observation.

Measures that are independent of therapy such as interviewing and counselling.

Behaviour therapeutical methods: coverant control, thought stopping, assertiveness training, contract management and individual strategies which are derived from behaviour analysis.

Case discussions

The seminar participants present cases from their own work: interrelating factors, which explain the origin and the maintenance of the symptomatology, will be discussed, and the therapy goals and a therapy plan will be derived from the information presented. The actual structure of individual intervention will be discussed and be examined with the aid of tape and/or video recordings which the participant has prepared from his therapy sessions. Discussion of cases will include the interaction between the patient and the therapist and the interaction plans of the patient which are derived from his behaviour in relation to the therapist. There will also be supervision by colleagues during the case discussions.

Organization of work

The conditions for the application of behaviour therapeutical methods at the participants' place of work will be discussed. Possible solutions will be worked out where there are difficulties in putting behaviour therapy into practice. The following are examples of such difficulties:

(1) In an outpatient clinic located in a small town, the number of patients whose symptomatology, age etc. are similar, is so small that it is difficult to form homogeneous groups for assertiveness training. How should self-assertiveness training be arranged?
(2) In the clinic of a seminar participant, work is done simultaneously on the basis of another theoretical concept (for instance psychoanalysis): how can the two therapy lines be reconciled with each other?

Teaching methods

The teaching of theoretical subjects and basic knowledge concerning clinical-psychological and behaviour-therapeutical methods is carried out by means of lectures, the reading of papers, brainstorming and discussions. The teaching of psychotherapy skills is much more difficult and there is much less relevant experience available. In the postgraduate training programme therapy methods are taught in three successive stages: role-playing, self-experience, supervision.

Role playing

In role playing, therapy situations are simulated. One participant acts as the patient, another participant as the therapist. Subsequent to the role playing the therapist receives feedback from the other seminar participants and from the group leaders. On the basis of the role playing different therapeutical methods will be discussed. The therapy situations which are simulated are drawn on the one hand from the daily practice of the participants (for example: therapeutical behaviour during the initial contact or if a patient starts to cry during the therapy session) and on the other hand from the behaviour therapeutical goals of the training (for example: the therapist explains to the patient the origin of his addiction based on theoretical learning aspects, the therapist trains thought stopping with a patient).

Self-experience

In the next step skills, which have been acquired in the course of role playing, will be put into practice in the self-experience phase and they will be further trained. In this phase, the seminar participants explore and modify undesired behaviour patterns (for instance disturbances relating to work, problems relating to self-confidence, excessive smoking). The self-experience phase has various objectives:

(1)   the participants improve their therapy skills in an almost realistic therapy situation by means of feedback from other seminar participants and the 'patient',

(2)   the seminar participants experience themselves the role of the patient and thereby heighten their perception regarding their own therapy procedures,

(3)   self-experience has a stabilizing effect upon the participants. Their own behaviour disturbances are reduced by it and their self-observation in regard to their problems and crises will be improved.

The personal stability of the therapist is considered to be a prerequisite for effective therapy. To avoid any misunderstandings: It is not expected — because this also would be unrealistic — that therapists are free from any psychic problems and that they are not influenced by personal crises. But therapists are expected to be able to observe themselves and reflect on the possible effects of their personal problems upon the therapy. As the following example will illustrate, even in the case of a so-called simple disturbance, negative effects may occur on account of unreflected behaviour on the part of the therapist: A therapist who is treating a patient for cynophobia, and who himself is afraid of dogs, may tend to increase the patient's fear by his verbal and non-verbal behaviour during their discussions. In addition, if he is not fully conscious of his own problems, he may make excessive or inadequate demands from the patient, if for instance he completes systematic desensitization at a level that is either too simple or too difficult. Similar factors inhibiting therapy can be imagined in the case of other disorders.

The therapist's communication behaviour may in particular have an inhibiting influence upon therapy. For example, if the therapist reacts to a juvenile alcoholic in a reproachful or demanding way as he would react to certain behaviour patterns in his own children, he then duplicates for the patient a problem father—child situation and thereby invokes the patient's resistance to the therapy. The communication behaviour of the therapist is therefore an important component of self-experience and of supervision.

Other standard therapy methods with which the seminar participants are involved during the training, are training in the building-up of social competence and a method for reducing disturbances relating to work.

Assertiveness training has been regularly included in the training programme, since it is one of the most frequently-used behaviour therapy methods and since the teaching of social competence requires personal social competence in the part of the therapist.

Instruction on the reduction of disturbances relating to work involves increased effect on the part of the seminar participants, in particular where the preparation required (for instance the reading of theoretical articles) for the individual seminars is concerned, since many of the participants have not practised such behaviour patterns for quite some time due to the volume of their practical work.

Additional behaviour patterns requiring modification are dealt with individually.

Supervision

In this phase, the seminar participants will apply the skills which they have acquired during the training to their dealings with their patients. Immediate supervision at their place of work is done by colleagues of the seminar participants who either simultaneously participate in the training, or who have already completed behaviour therapy training. Further supervision will also be carried out in these seminars. The seminar participants will present their cases there and tape recordings of selected therapy and counselling situations will be offered for discussion.

These three stages in the teaching of psychotherapeutic methods and skills are applied in addition to the teaching of theory in all of the seminars. The degree of difficulty of theoretical and practical tasks will increase progressively during the postgraduate training. Subjects and forms of teaching will vary considerably from seminar to seminar.

Organizational structure

The training will extend over 3 years and will consist of eight seminars each of a week's duration separated by intervals of 2–4 months.

The acquisition of competence in behaviour therapy will not be possible in eight week-long seminars. The theoretical and practical tasks which must therefore be completed between the seminars are of central importance. The time taken for these tasks will be approximately 8 hours per week.
The total time required for the training is:

seminars (8 weeks)	256 hours
supervision by colleagues	350 hours
theoretical and practical tasks	1000 hours
	1606 hours.

The time required according to the curriculum totals approximately 1600 hours. The actual time taken in acquiring competence in behaviour therapy will be much more, since during the period of training many of the subjects being dealt with may also be applied directly in the therapeutical and counselling practice of the participants who are working in the addiction field.

Individual training groups are comprised of a maximum of 14 members, since in the first place a number of learning goals are to be achieved by means of discussions on prepared texts, and in the second place all the participants should participate as often as possible in role playing. Small groups are also formed in the seminar.

The seminars will be headed by two psychologists with behaviour therapy training and experience in therapy in the addiction field.

The training will be held at a central conference place in order to keep it separate from the seminar participants' place of work and the possible work loads thereby involved. If the majority of the participants work in the same institution, however, the final practice-oriented seminars will be held if possible at their place of work. At the end of the training the participants sit for a final leaving examination, to which they will present two case reports in accordance with a set scheme (behaviour analysis scheme, see references 19–21). There will also be a written and an oral examination.

The Labour Exchange has recognized both the behaviour therapeutical training and the psychoanalytical training and participants may therefore apply for reimbursement of the training costs.

RESULTS

Postgraduate training in behaviour therapy was started in 1975. Since then nine groups ranging from a minimum of eight to a maximum of 13 persons have participated. For these participants the training extended over $2\frac{1}{2}$ years with a total of six 1-week seminars (192 seminar hours, 290 hours supervision by colleagues, about 850 hours theoretical and practical tasks). For current groups the training has been extended to 3 years and eight seminars.

Participants

Ninety-one persons have been admitted to the postgraduate training programme. Of the participants 58% were social workers, 9% were psychologists, 4% physicians and 29% from other professional groups such as nurses, educationalists and clergymen. The participants have been working in the addiction field for an average of 3.5 years (SD: 3.5).

The average age is approximately 32 years (SD: 6.7). Ten per cent of the participants are alcohol addicts, but have been abstinent several years. Fifty-five per cent of the participants work in an inpatient institution, 45% work in an outpatient institution.

Final examination

The results of the final examination provide an estimate of the effectiveness of the postgraduate training.

The examination is held 5 – 6 months following the final seminar and is based on two case reports, an oral and a written examination. The case reports follow the behaviour analysis scheme[19-21] and, in addition to diagnosis and selection of therapeutic measures, they contain a description of 12 treatment sessions, including data for the evaluation of the therapy. In addition, tape recordings of the treatment sessions are submitted. The oral and written examinations of the participants are graded according to a six-point scale. The participant's instructor and also a behaviour therapist who does not know the seminar participants are responsible for the final assessment.

During the training (for instance during the first, third and finally during the fifth seminar) nine persons (10%) dropped out of the course. Of the remaining 82 persons who attended the last seminar, 64 (78%) successfully completed their examinations. The average grade of the participants in the final examination is 2·2 ('1' signifies "very good", '6' signifies 'below standard'). In order to pass the examination, a grade of at least 4·0 is required.

Questioning of the participants after completion of the training

After the last seminar and 1 year after the final examination, a questionnaire is presented to the participants concerning their therapy activities and their evaluation of the postgraduate training. This survey has involved 25 persons, since the questionnaire has only been submitted during the last three training groups. Out of the 25, 16 participants completed the questionnaire.

One year after the final examination, the participants give their opinion as to how important they believe various methods to be in the addiction field and how confident they feel in applying these methods, using a 1 – 6 rating scale. They also state how many patients they have used the various procedures on during the last year (Table 26.1).

The sample size varies between the individual estimates of relevance and confidence and the indications of frequency of application since the participants did not always complete all the items. With regard to the frequency of application the sample size indicates how many of the participants have practised the individual methods.

According to the participants' evaluation, the most important behaviour therapeutical methods are assertiveness training, behaviour analysis, alcohol refusal training and communication training. Among the non-specific therapy methods, the information sessions on drugs and alcohol, seminars for family members and free discussion concerning the significance of addiction therapy are ranked highest.

Thought-stopping, covert sensitization and aversion therapy are considered to be the least important procedures. These methods are also ad-

Table 26.1   Assessment of treatment methods according to relevance, confidence and frequency of application

Methods	Estimation of						Frequency of application		
	relevance			confidence					
	N	M_R	SD	N	M_C	SD	M_F	SD	N
Assertiveness training	16	5·6	0·6	15	1·6	0·7	11·3	7·1	13
Information on drugs	15	5·5	0·9	15	1·6	0·7	62·4	87·8	13
Behaviour analysis	16	5·5	0·9	15	2·3	1·1	10·8	6·6	14
Courses for relatives	12	5·4	1·3	13	2·8	2·0	17·4	15·1	5
Communication training	15	5·3	0·9	15	2·7	1·0	12·1	6·0	11
Refusal training	15	5·3	0·9	13	2·2	1·4	9·5	10·0	11
Problem solving	14	5·2	0·7	13	3·5	1·7	15·5	19·4	11
.	.	.	.	.	.	.	.	.	.
.	.	.	.	.	.	.	.	.	.
.	.	.	.	.	.	.	.	.	.
Thought stopping	16	3·3	1·3	15	2·6	1·1	1·7	0·7	10
Covert sensitization	14	2·3	1·3	15	4·3	1·5	1·3	0·6	3
Aversion therapy	13	1·7	0·8	12	5·4	1·0	7·5	3·5	2

M_R: Mean scores in the estimation of relevance of treatment methods (1: totally irrelevant, 6: totally relevant)

M_C: Mean scores in the estimation of confidence in the application of treatment methods (1: totally confident, 6: totally unconfident)

M_F: Number of patients (mean), who were treated using the methods in one year

N: Number of participants who answered the item

SD: Standard deviation

ministered relatively rarely and the participants feel rather uncertain during their application (exception: thought-stopping). As expected, the procedures considered to be important are used frequently and in the participants' estimation with relative confidence. On the other hand it appears that with regard to problem solving there is no positive correlation between the frequency of application and the confidence in application of this method.

With regard to the indications of the frequency of application of the various methods, the nature of the individual procedures must be taken into account. Assertiveness training or behaviour analysis are much more time-consuming than contract management of thought-stopping. Indications of frequency must also be considered in relation to the extent of the participants' therapy work. One year after the final examination, only 31 % of the participants' working time is spent in the application of therapies; during the remaining time they are occupied with counselling, organizational tasks and other work. Whereas directly after the postgraduate training the proportion of therapy work increases to 42 %, by 1 year after the final examination it has fallen back to what it was before the beginning of the training.

Personality values

During the first and the last training seminars, the personality inventory, FPI[22] and the 'insecurity questionnaire' (U-questionnaire)[23] are distributed. The data given in Figure 26.2 apply to the last five training groups, in which 38 participants completed the questionnaires on both occasions when the surveys were conducted.

The average values of the U-questionnaire at the beginning of the postgraduate training are equal to the average values of a normal non-clinical group, which was used as a control group for the questionnaire. During the last seminar the values obtained for all items improved, considerably in spite of the good initial level at the beginning of the training (Figure 26.2).

The average values obtained in the FPI fall in the normal range at the beginning and at the end of the training (Figure 26.3). On completion of the postgraduate training, the participants show slight improvements within this normal range. That is, according to the FPI items they show fewer psychosomatic disturbances, they are more content and self-confident, more sociable and lively, less constrained and more approachable and they are emotionally stable.

DISCUSSION

The evaluation of the training of psychotherapeutical skills involves problems of method which are more numerous and difficult to cope with than the problems related to the evaluation of therapies. A postgraduate training programme is successful if the participants successfully apply the therapeutical skills taught. Since even the evaluation of therapies for addicts often proves difficult in practice, the evaluation of training courses in which these therapies are taught is still more difficult. Nevertheless an attempt will be made to examine the effectiveness of the postgraduate training programme, based on the results of the final examination, the questioning of the participants subsequent to the postgraduate training and the results of the personality questionnaires.

The number of enrolments for the two postgraduate training programmes – the psychoanalytically oriented programme and the behaviour therapeutically oriented programme – plus the data on the current situation, confirm the necessity for such time-intensive, high-level training courses for the teaching of psychotherapeutical skills.

Even though the postgraduate training has been planned primarily for social workers, psychologists and physicians, other professional groups (nurses, educationists, clergymen and others) are strongly represented in the training courses. However, the proportion of participants from the individual professional groups appears to correspond approximately to the distribution of those professions throughout the inpatient and outpatient institutions. Social workers and other non-psychological and non-medical professional groups are, taken as a whole, those who are engaged most frequently in the

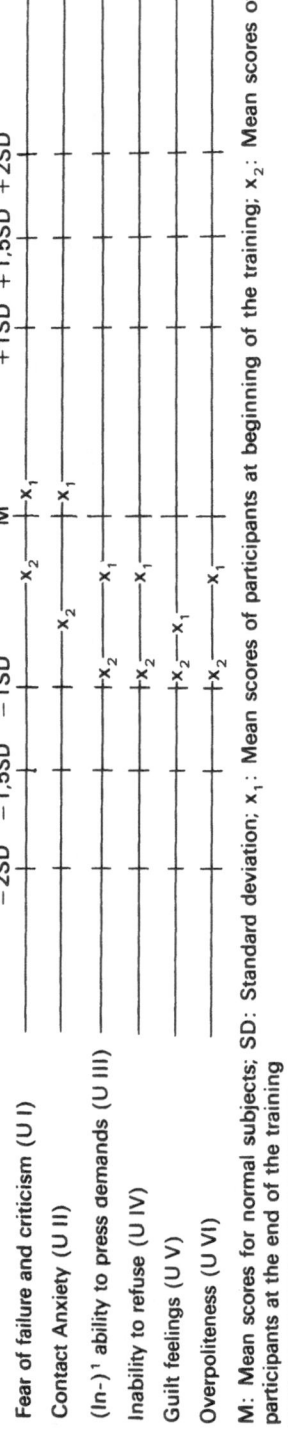

Figure 26.2   Insecurity Questionnaire. Mean scores of participants in the factors of the Insecurity Questionnaire (U-Fragebogen) at beginning and at the end of the training

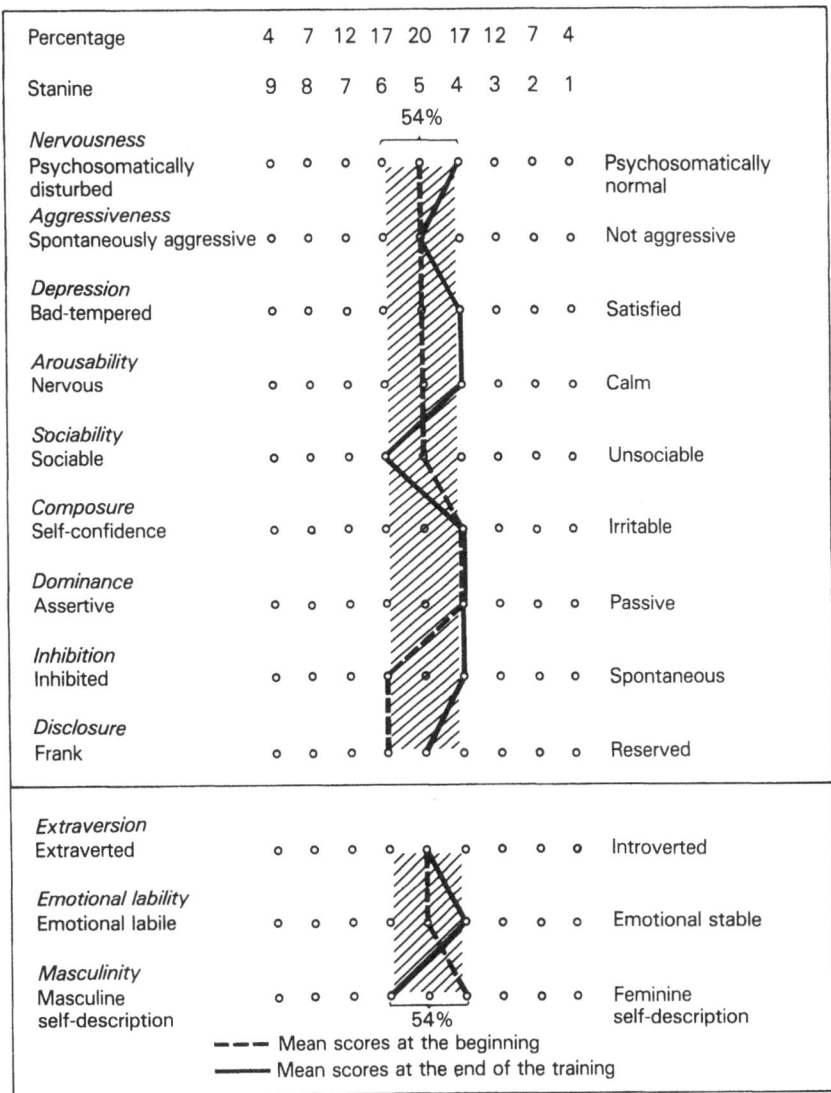

Figure 26.3 Mean scores of participants in the factors of the personality inventory (FPI)

care of addicts and their importance should be taken into consideration in the planning of the programmes.

The practicability of having a variety of professional groups participate in the training is confirmed by the results of the final examination. The majority of the participants receive good marks and important goals of the programme are thereby achieved. This result is especially pleasing when the high requirements of the final examination are considered.

It also appears that the participants are able to apply the behaviour-therapeutical methods taught in their practical work, and that they feel relatively confident with most of them (Table 26.1). With a few exceptions, there is a positive correlation between confidence and frequency of application of the methods. Assertiveness training, which ranks highest in the assessment of confidence, is one of the most frequently used methods in the training. Considerably less time is devoted to covert sensitization and thought-stopping during the training. It still has to be clarified whether the lower evaluation of confidence for these methods is due to less teaching or to a less relevance of the methods in practice. In this way appropriate conclusions may be drawn concerning the subjects of the postgraduate training. Since the participants believe that problem-solving is very important and since they also frequently use this method with their patients, even though their own confidence with it is low, the teaching of this method will be increased in subsequent courses by means of role playing and self-experience. Aversion therapy is not taught during the training, since the experts questioned during the preparation of the curriculum expressed the opinion that it had little practical relevance, and the efficiency of this method is in any case controversial.

An important goal of the training to be achieved under the heading of self-experience is the stabilization of the participant's personality. At the beginning of the training the average FPI- and U-questionnaire values of the participants were already within the normal range (Figures 26.2, 26.3). This group which has been accepted for the behaviour-therapy training therefore cannot be seen to confirm the hypothesis which is frequently stated in popular scientific literature: that many therapists themselves are suffering from neurotic disturbances. In accordance with the goals of the postgraduate training the participants improved in various aspects of their personality and their self-confidence by the end of the courses.

The proportion of therapy in the work with addicts remains constant, when a comparison is made between the amount of therapy carried out prior to the training and the amount 1 year after the final examination. This is in keeping with the objectives of the training, which do not aim to increase the amount of therapy and thereby reduce other important spheres of duty of social workers, psychologists or physicians. The training will, however, enable the professional groups working in the addiction field to work independently during the time available to them for therapy.

On the other hand, the training not only comprises closely defined teaching of therapeutical methods but also aims to improve qualifications in other areas of addiction work, since this work consists not only of assertiveness training, behaviour analysis and alcohol-refusal training etc., but also counselling, and the motivation etc., of addicts and their family members. Often these are important conditions for the actual commencement of therapy. Behaviour therapy in particular provides the opportunity to depart from the classical therapeutical setting prior to the therapy or also during the treatment.

Behaviour therapy allows the patient's social environment to be included in the care and/or the combination of the therapy and treatment activities of the individual professional groups (social workers, psychologists, physicians etc.). This can be illustrated by a case study, presented for the examination by a social worker.

Case Study. The patient is an alcoholic. She has made several suicide attempts, she is 20 years old, works as a barmaid, has no apartment, no identity papers, and she is in debt. The first contacts with the patient were made in the apartment of her aunt. After such talks, the patient was frequently taken by car to her place of work (a bar). The patient was also accompanied on some of her daily errands (shopping, visits to authorities etc.). While the patient was being observed in her social environment, several problematic forms of behaviour were observed, such as uneconomical behaviour when shopping and conspicuous behaviour in the street arousing aggression in passers-by etc. In a normal therapy setting in the counselling service such behaviour deficiencies would presumably not have been noted. On the basis of the discussions and behaviour observations, a therapy scheme was devised within the framework of behaviour analysis. This included termination of the work as a barmaid, a training course at the Labour Exchange, instruction in coping with money etc. Among the methods applied were contract management in small steps, operant conditioning, role playing, training in saying 'no'. During the first 3 months, the contact per week was about 8 hours. During this time the patient showed improvements in several aspects of her behaviour[24].

Even though such case reports — especially in detailed form (behaviour analysis) and including tape recordings — may be considered to be positive feedback for the postgraduate training programme, an evaluation of the training will only be possible on the basis of data from patients who had been treated prior to the training and after its completion. This would also have to be compared with a similar group involved with another postgraduate training programme. A field study of this nature would be hard to achieve, so the efficiency of the postgraduate training in behaviour therapy has had to be assessed in descriptive terms.

In addition to the modification of individual subjects in the programme on the basis of survey data, step-by-step improvement in the methods of evaluation of the training will be attempted during subsequent courses.

Acknowledgements

We should like to thank Ernst Knischewski (*Gesamtverband für Suchtkrankenhilfe im Diakonischen Werk der EKD*) for his support and for encouragement of the project and also Karin Höll and Charlotte Korintenberg for their first-class organization of the training.

References

1 Wittchen, H.-U., Fichter, M. and Dvorak, A. (1980). Ausbildungsund Berufssituation klinischer Psychologen. In Wittling, W. (ed.) *Handbuch der klinischen Psychologie*, pp. 142–176. (Hamburg: Hoffmann und Campe Verlag)

2 Bühringer, G. (1981). *Planung, Steuerung und Bewertung von Therapieeinrichtungen für junge Drogen- und Alkoholabhängige*. (Munich: Gerhard Röttger Verlag)

3 Hanel, E., Jauss, D. and Spies, G. (1981). *Ergebnisse der dritten Befragung in den Modelleinrichtungen des Psychosozialen Anschlussprogramms*. (Forschungsberichte der Projektgruppe Rauschmittelabhängigkeit. Bd. 36.) (Munich: Max-Planck-Institut für Psychiatrie)

4 Bühringer, G. (1982). Erste Konsequenzen aus der wissenschaftlichen Begleitung ambulanter Modellberatungsstellen für Abhängige und Gefährdete. In Vollmer, H. and Helas, I. (eds.) *Verhaltenstherapie in der Suchtkrankenhilfe*, pp. 3–13. (Munich: Gerhard Röttger Verlag)

5 Lindner, W. V. (1980). Prinzipien einer bedarfsgerechten Suchtkrankentherapie psychoanalytisch orientiert. In *Gesamtverband für Suchtkrankenhilfe* (eds.) *Sozialtherapie in der Praxis*, pp. 30–39. (Kassel: Nicol Verlag)

6 Triebel, A. (1980). Effekte psychoanalytisch orientierter Weiterbildung von Suchtkrankenhelfern. In *Gesamtverband für Suchtkrankenhilfe* (eds.) *Sozialtherapie in der Praxis*, pp. 40–50. (Kassel: Nicol Verlag)

7 Matarazzo, R. (1971). Research on the teaching and learning of psychotherapeutical skills. In Bergin, A. and Garfield, S. (eds.) *Handbook of Psychotherapy and Behavior Change*, pp. 895–924. (New York: Wiley)

8 Wolpe, J., Knopp, W. and Garfield, Z. (1966). Postgraduate training in behavior therapy. In *Proceedings of the IV World Congress of Psychiatry, Madrid*. Excerpta Medica International Congress Series No. 150. (Amsterdam: Excerpta Medica)

9 Davison, G. C. (1965). The training of undergraduates as social reinforcers for autistic children. In Ullman, L. P. and Krasner, L. (eds.) *Case Studies in Behaviour Modification*. (New York: Holt, Rinehart & Winston)

10 De Jong, R. and Bühringer, G. (eds.) (1978). *Ein verhaltenstherapeutisches Stufenprogramm zur stationären Behandlung von Drogenabhängigen*. (Munich: Gerhard Röttger Verlag)

11 Feldhege, F.-J., Krauthan, G., Schulze, B., Schneider, R. and Vollmer, H. (1977). Ein ambulantes Breitbandprogramm zur Behandlung jugendlicher Drogenabhängiger. *Wiener Z. Suchtforsch.*, **1**, 15

12 Kraemer, S. and De Jong, R. (eds.) (1980). *Therapiemanual für ein verhaltenstherapeutisches Stufenprogramm zur stationären Behandlung von Drogenabhängigen*. (Munich: Gerhard Röttger Verlag)

13 Schneider, R. (1982). Das Therapieprogramm der Fachklinik. In Schneider, R. (ed.) *Verhaltenstherapeutische Behandlung der Alkoholabhängigkeit in einer Fachklinik: Programm und Ergebnisse*. (Munich: Gerhard Röttger Verlag)

14 Vollmer, H. and Kraemer, S. (eds.) (1982). *Ambulante Behandlung des Alkoholismus. Erfahrungen aus der verhaltenstherapeutischen Arbeit mit jungen Alkoholikern*. (Munich: Gerhard Röttger Verlag)

15 Vollmer, H., Kraemer, S., Schneider, R., Feldhege, F.-J. and Schulze, B. (1982). Outpatient behaviour therapy for juveniles and young adults with alcohol problems. Second year treatment outcome. In Golding, P. (ed.) *Alcoholism: A Modern Perspective*, pp. 417–434. (Lancaster: MTP)

16 Schneider, R. (1976). Arbeitsbezogene Weiterbildung in Verhaltenstherapie für den Sozialarbeiter im psychosozialen Beratungsdienst. In Fiedler, P. and Hörmann, G. (eds.) *Therapeutische Sozialarbeit*, pp. 107–121. (Münster: DGVT)

17 Franks, C. M. and Wilson, G. T. (1979). *Annual Review of Behavior Therapy. Theory and Practice, 1978*. (New York: Brunner/Mazel)

18 Kazdin, A. E. (1978). *History of Behavior Modification*. (Baltimore: University Park Press)

19 Kanfer, F. H. and Saslow, G. (1969). Behavioral diagnosis. In Franks, C. M. (ed.) *Behavior Therapy: Appraisal and Status*, pp. 417–444. (New York: McGraw-Hill)

20 Schulte, D. (1974). *Diagnostik in der Verhaltenstherapie*. (Munich: Urban & Schwarzenberg)

21 Bartling, G., Echelmeyer, L., Engberding, M. and Krause, R. (1980). *Problemanalyse im therapeutischen Prozess*. (Stuttgart: Kohlhammer Verlag)

22 Fahrenberg, J. and Selg, H. (1970). *Das Freiburger Persönlichkeits-inventar, FPI*. (Göttingen: Hogrefe Verlag)

23 Ullrich, R. and Ullrich, R. (1977). *Der Unsicherheitsfragebogen — Testmappe U. Anleitung für den Therapeuten*. Teil II. (Munich: Pfeiffer Verlag)

24 Hautop, W. (1981). Verhaltensbeobachtungen und Verhaltensübungen ausserhalb der Beratungsstelle. In *Der VT-Sozialtherapeut*, **5,** 3—8.

27
Natal alcoholism and emotionality

H.-G. TITTMAR and T. S. McDADE

FAS AND BEHAVIOURAL AROUSAL

Contemporary writers on natal alcoholism have a tendency to credit Jones *et al.*[1] with the original description of the Fetal Alcohol Syndrome (FAS). Jones and Smith[2], however, acknowledge Lemoine *et al.*[3] to have provided the first inventory of growth deficiencies in such children, while two notable aspects of the FAS, namely fetal mortality and prematurity, had been referred to by much earlier writers (see reference 2).

When delineating the spectrum of disorders which characterize the FAS, associated behavioural disturbances have often been noted. In particular these consist of psychomotor retardation, agitation and 'character disturbances'[2-7]. While psychomotor retardation may be linked to reported cerebellar damage (e.g., see reference 8), and be associated with lowered IQ (compare references 7, 9), the reason for the existence of agitation is not so forthcoming, though it is implied[8] to have a neuronal foundation. Root *et al.*[10] found there to be no significant difference from normal levels in the hormonal activity of the hypothalamic–pituitary axis. Other aspects which may lead to FAS development, such as mineral imbalance, have also been investigated. Henderson *et al.*[11] found no zinc depletion in their alcoholized rat offspring, whereas Mendelson and Huber[12] did. Similarly, some human FAS cases may have associated hypoglycaemia and hypocalcaemia[13], while others are normal[14].

However, here it is much harder to decide whether the behaviour is due to an alcohol derived imbalance, or if it represents a secondary metabolic aspect, namely one of malnutrition (compare reference 15). Such malnutrition may be derived from errors in metabolism, distribution or absorption. It has been implied on occasions that neonatal nutrition may help aggravate the symptoms; especially noted here have been the weak suck and consequent failure to thrive[4, 5, 9, 16]. Equally, it has also been argued that nutritional attention may provide a means by which recovery is possible[17], and this has, on selected parameters, already been observed[12, 18] (and compare reference 19).

One alternative to the nutritional argument above, which has been presented to explain observed hyperactivity in FAS offspring, has focussed on the arousal system[20]. It was put forward that neurological insult at high levels of natal alcoholism would induce hyperactivity, while low levels of natal alcoholism may act to induce hypoactivity. The arousal system referred to in this context is necessarily the Arousal I system as described by Routtenberg[21], since it is this system which involves the cerebellum, damage to which from natal alcoholism has been reported[8]. Animal behavioural tests of arousal are limited, one of these being the Open Field test. For this test it may be argued that ambulation is more a reflection of arousal, whether elicited by exploration or by hyperactivity. A fearful situation may, on the other hand, be just as arousing, but be reflected by freezing (low ambulation) and defecation. This behaviour pattern has been termed Emotionality[22-24]. There is, as yet, no common consensus on what the Open Field measures[25], even though it has been investigated extensively[24, 26] and discussed[24, 27, 28].

Archer[28] points out the difficulties of relating measures of exploration (ambulation) and emotionality (defecation) to arousal state. Indeed, defecation was found to contribute to both factors, that of exploration and that for emotionality. An attempt has been made, however, to justify the use of behavioural measures as a reflection of arousal state[29]. It is worth noting that neither Abel[25] nor Archer[28] relate to this paper[29], even though Archer quotes Denenberg's work,[24] which occurs in the same journal! The argument presented[29] focusses away from discrete Drive concepts, such as exploration and fear, and recommends the use of a general motivational factor of behaviour, namely a non-specific excitability level (NEL). Utilizing an ethogram approach, the authors show that, when applying weights to different behaviours and summing these, the final behavioural index (NEL-score) shows a close correlation with the rat's hippocampal (theta) slow wave activity. When only using the sum of weighted scores for rearing and locomotion a good correlation is still attained, and hence one may utilize just these two measures to reflect arousal.

Lability, their second dimension, is taken to reflect the dynamic course of habituation (i.e. repeated trials), and summing this with defecation. Support for the utility of the Lability measure comes indirectly from Denenberg[24]. Certainly much of the contradiction existing between experimental findings (compare reference 28) could be due to the absence of these two measures.

On the other hand, the alternative implication is that NEL and Lability measures provide related information. Hippocampal theta activity (NEL) is a reflection of Arousal II system activity[21, 30], a reinforcement motivated system, which is operative during habituation (lability). Hence, animals with high NEL scores may be exploring (being generally motivated) rather than being non-specifically excited (compare reference 29). Since the two arousal systems are, however, reciprocally inhibiting[30], and a high NEL-score reflects Arousal II, then a low NEL-score could be reflecting Arousal I.

Animal experimentation, within its own rubric, has always been perceived as a useful tool to investigate natal alcoholism. It is unfortunately already obvious that such investigations can become shrouded in a morass of underlying theorizing. Accepting momentarily the simplified concept that the Open Field may be used to measure ambulation and defecation, then the apparatus itself needs to be considered next.

Tapp et al.[26] do in fact comment on the interaction between animal and equipment and the differential habituation that this may evoke. Archer[28] and Hill[31] review some of the work on the relationship between Open Field stimulus intensity (notably illumination level and noise), from which it may broadly be concluded that emotional responding occurs at higher stimulation levels[28, 31]. Despite a standard description of the Open Field (e.g., reference 22), there is little standardization between researchers[32]. The potential confounding by testing condition was ignored in a review of prenatal exposure to alcohol on offspring emotionality[25]. The assumed influence on habituation[26], is confounded further by a sex difference. High male scorers on the first day of testing habituated more rapidly, while for female rats rapid habituation occurred for low or moderate day 1 scorers[33]. Not only does an Open Field Sex difference show up with normal offspring (compare references 28, 34), but there is also a sex difference in respect of such behaviour to prenatal treatment[28, 35], and yet a large number of researchers will amalgamate data from both sexes (compare reference 28). Since it is possible to have a Treatment—Sex interaction in Open Field performance, here due to alcohol administered for the first 2 weeks post partum[34], it may conceivably be possible that a Treatment effect may be eliminated when amalgamating sexes. Indeed, there were no differences in defecation across treatment conditions, though there were in ambulation[36], but it is hard to interpret this finding since sexes had been pooled. And yet this study apparently does support the author's earlier findings of alcohol induced arousal, in which female offspring only were tested[37]. This earlier study[37] can however be criticized on statistical grounds (see discussion on degrees of freedom, below). It may be argued that any sex difference may have a genetic basis, which contributes to the phenotypic variation.

Genetic differences in testing for emotionality have been emphasized[38] and reviewed[28], and have been exemplified by the selective breeding of reactive and non-reactive sub-strains of rats[22] and dogs[39]. Consequently it has been suggested[40] that the strain of animal used and its behavioural characteristics should be regarded as a major variable. Only Morra[41] appears to have done this. His rat mothers were given a 1-minute trial in the Open Field, on which basis they were allocated to treatment conditions. Analysis of frequency of traversals and body weights showed that the groups were matched on these parameters. However, as is usual, not all rats mated or produced/maintained a viable litter. Having begun with 30 treated females, only 16 littered, of which one litter was completely cannibalized, while a further two were eliminated due to their smallness of litter size. Furthermore, out of the 128 offspring derived from the 13 litters, at day 30, only 123 survived to 45 days of age. Only 43.33 % of the treated females from the original matched-design therefore produced useable results. There is now no guarantee that the remaining 13 females (distributed amongst six treatment groups) were still equated for Open Field traversals, and no such further data were presented. This concept, taking account of maternal behaviour, has been discussed further[42]; in that discussion it is suggested that obtained data could be analysed by analysis of covariance, using the maternal data as the covariant. An additional/alternate way of including the maternal data is to consider a covariance−variance plot[38].

It appears, therefore, that when examining emotionality, as affected by natal alcoholism, one has to consider, beyond the treatment effect, the possible inclusion of variations due to genotype and dramatype (phenotype-environment interaction[43]). This may be confounded further by two aspects − the age of the animal being tested and the type of alcohol model being tested.

Age changes in Open Field behaviour have been documented[44, 45]; in these studies it was noted that Open Field activity is greater in juvenile rats (less than 70 days old), who also tend not to show habituation during repeated Open Field exposure. Since various authors have reported developmental delays in juvenile rats (compare Table 1 in reference 25), any suspected treatment effect on arousal in juveniles may equally be a reflection of maturational delay rather than a treatment effect on arousal *per se*. Perhaps it is such a delay in maturation which was being observed[36] at 28 and 56 days, but which had dissipated by 112 days of age. In fact, the tendency has been to test juvenile offspring at various ages rather than adult offspring (despite the title of Table 2 in reference 25 referring to adult emotionality), and, at that, invariably different ages were used, including 15 days of age[46], when offspring naturally tend to be hyperactive[46]. Despite these comments, a common finding does appear to be some increase in activity (decrease in emotionality). This, in juveniles, may merely be reflective of delayed maturation, rather than a direct enhancement of arousal *per se*.

Research on natal alcoholism induced emotionality may be divided into two groups according to the treatment phase: (1) those experiments in which alcohol is administered during gestation only and (2) those experiments which also provide alcohol before and/or after gestation. Respectively, these two groups are equivalent to Phase II, and Phase I (sometimes also Phase III) of the guidelines for reproduction studies for the safety evaluation of drugs for human use[47]. In line with such evaluation, experimental procedures have been derived to reflect Phase II[48], and Phase I[49] respectively, and their attributes have been discussed[20, 42]. Effectively, Phase II tests for effects of alcohol, while Phase I tests for effects due to alcoholism. As many other variables, due to alcoholism, may become intervening[43], results between these two procedures are not equivocal, and may indeed be contraindicative.

Even when taking account of the above aspects, data interpretation may still become biased, according to the statistical procedures involved. While this has been discussed at length elsewhere[42], one aspect of that discussion is pertinent here, namely that the litter should be considered as the treatment unit (treatment being maternally derived), rather than individual offspring (within litter variation tends to be smaller than between litter variation). If this is not done so, an overstating of the degrees of freedom occurs, which may lead to spurious significance. Such an inflated degree of freedom can be found in various publications (e.g., references 34, 36, 37, 41, 50). Recalculation of probability values, where this is feasible from the information presented[50], induces a change in p from <0.025 to $= 0.1943$! One of the examples[37] presents probability values only. However, it can be calculated that the degrees of freedom should not have been 25, but only 5! While the remaining examples do not supply sufficient information to estimate their true degrees of freedom, one can nevertheless calculate association values for their results[42], from which their worthiness may be estimated. Thus, one[41] shows at best 2.8 % of association, implying that the significant result was achieved solely by inflating the degrees of freedom; another[34] appears to have only a Treatment × Sex interaction as significant (est. $\omega^2 = 0.1656$); while in the final example[36] all three main effects should be discounted, even though one does reach 13 %, due to sexes being pooled.

In conclusion it must be evident that errors may be derived in animal research and that these may be controlled to various degrees. If this is not always possible, then their potential must be born in mind in any interpretation of obtained results. The major variables that may contribute to variations in results on emotionality are: genetic endowment (maternal behavioural characteristics), treatment administration, age of tested subject, sex of tested subject, testing environment and data manipulation. Perhaps, through a closer consideration of these variables, Open Field studies will help to elucidate hyperactivity in the Fetal Alcohol Syndrome.

NATAL ALCOHOLISM AND TIMIDITY

Pharmacological researchers tend to investigate those behavioural variables which they feel may be affected by the drug under investigation. Consequently, for drugs acting on the central nervous system, tests are generally chosen which investigate a rat's startle response, exploratory behaviour, learning ability etc. Many such tests have been detailed or mentioned[51-54]. For this research programme several tests were chosen, the pertinent one here being the Home Cage Emergence test (HCE). This test is classified as a test of timidity (of emotionality[40]), and measures the latency of a rat leaving its cage once the front of the cage has been opened. To facilitate emergence, the front door of the cage was held in a horizontal position by a hook.

The door was opened and suspended. Timing began when the rat's nose crossed the 'doorstep'. The time taken by the rat to place both front paws over the 'doorstep' as well as the total emergence time (four paws) was recorded. In addition, the number of times the animal attempted to emerge was noted — this being indicated by the number of times both front paws passed the 'doorstep' prior to full emergence — from which a time score, using the time difference between the first (initial) and final (full) emergence, was calculated. If the animal had not emerged fully after 400 seconds, testing was discontinued.

Method

Sixty albino Wistar female rats were used in this experiment, along with 15 pairs of males (for breeding), who were all obtained from Olac. The housing conditions and the procedure for mating are reported[55], as well as the details of the intermittent fasting schedule[48], which served to administer the alcohol (10 % v/v)[56]. The rats were allowed more than 3 weeks to adapt to the laboratory conditions and its routine. One of the routines observed was weekly weighing of all female rats. At the end of the adaptation period, the females were given a Home Cage Emergence Test, and their Home Cage Activity was sampled. Female rats were allocated to the treatment groups according to the HCE scores, so that equal proportions of early and late emergers were in each group, which at this stage were of equal size. As a final check on group allocation, the HCE was repeated prior to mating. The three groups were:

C   Control group: This group received a similar amount of disturbance and handling as the other groups, but was not subjected to any experimental manipulation.

W   Water control group: Animals in this group received their food and water intermittently[48], and the tap water was replaced by distilled water during days 5—19 of gestation.

A   Alcohol group: The rats in this group differed from W animals in so far as they received 10 % ethanol during days 5—19 of gestation.

Food and water intakes were monitored throughout, because a subsidiary investigation was being made into catabolic metabolic rate. On day 19 of gestation, rats were supplied with hay for bedding. After birth, litters were weighed daily and developmental indices were noted[20], until vaginal opening. Weaning was at 22 days of age, and sexes were segregated on vaginal opening. Offspring had been raised as three males and females per litter, and, as far as possible, one from each sex per litter was selected at 100 days for HCE testing. In all cases, the offspring of intermediate weight (out of each set of three) were used. They were caged individually in MRC-type cages and their Home Cage Activity was recorded for 2 weeks, at the end of which HCE testing was done.

Results

The mothers did the HCE test four times. Twice during the adaptation period, once before mating, and again 6 days after having weaned their pups. The results from the third and fourth test were averaged and used as covariant score when analysing the offspring results. Since latency data has the tendency to be [-shape distributed, all data was checked for skew. Transformations were applied to normalize the data, within the skew range of ± 1.0. Utilizing maternal data from only those rats whose offspring contributed to the analyses, ANOVA on maternal HCE scores showed no difference between treatment groups ($p > 0.05$) on any of the four testing occasions − i.e. treatment groups were equated for HCE scores.

Analysing the results from male and female offspring separately (Tables 27.1 and 27.2), there is no difference in HCE scores among treatment groups, either in terms of significance ($p > 0.05$) or in terms of association (est. $\omega^2_{Max} = 0.0694$). There thus appears to be no treatment effect in terms of timidity.

However, when using offspring data only, a strong sex difference emerges on the first two HCE measures (Table 27.3), which is detailed further in Figures 27.1 and 27.2, where the influence of natal alcoholism, at best, amounts only to 6.22%. It does confirm, though, that in research on emotionality, sex differences may occur, and for this reason sexes should not be pooled in an analysis.

Conclusions

No statistically significant differences in adult timidity, in relation to natally experienced alcohol, were observed. While this may mean that natal alcoholism bears no relevance on this measure of emotionality, it may equally

Table 27.1   Home Cage Emergence Test: female offspring

		ANOVA		ANCOVA
		Mother's score	Offspring's score	Offspring's score
Time elapsed to first emergence	Transformation applied	Log X	Log X	
	$f(2,27)$	2.5386	0.0917	0.1881
	p	0.0977	0.9127	0.8296
	est. ω^2	0.0930	0.0000	0.0000
Time elapsed between first and final emergence	Transformation applied	Log $1/X$	Log X	
	$f(2,27)$	0.0084	0.2123	0.2189
	p	0.9916	0.8101	0.8049
	est. ω^2	0.0000	0.0000	0.0000
Number of emergence attempts	Transformation applied	Log X	Log X	
	$f(2,27)$	0.2787	0.3036	0.2853
	p	0.7589	0.7406	0.7541
	est. ω^2	0.0000	0.0000	0.0000

Table 27.2   Home Cage Emergence Test: male offspring

| | | ANOVA | | ANCOVA |
		Mother's score	Offspring's score	Offspring's score
Time elapsed to first emergence	Transformation applied	Log X	Log X	
	$f(2,29)$	2.2191	0.5010	1.2085
	p	0.1282	0.6114	0.3149
	est. ω^2	0.0752	0.0000	0.0142
Time elapsed between first and final emergence	Transformation applied	Log ^{1}/X	Log X	
	$f(2,29)$	0.3449	1.3759	2.0602
	p	0.7112	0.2686	0.1463
	est. ω^2	0.0000	0.0229	0.0640
Number of emergence attempts	Transformation applied	Log X	Log X	
	$f(2,29)$	0.3626	1.9789	2.1556
	p	0.6990	0.1565	0.1347
	est. ω^2	0.0000	0.0577	0.0694

mean that by this age (100 days plus) any difference has disappeared. Certainly, it has been highlighted[4] that some catch-up is possible, which has been explained as being possible at low treatment levels, but not for high dosages[58]. Since a sex difference in Home Cage Emergence can be demonstrated to exist (Figures 27.1, 27.2), this type of test of timidity appears to be sufficiently sensitive as a behavioural discriminant. Two main alternative conclusions are possible: (1) the dosage imbibed (compare reference 48) may be below effective threshold for this behaviour and (2) any effect, being due to low dosage, has been eradicated over time.

NATAL ALCOHOLISM AND THE OPEN FIELD

It has been pointed out here, and elsewhere[59], that empirical results of Open Field activity can be contradictory and are difficult to interpret if the intervening variables are not controlled. Despite theoretical discussions[24, 27, 29] concerning the meaning of the Open Field activity, writers[25, 59] still question the meaning of such activity. Even when attempting to take adequate precautions in this kind of research, actually to utilize one pup per sex per litter may be an arbitrary mode of seeking results. It is quite possible that differential effects may be incurred within a litter[42]. Differential susceptibility in twins to the same dysmorphogenic influence may be attributed to not only genetic but also intrauterine factors[60]. Because of the

Table 27.3 Home Cage Emergence Test: female and male offspring; 2-way ANOVA

		Treatment (2,30)	Sex (1,30)	Treatment × sex (2,30)
Time elapsed to first emergence	f	0.1711	20.8162	0.1321
	p	0.8436	0.0001	0.8768
	est. ω^2	0.0000	0.2356	0.0000
Time elapsed between first and final emergence	f	1.3551	11.0537	1.3072
	p	0.2733	0.0003	0.2855
	est. ω^2	0.0098	0.1229	0.0075
Number of emergence attempts	f	2.5873	0.1886	3.7293
	p	0.0919	0.6672	0.0358
	est. ω^2	0.0490	0.0000	0.0643

All data were transformed (Log X); missing data were represented by mean values[57]

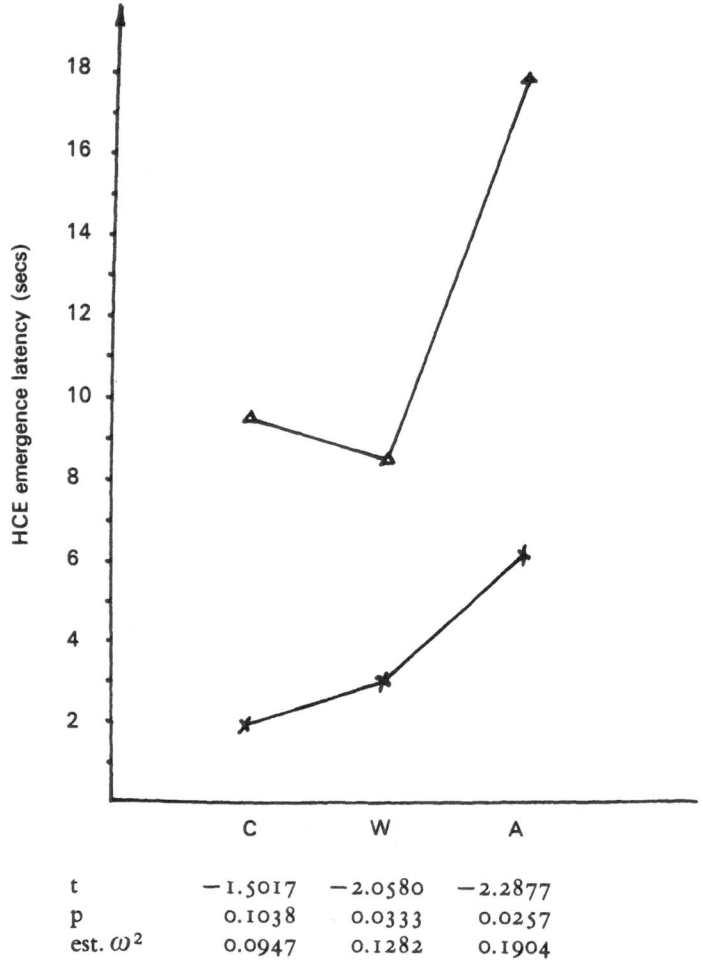

	C	W	A
t	−1.5017	−2.0580	−2.2877
p	0.1038	0.0333	0.0257
est. ω^2	0.0947	0.1282	0.1904

Figure 27.1   Mean latency to first emergence for male (◄———►) and female (×——— ×) offspring in the Home Cage Emergence test

potential FAS modulation by intrauterine factors[42], this second study was to incorporate a comparison of heavy and light offspring obtained from the same litter.

Method

This experiment followed the procedure of the previous one (p. 328), where females were equated for body weight and Open Field activity prior to mating, when 3-months old. Their offspring were tested at 8 weeks of age. Offspring had been raised in litters of six (three of each sex), and were segregated by sex on reaching vaginal opening. Prior to testing, the offspring

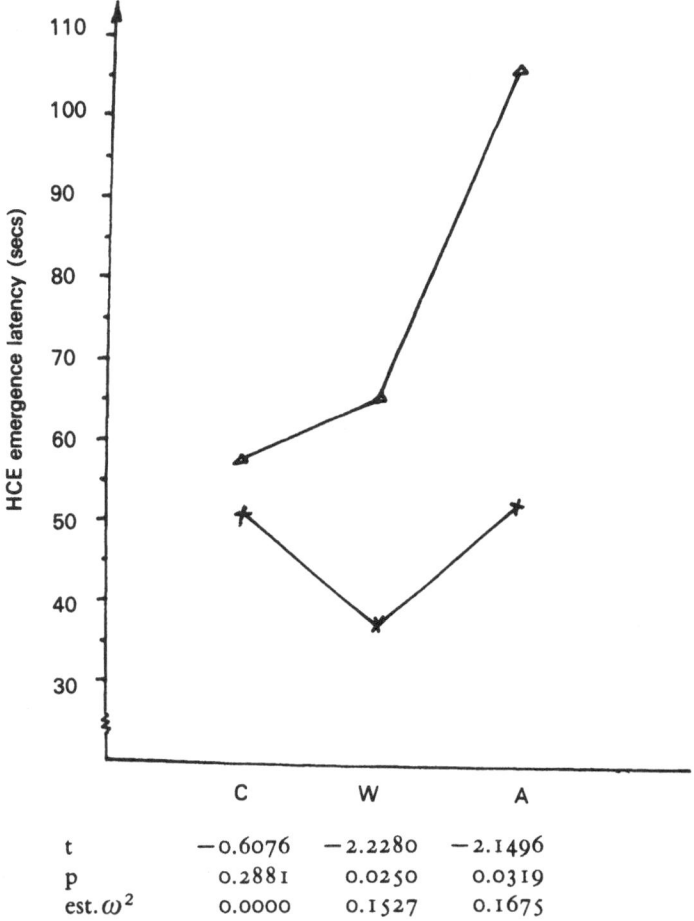

	C	W	A
t	−0.6076	−2.2280	−2.1496
p	0.2881	0.0250	0.0319
est. ω^2	0.0000	0.1527	0.1675

Figure 27.2 Mean latency between first and final emergence for male (◁——————▷) and female (——————×) offspring in the Home Cage Emergence test

were weighed, to allow selection of the heaviest and lightest of each sex from each litter for Open Field testing.

The Open Field was constructed on supplied dimensions[22], but was used without the presence of white noise. Testing was randomized over time of day, and was repeated several times for the mothers (as with the HCE), and for offspring was repeated over three consecutive days. Four behavioural activities were scored.

(1) *Walking.* The number of segments entered by an animal. A new segment was counted when both front paws had been placed into it.

(2) *Rearing.* This was scored when the rat lifted both front paws off the horizontal surface (floor). No distinction in vertical raising was

otherwise made. Self-supporting against the vertical wall was included, providing the above criteria were satisfied.

(3) *Defecation.* This was a numerical count of the number of bolusses deposited by the test animal during Open Field trials.

(4) *Grooming.* Any kind of grooming was scored, though not analysed due to its infrequent occurrence.

Each testing trial lasted for three minutes and was conducted in the room which housed the animals. This was to minimize antecedents to the testing, which may interfere with testing outcome.

Results

Open Field activity analyses have been summarized in Tables 27.4−6. Because of uneven treatment groups, separate analyses by sex and by weight were conducted, with transformations applied where appropriate, and incorporating maternal scores as covariate. Only one analysis (light males, Table 27.5) is significant ($f_{2,27} = 3.3779$; $p = 0.0496$; est. $\omega^2 = 0.1409$). There being a slight difference among sample sizes of the treatment groups, a common suggestion is that the acceptance level ought to be increased[61]. This, of course, would make the result non-significant. The association value, on the other hand, implies that some difference may exist, provided a larger sample were to be chosen[42, 62].

Table 27.4 Open Field activity: rearing

Sex/Relative weight	Statistic	ANOVA Mother	ANOVA Offspring	ANCOVA Offspring
Male				
Heavy	$f(2,27)$	2.4806	0.6154	0.4267
	p	0.1026	0.5454	0.6551
	est. ω^2	0.0898	0.0000	0.0000
Light	$f(2,27)$	2.4806	1.5528	0.8211
	p	0.1026	0.2305	0.4515
	est. ω^2	0.0898	0.0355	0.0000
Female				
Heavy*	$f(2,29)$	1.6454	0.6701	0.1168
	p	0.2104	0.5194	0.8902
	est. ω^2	0.0388	0.0000	0.0000
Light	$f(2,29)$	1.6454	0.8167	0.5223
	p	0.2104	0.4518	0.5988
	est. ω^2	0.0388	0.0000	0.0000

* Log X transformation applied

A tentative way of exploring this weight dependent result further is by means of a three-way ANOVA with repeated measures on sex and weight.

A treatment effect on walking can be observed, with alcohol offspring walking significantly less than offspring from either control group (Figure

Table 27.5 Open Field activity: walking

| Sex/Relative weight | Statistic | ANOVA | | ANCOVA |
		Mother	Offspring	Offspring
Male				
Heavy	f (2,27)	0.3075	2.4733	2.4750
	p	0.7360	0.0951	0.1042
	est. ω^2	0.0000	0.0947	0.0923
Light*	f (2,27)	0.3075	3.1899	3.3779
	p	0.7378	0.0571	0.0496
	est. ω^2	0.0000	0.1274	0.1409
Female				
Heavy	f (2,29)	0.1970	2.0812	2.1252
	p	0.8199	0.1430	0.1383
	est. ω^2	0.0000	0.0633	0.0677
Light*	f (2,29)	0.1970	0.9845	0.9183
	p	0.8223	0.3858	0.4109
	est. ω^2	0.0000	0.0000	0.0000

* Log X transformation applied

Table 27.6 Open Field activity: defecation

| Sex/Relative weight | Statistic | ANOVA | | ANCOVA |
		Mother	Offspring	Offspring
Male				
Heavy	$f(2,27)$	0.7534	1.7308	1.6864
	p	0.4804	0.1962	0.2048
	est. ω^2	0.0000	0.0465	0.0452
Light	$f(2,27)$	0.7534	0.1314	0.0084
	p	0.4804	0.8774	0.9916
	est. ω^2	0.0000	0.0000	0.0000
Female				
Heavy	$f(2,29)$	0.7514	0.0275	0.0340
	p	0.4807	0.9729	0.9666
	est. ω^2	0.0000	0.0000	0.0000
Light	$f(2,29)$	0.7514	2.3401	2.8363
	p	0.4807	0.1142	0.0756
	est. ω^2	0.0000	0.0773	0.1059

27.3). This, however, is a pooled result. Since in the analysis on walking no other significant result is obtained, pooling becomes admissable. In the case of defecation and rearing, however, sex differences exist instead (Defecation: $f_{1, 11} = 6.3269$; $p = 0.028$; est. $\omega^2 = 0.0452$. Rearing: $f_{1, 11} = 6.4763$; $p = 0.026$; est. $\omega^2 = 0.0182$). Not only that, but an interaction of sex with weight also exists in the case of rearing (Table 27.7). This sex/weight interaction can be traced to a derivation entirely from the alcohol offspring group (Table 27.7), where a significant reduction in rearing is found with light males and heavy females, when contrasted with light females (Figure 27.4)

Table 27.7 Summary of ANOVA analysis of sex × weight interaction of offspring rearings in the Open Field test

	f	p	est. ω^2
All groups	5.57	0.036	0.0182
C	1.79	0.197	0.0227
W	0.32	0.581	0.0000
A	7.01	0.014	0.1502

Discussion

Because this paper is concerned with difficulties in Open Field interpretation rather than with Open Field performance, only a limited amount of available data was analysed in order to bring out some relevant points.

Two aspects should now be clear, however. Even when using the appropriate statistical test, the outcome of an analysis may depend on the degree of data transformation, i.e. not only may a numeric transformation be required, but an allowance for maternal behaviour may also have to be made (Table 27.5: light male offspring). Secondly, not only do sex differences hold true on some behavioural parameters (Table 27.3; Figures 27.1 and 27.2), but this may be confounded further by offspring size (Table 27.7; Figure 27.4).

Earlier, research[36] was criticized for the pooling of data from offspring of both sexes, and yet this is exactly what occurs in Figure 27.3. However, the pooling in reference 36 is prospective (i.e before an analysis), while in this example it is of a retrospective type (i.e. only on grounds that no sex difference, nor a sex/treatment interaction exists). Furthermore, unlike previous studies[34, 36, 37, 41, 50], offspring here were not treated as independent units, but those who were derived from the same litter were treated as repeated measures. The consequence of such a lowering of degrees of freedom is a fewer number of significant results[42], but the advantage of this is a lowered likelihood of attaining results due to Type I errors[62].

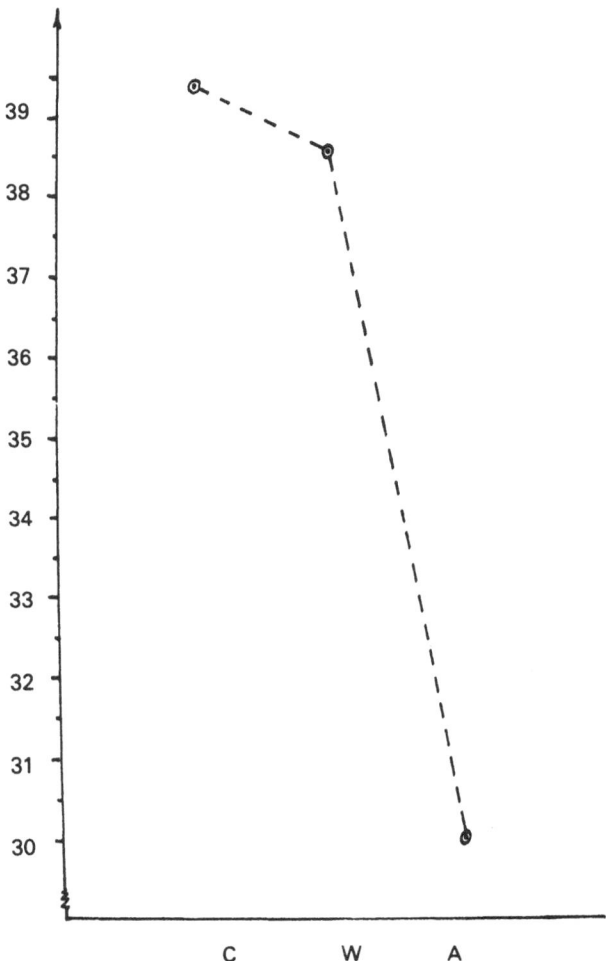

Figure 27.3   Number of Open Field segments entered by rat offspring

While a sex difference has been demonstrated in behavioural arousal, which may be associated with the natal treatment, it is important to recognize that such a difference is not common to all parameters of behaviour. Moreover, the sex/weight interaction observed (Table 27.7; Figure 27.4), is fairly restricted. One could conclude that light females are least affected by natal alcoholism, and, perhaps, that low birth weight does not necessarily have to be a detriment in natal alcoholism — but any such conclusion may be inappropriate, as the categorization by weight is entirely relative. This makes it a classification at the nominal level, and, having found a weight interaction, any future analyses may need to incorporate actual body weights as a covariant.

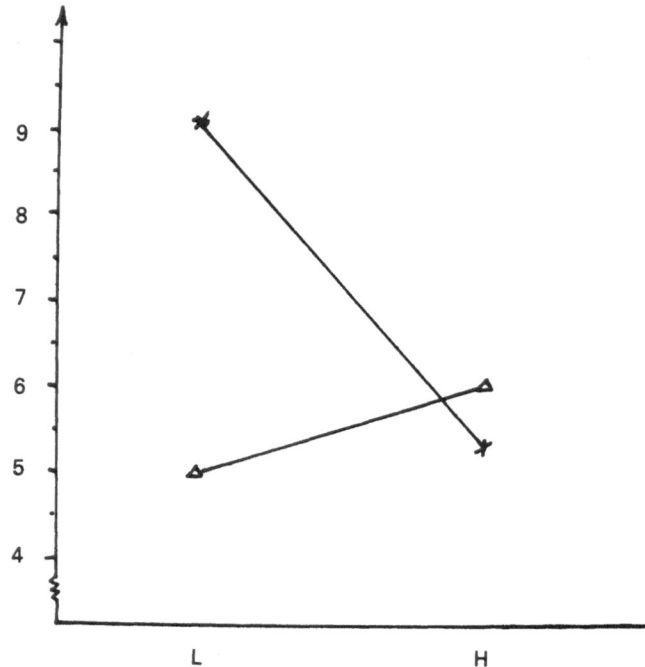

Figure 27.4   Mean number of rearings by light (L) and heavy (H) male (◁——▷)
and female (×———— ×) offspring in the Open Field test

A supplementary point to this is that of choice of test subject. It has been
shown that when 'randomly' picking rats and mice from stock cages, there
can be a tendency to select larger animals first. Consequently, if 'randomness'
is the criterion for selecting one representative from each litter, there can be a
bias not only in such a selective process, but also an additional bias in test
results. Equally, by selecting an 'average' weight animal from litters (as was
done for the HCE; see p. 328), there may possibly be a dilution of treatment
effects.

A further, moot, point is, of course, does the treatment cause the change in
behaviour, or is it a (non-causal) association of weight/sex?

In terms of arousal, it is interesting to note that, contrary to the FAS-
associated hyperactivity, there appears to be instead a certain degree of
hypoactivity. Although not significant, HCE scores for alcohol offspring
show a greater degree of timidity (Figure 27.2), and a significantly lower
degree of Open Field exploration (Figure 27.3). Induced hypoactivity was
postulated[20] for low dosage application. The important conclusion here has
to be that in using the Open Field to study natal alcohol effects on offspring,
account of sex and weight should be taken.

Acknowledgements

This research was funded by the Medical Council on Alcoholism (MCA), whose encouragement is greatly appreciated. The HCE experiment was accomodated by the Zoology Department of Queen's University, and the Open Field experiment was supported by the Ulster Polytechnic. My thanks to Mr J. O'Neill for his photographic expertise and help in this project, and to Dr T. McDade for his sterling work with the Open Field experiment.

References

1 Jones, K. L., Smith, D. W., Ulleland, C. W. and Streissguth, A. P. (1973). Pattern of malformation in offspring of chronic alcoholic women. *Lancet*, **1**, 1267
2 Jones, K. L. and Smith, D. W. (1975). The Fetal Alcohol Syndrome. *Teratology*, **12**, 1
3 Lemoine, P., Harousseau, H., Borteyru, J. P. and Menuet, J. C. (1967). Les enfants de parents alcooliques: anomalies observées à propos de 127 cas. *Arch. Fr. Pédiatr.*, **25**, 830
4 Bierich, J. R., Majewski, F., Michaelis, R. and Tillner, I. (1976). Über das embryo–fetale Alkoholsyndrom. *Eur. J. Pediatr.*, **121**, 155
5 Streissguth, A. P. (1978). Fetal Alcohol Syndrome: An epidemiologic perspective. *Am. J. Epidemiol.*, **107**, 467
6 Sandor, S. (1979). The prenatal noxious effect of ethanol. *Rev. Roum. Morphol. Embryol. Physiol. (Morphol. Embryol.)*, **25**, 211
7 Olegård, R., Sabel, K.-G., Aronsson, M., Sandin, B., Johansson, P. R., Carlsson, C., Kyllerman, M., Iversen, K. and Hrbek, A. (1979). Effects on the child of alcohol abuse during pregnancy. *Acta Paediatr. Scand.*, **275** (Suppl.), 112
8 Jones, K. L. (1975). Aberrant neuronal migration in the Fetal Alcohol Syndrome. *Birth Defects: Original Article Series*, **11**, (7), 131–132
9 Streissguth, A. P., Herman, C. S., and Smith, D. W. (1978). Intelligence, behavior, and dysmorphogenesis in the fetal alcohol syndrome: A report on 20 patients. *J. Pediatr.*, **92**, 363
10 Root, A. W., Reiter, E. O., Andriola, M. and Duckett, G. (1975). Hypothalamic-pituitary function in the fetal alcohol syndrome. *J. Pediatr.*, **87**, 585
11 Henderson, G. I., Hoyumpa, A. M., McClain, C. and Schenker, S. (1979). The effects of chronic and acute alcohol administration on fetal development in the rat. *Alcoholism Clin. Exp. Res.*, **3**, 99
12 Mendelson, R. and Huber, A. (1979). Maternal alcohol consumption: effect of alcohol on trace element deposition in the fetus. *Alcoholism Clin. Exp. Res.*, **3**, 186
13 van Biervliet, J. P. (1977). The Foetal Alcohol Syndrome. *Acta Paediatr. Belg.*, **30**, 113
14 Pierog, S., Chandavasu, O. and Wexler, I. (1977). Withdrawal symptoms in infants with the fetal alcohol syndrome. *J. Pediatr.*, **90**, 630
15 Lieber, C. S. (1979). Alcoholism and nutrition: A Seminar. *Alcoholism Clin. Exp. Res.*, **3**, 125
16 Streissguth, A. P., Barr, H. M., Martin, D. C. and Herman, C. (1979). Effects of maternal alcohol, nicotine, and caffeine use during pregnancy on infant development at 8 months. *Alcoholism Clin. Exp. Res.*, **3**, 197
17 Tittmar, H. -G. (1980). The elusiveness of the British Fetal Alcohol Syndrome. Presented at the *N. Ireland Branch Meeting of the British Psychological Society*, 11 December, Belfast
18 Rosman, N. P. and Malone, M. J. (1977). Reversal of delayed myelinogenesis in the Fetal Alcohol Syndrome. *Neurology*, **27**, 369
19 Charlebois, A. T. and Fried, P. A. (1980). Interactive effects of nutrition and cannabis upon rat perinatal development. *Dev. Psychobiol.*, **13**, 591
20 Tittmar, H.-G. (1978). Some effects of alcohol, presented during the prenatal period, on

the development and behaviour of rats. Paper read at the *4th International Conference on Alcohol and Drug Dependence*, 9–14 April, Liverpool

21 Routtenberg, A. (1968). The two-arousal hypothesis: reticular formation and limbic system. *Psychol. Rev.*, **75**, 51

22 Joffe, J. M. (1969). *Prenatal Determinants of Behaviour.* (London: Pergamon)

23 Denenberg, V. H. (1964). Critical periods, stimulus input and emotional reactivity: A theory of infantile stimulation. *Psychol. Rev.*, **71**, 335

24 Denenberg, V. H. (1969). Open Field behavior in the rat: What does it mean. *Ann. NY Acad. Sci.*, **159**, 852

25 Abel, E. L. (1980). Fetal Alcohol Syndrome: behavioral teratology. *Psychol. Bull.*, **87**, 29

26 Tapp, J. T., Zimmerman, R. S. and D'Encurnacao, P. J. (1968). Intercorrelational analysis of some common measures of rat activity. *Psychol. Rep.*, **23**, 1047

27 Halliday, M. S. (1966). Exploration and fear in the rat. In Jewell, P. A. and Loizos, C. (eds.) *Play, Exploration and Territory in Mammals*, Symposia of the Zoological Society of London, No 18, pp. 45–59. (London: Academic Press)

28 Archer, J. (1973). Tests for emotionality in rats and mice: A review. *Anim. Behav.*, **21**, 205

29 Lát, J. and Gollová-Hémon, E. (1969). Permanent effects of nutritional and endocrinological intervention in early ontogeny on the level of nonspecific excitability and on lability (Emotionality). *Ann. NY Acad. Sci.*, **159**, 710

30 Birbaumer, N. (1975). *Physiologische Psychologie*, p. 55. (Berlin: Springer)

31 Hill, O. (1971). The effects of post-natal maternal stress on offspring tested for emotionality in adulthood in the Wistar albino rat. *BSc Thesis*, Queen's University, Belfast

32 Crnic, L. S. (1976). Effects of infantile undernutrition on adult learning in rats: Methodological and design problems. *Psychol. Bull.*, **83**, 715

33 Becker, G. (1969). Initial and hábituated autonomic reactivity in the male and female rat. *J. Comp. Physiol. Psychol.*, **69**, 459

34 Abel, E. L. (1975). Emotionality in offspring of rats fed alcohol while nursing. *J. Stud. Alc.*, **36**, 654

35 Thompson, W. R. and Quinby, S. (1964). Prenatal maternal anxiety and offspring behavior: Parental activity and level of anxiety. *J. Genet. Psychol.*, **105**, 359

36 Bond, N. W. and Di Giusto, E. L. (1977). Prenatal alcohol consumption and Open-Field behaviour in rats: Effects of age at time of testing. *Psychopharmacology*, **52**, 311

37 Bond, N. W. and Di Giusto, E. L. (1976). Effects of prenatal alcohol consumption on Open-Field Behaviour and alcohol preference in rats. *Psychopharmacology*, **46**, 163

38 Broadhurst, P. L. (1969). Psychogenetics of Emotionality in the rat. *Ann. NY Acad. Sci.*, **159**, 806

39 Murphree, O. D. and Dykman, R. A. (1965). Litter patterns in the offspring of nervous and stable dogs. I: Behavioural tests. *J. Nerv. Ment. Dis.*, **141**, 321

40 Archer, J. E. and Blackman, D. E. (1971). Prenatal psychological stress and offspring behaviour in rats and mice. *Dev. Psychobiol.*, **4**, 193

41 Morra, M. (1969). Ethanol and maternal stress on rat offspring behaviors. *J. Genet. Psychol.*, **114**, 77

42 Tittmar, H.-G. (1982). Statistical considerations in the analysis of data in teratology. In Abel, E. L. (ed.). *The Fetal Alcohol Syndrome*. Vol. III: Animal Studies, pp. 15–37. (Boca Raton, FL: CRC Press)

43 Tittmar, H. -G. (1982). Some problems inherent in natal alcoholism. *J. Psych. Treat. Eval.*, **4**, 165

44 Bronstein, P. M. (1972). Cross-sectional and longitudinal investigations. *J. Comp. Physiol. Psychol.*, **80**, 335

45 Bronstein, P. M. (1972). Repeated trials with the albino rat in the Open Field as a function of age and deprivation. *J. Comp. Physiol. Psychol.*, **81**, 84

46 Campbell, B. A. and Raskin, L. A. (1978). Ontogeny of behavioural arousal: the role of environmental stimuli. *J. Comp. Physiol. Psychol.*, **92**, 176

47 Schardein, J. L. (1977). *Drugs as Teratogens*, p. 9 (Cleveland, Ohio: CRC Press)

48 Tittmar, H.-G. (1974). Alcohol intoxication: A method for obtaining increased ethanol intake in gravid rats. *IRCS (Med. Sci.)*, **2**, 1079

49 Chernoff, G. F. (1977). The Fetal Alcohol Syndrome in mice: an animal model. *Teratology*, **15**, 223

50 Branchey, L. and Friedhoff, A. J. (1976). Biochemical and behavioral changes in rats exposed to ethanol *in utero*. *Ann. NY Acad. Sci.*, **273**, 328

51 Kreezer, G. L. (1967). Techniques for the investigation of behavioural phenomena in the rat. In Farris, E. J. and Griffith, J. Q. (eds.) *The Rat in Laboratory Investigation*, pp. 203–277. (New York: Hafner)

52 Hutt, S. J. and Hutt, C. (1970). *Direct Observation and Measurement of Behaviour.* (Springfield: Thomas)

53 Laurence, D. R. and Bacharach, A. L. (1964). *The Evaluation of Drug Activities: Pharmacometrics.* Vol. I. (London: Academic Press)

54 Mikhel'son, M. Y. and Longo, V. G. (1965). Proceedings of the Second International Pharmacological meeting. Vol. I. *Pharmacology of Conditioning, Learning and Retention.* (Oxford: Pergamon)

55 Tittmar, H.-G. and Farry, K. (1974). Synchronised mating by albino rats. *IRCS (Med. Sci.)*, **2**, 1568

56 Tittmar, H.-G. (1977). Some effects of ethanol, presented during the pre-natal period, on the development of rats. *Br. J. Alc. Alcoholism*, **12**, 71

57 Hays, W. L. (1963). *Statistics.* (London: Holt, Rinehart & Winston)

58 Abel, E. L. and Greizerstein, H. B. (1982). Growth and development in animals prenatally exposed to alcohol. In Abel, E. L. (ed.) *Fetal Alcohol Syndrome.* Vol. III: Animal Studies, pp. 39–57. (Boca Raton, FL.: CRC Press)

59 Abel, E. L. (1982). Behavioral teratology of alcohol (Animal model studies of the Fetal Alcohol Syndrome). In Abel, E. L. (ed.) *Fetal Alcohol Syndrome.* Vol. III: Animal Studies, pp. 59–81. (Boca Raton, FL: CRC Press)

60 Riley, E. P. and Lochry, E. A. (1982). Genetic influences in the etiology of Fetal Alcohol Syndrome. In Abel, E. L. (ed.) *Fetal Alcohol Syndrome.* Vol. III: Animal Studies, pp. 113–130. (Boca Raton, FL: CRC Press)

61 Lindquist, E. F. (1956). *Design and Analysis of Experiments in Psychology and Education.* (Boston: Houghton Mifflin)

62 Tittmar, H. -G. (1975). Fetal units or litter units? – A possible solution. *Teratology*, **12**, 89

63 Rümke, Chr. L. and De Jonge, H. (1964). Design, statistical analysis and interpretation. In Laurence, D. R. and Bacharach, A. L. (eds.) *Evaluation of Drug Activities: Pharmacometrics.* Vol. I. Chap. 3. (London: Academic Press)

28
Object relationships and substance abuse: self-object and alcoholism

M. H. WETHERHORN

Alcohol abuse reflects a personal failure in capacity for intimacy in object relations. Intimacy is defined as the capacity for personal disclosure, i.e. frankness, honesty, sincerity and especially the capacity to share a broad spectrum of feelings involving ambivalence with significant objects. This chapter addresses the treatment of those patients suffering from narcissistic and borderline conditions and who may be perceived as suffering from epigenetic disorders described as early pre-oedipal.

The need for unconditional positive regard from significant objects, the inability to deal with 'uncomfortable' feelings, the splitting of objects into good object and bad object on the basis of hedonic tone, is central. The incorporation of the object as part of the self, as a commodity whose mission to supply admiration and unconditional affectional and nurturential regard, is then the impossible contract imposed on the self-object. Failure of the self-object to fulfill the unconscious contract results in rage, outrage, feelings of abandonment, helplessness, and 'emptiness', then setting the stage for turning to substance abuse as a means of tranquillizing the rage and overcome the feelings of 'void' and helplessness. Turning to an attainable commodity, such as alcohol, relieves the patient of repeated interpersonal failure in the search to overcome profound feelings of alienation, horror vacui and the perception of self as quintessentially 'unloveable.'

The scope of this presentation allows only the articulation of the treatment process silhouette with pre-oedipal disorders. No map covers all the territory. This semantic principle is most applicable since elaboration is obviated. It is proffered that the core stages of treatment with narcissistic and borderline condition alcoholism involve the following sequence:

(1)   development of the therapeutic alliance
(2)   analysis of the narcissistic mirror transference
(3)   replacement of the pathic maternal introject or object representation

Stage one, the development of the therapeutic alliance, involves the establishment of an empathic relationship. The empathic relationship is the *sine qua non* of the entire therapeutic process. Empathy is defined as the capacity for participating in another's feeling and thinking. Further, it is posited that the lack of this empathic relationship, especially during the first 36 months of life, has been the single most pathic influence on development of an autonomous well-integrated self which possesses reasonably adequate self-esteem. Empathy does not presume the participation by the therapist in all of the patient's thinking and feeling. Even the most empathic therapist does not possess perfect coenaesthetic empathy. Rather, the therapist strives to participate in the patient's inner life. It is only necessary that the patient recognize the therapist's willingness and striving to participate. Here, Winnicott's[8] 'reasonably good enough mother' becomes a paradigm and metaphor for the 'reasonably good enough therapist'. During this stage of treatment, fears of identity diffusion (loss of autonomous self) may be evoked in the transference. Similarly, fears of abandonment by the therapist are conspicuous at this stage. These conflicts, I submit, are a shadow-play of the separation—individuation conflicts of pre-oedipal development. It is the lack of the empathic relationship with the coterminal positive hedonic tone which leads to the child's inability to evoke a positive object representation when not in the presence of the mother. Narcissistic and borderline patients report emptiness and horror vacui experiences which are the developmental sequelae. Stated somewhat differently, the empathic relationship at this stage of treatment involves unconditional positive regard.

Following the establishment of the empathic relationship, the therapeutic alliance allows the patient to perceive the dyadic subculture as markedly different from his usual experiences. Only then is the exploration of the self reasonably safe. The mirror transference results (admiration, love, exaltation of the therapist and exhibitionism through performance) denote the entrance to this stage. Simply stated, the patient relates to the therapist in precisely the fashion the patient craves the therapist to relate. It is centrally important at this stage of treatment to develop a treatment contract with the patient whereby the therapist is allowed to make up his own mind about many issues in treatment which reciprocally allows the patient to separate and individuate without a feeling of abandonment.

Again, a shadow-play occurs in therapy of former splitting phenomena. The patient's low self-esteem does not allow him to feel worthy of the craved-for emotional supply and a compensatory self develops. Whether or not the compensatory self is grandiose or merely expansive is a moot question. Perhaps, grandiose is descriptive hyperbole for many patients. The existence of low self-esteem has led historically to the perception that success is not real, plastic and undeserved. It is very common for depression and feelings of unworthiness to follow success — both success in the acquisition of affectional supplies and vocational success. These patients often experience paradoxical depression, emptiness, and even anhedonia following 'success'.

The compensatory self is a personal construct not based on interpersonal experience but, rather, on personal need. The patient attempts to provide himself with the needed affectional supply without recourse to others, hence the term 'narcissistic'. Recall of self-rocking and self-stroking in childhood are replete. The self is taken as a love object and the disorders of schizophrenia, borderline state manic depressive illness, addiction, and most probably severe character disorders are coterminally related in reference to the narcissistic dimension. The narcissistic-compensatory self as an adaptive-defensive ego manoeuvre becomes an anachronism of the adult mature ego. It is thus dissembled or discarded in the therapeutic process. It is replaced by a real self capable of developing empathic relationships both within and outside of the treatment relationship.

For many patients it is necessary to forego the established psychoanalytic model regarding countertransference and permit the expression of a caring attitude provided it is genuine. It is precisely the caring attitude *vis-a-vis* the care-taking attitude that provides the necessary therapeutic impact. In other words, an existential rather than standard psychoanalytic approach is proposed. The non-empathic introject needs to be replaced with a caring introject. The positive hedonic tone of this therapeutic alliance and the resolution of the conflicts that led to the compensatory self may lead to the analysis of oedipal conflicts, but not necessarily so. Whether or not analysis of oedipal conflicts is necessary is an issue for the polemic arena.

Bibliography

1 Goldberg, A. (1978). *The Psychology of the Self.* (New York: International University Press)
2 Hartocollis, P. (ed.) (1977). *Borderline Personality Disorders.* (New York: International University Press)
3 Kernberg, O. (1975). *Borderline Condition and Pathological Narcissism.* (New York: Aronson, Jason)
4 Kohut, J. (1977). *The Restoration of the Self.* (New York: International University Press)
5 Nelson, M. (ed.) (1977). *The Narcissistic Condition.* (New York: Human Science Press)
6 Spotnitz, J. and Meadows, P. (1976). *Treatment of the Narcissistic Disorders.* (New York: Manhatten Center for Advanced Psychoanalytic Studies)
7 Volkan, V. (1975). *Primitive Internalized Object Relations.* (New York: International University Press)
8 Winnicott, D. W. (1958). The Capacity to be Alone. *Int. J. Psychoanal.*, **39,** 416

Part 7:
ALCOHOLISM – SPECIAL GROUPS

29
Alcoholism and doctors:
Some characteristics of 50 male (recovering) alcoholic doctors: results of a questionnaire enquiry 1982

M. M. GLATT

RESULTS OF A *1979* ENQUIRY

Three years ago, in June 1979, two members of the British Doctors Group[1] for recovering alcoholics (which by then had been in existence for 5 years), sent a letter to *The Lancet* briefly describing the preliminary results of a questionnaire enquiry among members of the Group. (*The Lancet* did not publish the letter.) Replies had been received from 59 doctors out of 120 members to whom the questionnaire was sent (by the time the letter was written); several further replies arrived too late for the results to be considered so that the preliminary response rate was taken as 50 %. Of the 59 individuals, three had filled in their forms incompletely.

Of the remaining 56 doctors, 37 had been sober for more than 1 year; of these 37, 75 % (28 doctors) admitted that in the past they had tried unsuccessfully to control their drinking without any form of treatment. This admission was taken as indicating that their alcoholism had reached the stage of 'loss of control'.

The mean period of sobriety was 4.1 years (range 1 – 26 years); 54 % of the sober 37 doctors (20) had been sober for over 3 years.

Eighty-four per cent of the sober 37 doctors (31 individuals) had received inpatient treatment at some stage.

Fifty-four per cent (20 individuals) had been treated in a National Health Service alcoholism treatment unit, or in a private unit encouraging group therapy.

As regards regular follow-up (usually regarded as an essential part of the treatment of alcoholism), only two (5% of the 37 sober doctors) had no follow-up. Many attended AA meetings (28 doctors – 76%) and/or the Doctors' Group (28 doctors – 76%); some were also followed up by the unit at which they had been treated or by such organizations as 'Accept'. It was usual for the individual doctor to have more than one follow-up.

Drs K. and H. – co-chairmen at the time of the Doctors' Group – concluded that the high proportion of sober alcoholic doctors in the survey for whom inpatient care had been required to achieve sobriety (after attempts at control by their own had failed), was important – indicating that inpatient facilities for the treatment of alcoholism are needed at the present time and for the foreseeable future. Obviously these doctors had not presented themselves for treatment at a stage so early in their condition that their treatment could have been carried out on an outpatient basis.

RESULTS OF THE PRESENT (1982) ENQUIRY: 50 MALE BRITISH ALCOHOLIC DOCTORS

In March 1982 a further, more detailed questionnaire was mailed to the members of the British Doctors' (and Dentists') Group. The following analysis presents the replies from the first 50 male doctors answering the questionnaire. Not all of these replied to all questions; replies from the few female members and dental surgeons were not included in the following analysis.

(1) *Age* distribution: 45–72

(2) *Birthplace*: English, 26; Scottish, 15; Irish, 7; Welsh, 2.

(3) *'Specialty'*: GPs, 32; specialists, 17: community medicine 4, Psychiatry 3.

(4) *Medical school* situation: England, 24; Scotland, 17; Eire, 2.

(5) Place of *practice*: England, 34; Scotland, 8; Eire, 2.

(6) Average *time of practice* as a doctor: 20 years.

(7) *Religion*: Church of England, 16; Church of Scotland, 10; Roman Catholic, 8; 'no religion', 11; Jewish, 1; Muslim, 1.

(8) *Education about alcohol in medical school*: none, 38; little, 11; 'a lot', 1.

(9) A. Main *Reason* ('excuse') *for drinking*:
    (a) as *undergraduates*:
        (i)   peer group, 24 (48%)
        (ii) stress of study, 1 (2%)
        (23 doctors (46%) did *not* drink heavily as students).
    (b) as *postgraduates*:
        (i)   drinking with others 30 (62%)

    (ii)   stress of work, 29 (58 %); (mainly long hours, 20 (40 %))

    (iii) domestic stress, 19 (38 %)

    (iv) depression, 15 (30 %)

    (v)   economic stress, 6 (12 %).

B. Main *reason*: 'Host'? or 'Environment'?

  (a)   *'vulnerability'* of personality, 34 (68 %)

    (i)   insecure, anxious etc., 33 (66 %)

    (ii) workoholic, 18 (36 %)

  (b)   *socioeconomic* reasons: exposure, 'subculture', economic, 18 (36 %).

(10) *Age of onset of drinking*:

  (a)   regular *'moderate'* drinking (4 pints, or 4 doubles, or 1 bottle of wine/day), 25 years

  (b)   regular *'heavy'* drinking (more than 4 pints/4 doubles/1 bottle of wine), about 36 years

  (c)   regular *'excessive'* drinking (more than 8 pints/8 doubles/2 bottles of wine), about 41 years.

(11) Certain important events/experiences in *Drinking history*[3]

  (a)   amnesia, 43 (expressly denied by 7)

  (b)   loss of control, 48 (expressly denied by 2)

  (c)   fits, 8

  (d)   DT, 11

  (e)   liver damage, 18 (as reflected in LFT, or clinical features)

  (f)   polyneuropathy, 9

  (g)   peptic ulcer, 3 (no case of gastrectomy)

  (h)   hospitalized, 36.

(12) Duration of *abstinence* by the time of replying to the questionnaire:

  (a)   the majority had been continually sober for less than 6 months (most were newcomers to the Group, a few had relapsed)

  (b)   2–14 years of abstinence, 11

  (c)   6–18 months of abstinence, 8.

(13) *Reasons* given *for doing something* about one's drinking:

  (a)   mental complaints, 17

  (b)   physical complaints, 11

  (c)   breathalysed, 8

  (d)   car accidents, 8

  (e)   Court appearance, 7 (for car offences, 6)

  (f)   appearance before General Medical Council, 5

  (g)   (threat of) wife walking out, 6

  (h)   loss of job, 5.

Note: 3 doctors were breathalysed after car accidents – thus in at least 15 doctors, car offences led to 'doing something.'

(14)   *Abstinence was accompanied in sphere of*:

	domestic	*work*	*social*	*eating*	*sleep*	*contentment*
by *improvement*	35	39	40	39	34	38
by *deterioration*	2	2	3	1	3	1
by *no change*	13	9	6	11	11	9

(15)   *Abstinence was accompanied by*:

	in *Spouse*		*Children*	
	attitude	*mental health*	*attitude*	*mental health*
improvement	24	28	33	30
deterioration	2	2	1	—
no change	10	13	4	9

(16)   *Treatment* for alcoholism received *by* (*in*):
    (a)   alcoholic unit, 30
    (b)   other inpatient treatment, 13
    (c)   OP only, 2
    (d)   GP, 4 (of whom 3 were also in a unit).

(17)   Members of *AA*: 37.
    AA found very helpful by 33 (of the 37).

(18)   *Controlled drinking in the past*:
    never tried: 18 drs.
    tried: 30 drs.
    result regarded as:
        "disaster" in 25 drs.
        OK (for 3 months) 1
        "not good" (weeks) 1
        "no benefit" 1

(19)   *Delay between your recognition* of problem *and 'doing something'*: over 4 years average in 40 doctors.
    Reason for delay: denial of problem by 15 doctors. Other reasons given: 'I thought I could control it'; pride; 'I could not find treatment'.

(20)   *Cooperation* with treatment:
    (a)   cooperating fully, 35
    (b)   'a bit', 8
    (c)   'not at all', 1
    (d)   taking premature discharge, 2

(21)   History of *suicidal attempts*: 5

(22)   *Habitual drug misuse*: 14 (barbiturates, amphetamine, Valium, Heminevrin, Mandrax, amitryptiline, Distalgesic, codeine).

(23)   How do you compare your *functioning during abstinence period and drinking period*?

    (a)   improved during abstinence, 41
    (b)   worse during abstinence, 1
    (c)   no difference, 1
    (d)   no clear answer, 5.

(24)   *Family reaction* to:
    (a)   *controlled drinking*: (total: 30)
        (i)   sceptical, disappointed in case of 13
        (ii)   'well' received, 4
        (iii)   doubtful reaction, 4
    (b)   *abstinence*:
        (i)   'delighted', 41
        (ii)   'edgy', 1
        (iii)   no reaction, 3.

(25)   Were you mainly a *gamma* (LoC, bout) or a *delta* (plateau, intermittent) drinker, or both?
    (a)   gamma, 3
    (b)   delta, 20
    (c)   both, 26.

(26)   Your *favourite drink*?:
    in 42 doctors, spirits (sometimes together with beer).

(27)   Your *follow-up* after finishing inpatient treatment:
    (a)   AA, 27
    (b)   Doctors' Group, 22

(28)   '*Cover-up*' for one's drinking by colleagues?
    (a)   Yes, 33
    (b)   No, 10.

DISCUSSION OF 1982 ENQUIRY RESULTS

Alcoholism is one of the most important social problems of our time. At the same time, whilst it is, or should be, the concern of various professional disciplines, it is of course also an important medical problem. Unfortunately, however, throughout history the medical profession as a whole has taken little notice of the problem[2].

How much, in fact, does the average medical practitioner know about alcoholism and alcoholics? In the past, medical students learnt very little about the condition[3], as clearly reflected in the replies to question 8 in the present questionnaire: of these 50 doctors, 49 received no or little education about alcohol at their medical school (referring to the period about 30 years ago or so), although matters have undoubtedly improved to a certain degree in the meantime[3].

At any rate, certain doctors do know about alcoholism — from their own experience both as sufferers from the disorder and later on from their efforts in trying to recover, and in sharing their experiences with other medical men who are fellow sufferers. Some of these in Britain, in 1973, formed the British Doctors' Group[4, 5] whose members originally met regularly only in London but now also in a few other English towns, as well as in Glasgow, and in Eire. Among them these recovered and recovering alcoholic doctors have a large fund of experience and knowledge about alcoholism. The questionnaire was an attempt to tap this fund of knowledge.

It is, of course, clear that these recovering alcoholic doctors and their replies cannot be taken as representative of the views of alcoholic doctors in Britain in general. Of the 2000 or 3000, or more, alcoholic medical men in Britain[3], unfortunately only a small proportion seem to take active steps to overcome their problem or join AA, whereas the members of the British Doctors' Group largely adopt attitudes to alcoholism and its management which are identical with, or very similar to, the AA approach. Initially such doctors often fight shy of joining local AA groups, for example because of the fear that they might there come face to face with their own patients. They find it much easier to join the Doctors' Group in the knowledge that all the others are professional men and women who had, or still have, to face similar problems[3, 4, 5]. The great majority, however, soon derive so much benefit from sharing their problems with fellow sufferers that they also start attending AA meetings in their home towns. Replies to questions 17 and 27 show that four out of five recovering doctors have become members of AA and that almost all of these find AA very helpful. Their approval of abstinence as treatment goal for alcoholics (Q. 14, 15) and disapproval of controlled drinking (Q. 18) − whilst based on their own personal experiences (Q. 14, 15, 18, 23) and on the reactions of their families to their abstinence and controlled drinking attempts respectively (Q. 24) − has undoubtedly been reinforced by the AA philosophy. Many still drinking alcoholic doctors, on the other hand, probably nourish the belief and hope that − in spite of many disastrous experiences and the doubts of their families − they may still 'regain the lost willpower' and learn to control their drinking (Q. 19 shows that it took the recovering doctors an average period of 4 years between their recognition of having a drink problem and their decision actively to do something about it). Their denial of the problem probably largely reflects the intensity and degree of their psychological dependence. Moreover, in a high proportion of these doctors it took definite physical or mental complaints or threatening court appearances, loss of wife or job to persuade them finally to 'do something'. Clearly the attitudes of these recovering doctors are unlikely to be representative of British doctors in general or even of that great majority of British alcoholic doctors who still 'practise' their alcoholism − painfully but yet living in hope that some day they may yet master the art of drinking in a controlled way.

In another aspect the composition of the Doctors' Group may be more representative of British alcoholic doctors in general, i.e. in the relatively high proportion of *Scottish and Irish doctors* among them (Q. 2, Q. 4). Several observers have found relatively high proportions of Irish and Scottish doctors among their alcoholic medical patients[3]; these higher proportions may reflect the relatively higher rates of alcoholism in Ireland (when making allowances for the relatively large numbers of teetotallers — 'pioneers' — there[4]) and Scotland. Compared to the finding that at present 34 of these doctors practised in England as against 8 practising in Scotland and 2 in Eire (Q. 5), a much lower proportion were English-born (26), a higher proportion born in Scotland (15) or Eire (7) (see Q. 2); and as regards their medical school, only 24 of 43 doctors had been at an English medical school, compared to 17 who were trained in Scotland (Q. 4), whereas now 34 practise in England and only 8 in Scotland (Q. 5). (Incidentally, the fact that the questionnaire was distributed in Glasgow directly by the Glasgow chapter of the Doctors' Group very likely has a bearing on the finding that 7 of the 17 doctors trained in Scotland had been at the Glasgow medical school).

The *hypothetical average recovering British alcoholic doctor* — as reflected in the replies to the questionnaire — was male (the Group has relatively few female members so far), middle-aged (Q. 1), likely to be born in England but quite possibly in Scotland or Ireland and possibly trained at a Scottish medical school; mostly Church of England or Church of Scotland, and sometimes Roman Catholic; surprisingly often he gives his religion as 'none' (Q. 7). He has been in medical practice for about 20 years and is most likely to be a GP though often a specialist (Q. 3); either way he has received no education about alcohol in medical school (Q. 8). Equally often he may or may not have been a heavy drinker already as a medical student (Q. 9). He started regular moderate drinking in his mid-twenties, regular heavy drinking 10 years later and regular excessive drinking in his early forties (Q. 10): soon afterwards he showed prodromal features of alcoholism (amnesias) and a few years later 'lost control' over alcohol[3, 6] (Q. 11). Surprisingly often he had suffered from physical withdrawal symptoms (fits or DT) (Q. 11.). Often he may have been sober for several years, more often for several months only in the immediate past (Q. 12), and there was usually some definite factor — such as a medical complaint or pressure from some outside source — that triggered off his final decision to do something about his drinking (Q. 13). This step was, however, only taken after he had 'denied' the existence of his problem, in spite of being at least vaguely aware of its existence, for over 4 years (Q. 19); and quite likely he may have tried to control his drinking, usually with 'disastrous' results (Q. 18). His family was frequently sceptical or disappointed about his attempts to control his drinking, whereas they were usually delighted when he decided to abstain from drinking altogether (Q. 24). Not infrequently he had also habitually misused other psychotropic drugs (Q. 22), but suicidal attempts were surprisingly uncommon (Q. 21). As expected, spirits was the favourite drink, sometimes beer was also taken (Q. 26). At first glance, perhaps surprising is the finding that many of these alcoholic doctors regarded themselves as 'delta'[3, 6] ('inability to abstain', plateau or intermittent) drinkers and only very few as 'gamma'[3, 6] ('loss of control' or bout) drinkers; and that over 50 % regarded themselves as a combination of gamma and delta drinkers (Q. 25). This may seem unexpected because the earlier World Health Organization publications on alcohol and alcoholism in the 1950s[3] and

Jellinek (1960)[6] stated that in the Anglo-Saxon countries — with spirits the popular drink among alcoholics — the gamma type was the predominant type of alcoholism whereas delta was more common in wine-drinking countries. However, the finding that among these British doctors a combination of gamma and delta seemed to be the most common manifestation of alcoholism is very much in line with our observations among British alcoholics in general[3].

As could be expected, the doctor's drinking had been known to his colleagues who 'covered up' for him (Q. 28). In the long run this is obviously a course of behaviour that is as unhelpful to the sick colleague as it is dangerous to his patients. It is a vital issue that at present exercises the ingenuity of the General Medical Council in Britain.

Ultimately the great majority of these doctors required residential treatment, mostly in alcoholic units (Q. 16); and contrary to the view sometimes expressed that medical men are unco-operative patients, the great majority co-operated fully (Q. 20) — as has indeed been the case with those alcoholic doctor patients observed by us in alcoholic units[3]. Most doctors after finishing treatment attended meetings of their local AA or the Doctors' Group (Q. 27). It is often claimed by those observers who are in favour of the 'controlled drinking' goal in alcoholics that abstinence not infrequently may be accompanied by lack of improvement or even deterioration in other important areas of the drinker's adjustment, including for example in the domestic sphere. This view is not supported by the results of this enquiry. Certainly by itself abstinence is not the goal of treatment of alcoholics but 'the best and usually only means towards (a happy, harmonious life)'[3]: as again shown in the present study, in most cases abstinence is accompanied by improvement in other spheres of the drinker's adjustment (Q. 14) and in the attitude and state of mental health of his family (Q. 15). As regards the doctors' own assessments, 70–80 % noted an all-round improvement in other spheres accompanying their abstinence, about 20 % noted 'no change', 2–6 % of doctors felt that their abstinence was accompanied by a deterioration in other areas of adjustment (Q. 14). Similarly 50–60 % considered attitude and mental health of wife and children to be improved, 5–25 % saw no change, and only 2–4 % noted a deterioration (Q. 15). Similarly 82 % of these doctors noted an overall improvement of their general functioning during their abstinence as compared to their performance during their drinking periods (Q. 23).

Obviously — as pointed out above — the continuing influence of the prevailing AA philosophy among the members of this group must to a certain extent have coloured their views about the value of abstinence as against controlled drinking. A corresponding 'bias' may be reflected in the finding that quite a few doctors altered the question (9) as to the 'main reason for drinking' into 'excuse' — indicating their view that there is no adequate 'reason' for an alcoholic's drinking, only excuses. Whilst obviously an alcoholic's continued (heavy) drinking cannot improve the situation but must make it worse, a non-alcoholic observer who has observed a great many alcoholics will surely often ask himself how many average non-alcoholic individuals would have weathered some of the problems that alcoholics encounter, without attempting some form of escape. Nonetheless to counsel and to help alcoholics to face such problems without recourse to drink or other psychotropic drugs (Q. 22) is a main task of the treatment[3]. The task confronting such patients would seem even more difficult for the high proportion of doctors (68 %) who felt that personality vulnerability (such as insecurity, anxiety etc.) may have contributed to their excessive drinking; and that sometimes an added tendency to 'workoholism' (itself possibly often a consequence of their insecurity) may have acted as a further stress factor (Q. 9A, B). The importance of social factors, however, is evident both at the undergraduate and the postgraduate stage (Q. 9A). Domestic stress was often given as an important factor; as is well known, often the spouses of alcoholic doctors themselves show clear evidence of a disturbed state of mental health[3]. It is the more gratifying and an important hopeful feature − as well as an encouragement to diagnosis and the institution of treatment − to note the all-round improvement in the great majority of these doctors who accepted the abstinence philosophy − an improvement in spite of their longstanding (Q. 10), and severe degree (Q. 11) of, alcoholism: virtually all admitted loss of control over alcohol (Q. 11) and had therefore reached (at least) the middle or crucial phase[3]; and a considerable proportion had shown evidence of liver or nervous system affection (Q. 11). Quite astounding is the high proportion of doctors who seemed to have so little insight into their condition as to precipitate epileptiform fits or DT (Q. 11), presumably by just suddenly stopping their heavy drinking without asking for help. This again reflects the lamentable lack of training of medical students in this field and highlights the need for marked improvement of medical undergraduate and postgraduate training[3]. This has been one of the main aims of the British Medical Council[3].

Hopefully the work of the British Doctors' Group in itself and its successes will alert the medical profession to the fact that alcoholism is an occupational hazard among doctors, to the need for preventive steps (such as adequate specific medical training in this area) and for early diagnosis and adequate treatment, and finally give hope to sufferers that adequate treatment and follow-up is likely to lead to marked improvement or full recovery.

CONCLUSION

A questionnaire enquiry among male members of the British Doctors' Group (formed by recovering alcoholic men and women) elicited many findings confirming results found in other studies but also some more surprising replies. The well-known, deplorable lack of medical education in this field (hardly anyone had had any undergraduate education on alcohol or alcoholism) was reflected in the very high proportion of alcoholic doctors who had suffered serious physical withdrawal manifestations, i.e. epileptiform fits or DT; and in the serious state of alcohol dependence and of physical complications reached by these doctors before they finally were virtually forced (by their poor state of health, or threats by wife, employers or the Court) into treatment. On the other hand, a promising result of the enquiry is the finding of the marked improvement in state of health and functioning (not only of the drinker himself but also of wife and children) of these men after accepting, and co-operating with, treatment, the need for follow-up and the need for abstinence.

Acknowledgements

I should like to express my thanks to the Hon. Secretary of the British Doctors and Dentists' Group, Dr S. M. N., and to his wife, for despatching the questionnaires, and to the members of the Group for their keen co-operation.

References

1 M. G. K. and S. H. (1979). Personal communication
2 Glatt, M. M. (1958). The British Drink Problem, its rise and decline through the ages. *Br. J. Addict.*, **54,** 51
3 Glatt, M. M. (1982). *Alcoholism*, Chaps. 3, 11, 18. (London: Hodder & Stoughton, Teach Yourself Books)
4 Glatt, M. M. (1975). Doctors with a drink problem. *Lancet*, **1,** 219
5 M. G. K. (1980). The British Doctors' Group. *Br. J. Alc. Alcoholism*, **15**(1), 13
6 Jellinek, E. M. (1960). *The Disease Concept of Alcoholism.* (New Haven: Hillhouse)

30
Treatment of gay alcoholics – separate but equal

A. B. CECCONI

The goal of this chapter is to point out the reasons 'why existing heterosexually oriented programmes fail in their treatment of gay alcoholics, as well as to encourage the establishing of openly gay treatment facilities for the approximately 2–3 million gay alcoholics in the United States[1].

Traditional treatment programmes lack three essential ingredients for the successful treatment of gay alcoholics. The first is that they are staffed primarily by heterosexually oriented individuals with very few having openly gay staff members. The gay/lesbian alcoholic entering a heterosexually staffed treatment facility immediately feels alienation/isolation. He/she may contemplate the following questions: Do I tell the staff that I'm gay? How will they accept it? Will they accept me? . . . These feelings of isolation or separateness establish a barrier that, unless overcome, will hinder the client's progress. A second problem arises: will the client function in group or individual counselling? Can he freely discuss personal issues of intimacy, sexual dysfunctioning, feelings of rejection by parents or 'lovers'? The issue of a same-sex 'lover' cannot be handled by staff who have no conceptual frame of reference to this unique position[2]. Secondly, these facilities are deficient in their knowledge of gay support services available to their clients in the community. Very few treatment facilities know about, or have as referral sources, directories of facilities and services for gay alcoholics and drug abusers. Heterosexually oriented treatment facilities are not tuned into the gay community, so they are unaware of activities that the recovering gay/lesbian alcoholic can become involved with upon re-entry into the day community. Thirdly, the staff is working without the 'key' to successful treatment of gay alcoholics. This is the need for self-acceptance of being gay, along with the ability to function within a subculture that is rejected by the majority of people with whom the gay man or lesbian comes into daily contact[3].

All alcoholism treatment programmes have as their goal the breaking or interrupting of the cyclical lifestyle pattern surrounding the client's drinking. Effective treatment for gay alcoholics requires special considerations. First, any intervention must be brought to the gay community to reach gay alcoholics who often are socially isolated. Feelings of isolation, rejection and differentness are common to alcoholism and homosexuality. It is through locating the treatment facilities in the 'gay ghettos' that exist in most large cities in the United States that gay/lesbian alcoholics can be given a gay identity. Treatment programmes should be clearly identified as being staffed by openly gay and gay-oriented individuals to remove the fear of 'coming out'. This fear often has paralysed the gay alcoholic into not utilizing available treatment modalities.

Secondly, alcoholics, gay or not, need a place where they can break the pattern of a drinking lifestyle — whether bar or closet drinking. This can be accomplished through involvement in a programme that (1) lifts the alcoholic out of his/her existing environment for a short term (20–28 days), (2) treats any accompanying physical illness, e.g., pancreatitis, cirrhosis, malnutrition, (3) educates the alcoholic to the disease process through seminars, films, group discussion, and counselling in groups and/or individually and (4) provides an accepting environment that allows the sober person to feel and act on a whole spectrum of emotions arising out of interpersonal and intrapersonal relationships (perhaps for the first time). Finally, the programme should provide alternatives to the parties, bar scenes and isolation that are often associated with being gay. The clients need an introduction to gay Alcoholics Anonymous meetings along with other support services (e.g. Dignity, M.C.C.) which become an essential part of re-entry into the homosexual community.[4]

Thirdly, recovery of the gay alcoholic depends on his/her self-acceptance as a homosexual and as a part of a subculture that can function within a larger culture. This is where an openly gay staff as well as gay-oriented heterosexuals (non-homophobic) play an important role. For it is through role models and interaction in group and individual therapy that the gay/lesbian alcoholic first learns self-acceptance and functioning as a member of a homosexual subculture.

The gay alcoholic develops a unique denial pattern which admission to a heterosexually oriented treatment programme can reinforce. This 'I've got a secret . . .' concept fits right into this pattern that gay alcoholics develop; 'If I don't have to admit to being gay to you or myself, then I don't have to admit to being an alcoholic'. A definite lose-lose situation emerges. A two-person (gay/straight) counselling team provides the catalyst for self-acceptance through their interactions with the client; in partnership with self-acceptance comes the acceptance of being powerless over alcohol. Self-acceptance of being gay increases the chances of acceptance of one's alcoholism. Being placed in a double bind — not being able to accept being different, masking the subsequent emotions with alcohol until the denial of one melts into the denial of the other — the gay alcoholic becomes lost in a 'divided world'[5]. Providing survival tools, as well as opportunities for the client to sort out his/her 'divided world', and confronting psychic pain of being different must be the goals of a gay alcoholics' treatment centre.

References

1 Kinney, J., and Leaton, G. (1978) *Loosening the Grip: A Handbook of Alcohol Information*. (St. Louis; Mosby)
2 Stahman, R. F., and Hiebert, W. J., (1977). *Counseling in Marital and Sexual Problems; A Clinician Handbook*. 2nd Edn. (Baltimore: Williams and Wilkins)
3 Ziebold, T. O. (1979). *Alcoholism and Recovery, Christopher Street*, (January 1979).
4 *Alcoholics Anonymous, Third Edition*. (1977). (New York: A.A. World Services Inc.)
5 Fleming, M. (1978). Paper presented to the *Gay Caucus Group of the American Psychiatric Association*.

Further reading

1 Bell, A. P. (1978). *Homosexualities*. (New York: Simon & Schuster)
2 Cory, D. W. (1960). *The Homosexual in America*. 2nd Edn. (New York: Castle Books)
3 Fifield, L. (1975). *On My Way to Nowhere: Isolated, Alienated and Drunk*. (Los Angeles: Gay Community Services Center). (Summarized by Shilts, R., in the *Advocate*, 25 February, 1976)
4 Hooker, E. (1961). The homosexual community. In *Proceedings of the XIV International Congress of Applied Psychology* (Copenhagen: Munksgaard) (Reprinted (1969) in Weltge, R. W. (ed.) *The Same Sex* (Philadelphia: Pilgrim Press))
5 May, R. (1977). *The Meaning of Anxiety*. Revised Edn. (New York: Norton)
6 Snyder, C. R. (1959). *A Sociological View of the Etiology of Alcoholism*. In Pittman, D. J. (ed.) *Alcoholism: An Interdisciplinary Approach*. (Springfield: Thomas)
7 Szasz, T. S. (1970). *The Manufacture of Madness*. (New York: Harper & Row)
8 Weinberg, J. R. (1974). *Ten Tips for Counseling Recovering Alcoholics*. (Center City, MN: Hazelden Foundation)
9 Weinberg, M. S. and Williams, C. J. (1974). *Male Homosexuals*. (New York: Oxford UP)

31
Chemical dependency within the university communities

W. D. WYSS

THE CHEMICAL DEPENDENCY PROBLEM

Health care professionals and sociologists generally agree that chemical dependency is the leading health and social problem in the United States today; it affects approximately 10–15% of the population. The US Department of Public Health estimates that chemical dependency costs industry between $50 and $100 billion dollars annually for absenteeism, tardiness, related accidents, decreased production and training of replacements.

THE PREVALENCE AND TREATMENT OF CHEMICAL DEPENDENCY AT THE UNIVERSITY OF MINNESOTA

Of the employees of the University of Minnesota, between 2060 and 3090 may be chemically dependent. To identify and serve this clientele, the Director of the University's Chemical Dependency Awareness and Assistance Programme:

(1) Makes Supervisors aware that the programme exists by distributing brochures and conducting ongoing inservice awareness sessions.

(2) Contacts employees who have identified themselves or who have been referred by supervisor, spouse or concerned person for possible alcohol or drug abuse.

(3) Contacts immediate supervisor to check effect of problem on attendance and work performance.

(4) Schedules meetings with supervisor and/or union representative making

employee aware of his/her options. The options could be one or more of the following:

(a)   dependency evaluation
(b)   inpatient treatment facility
(c)   outpatient treatment facility
(d)   other support services
(e)   termination if referral or recommendations are refused.

(5)   Has contact with facility counsellor (if employee is in a treatment facility) and acts as liason between supervisor, employee and facility counsellor.

(6)   Holds follow-up meetings with supervisors and/or union representative of assisted employee to determine employee's progress in the work setting, or in treatment.

(7)   Helps coordinate the employee's schedule and University facilities so that the employee can attend on-campus AA meetings. Is available after meetings for individual needs.

(8)   Contacts employee on return from treatment facility and offers assistance and support.

(9)   Recommends to the appropriate supervisor that the employee be terminated if every available resource − treatment, support groups etc. − has been utilized and the employee's work performance is still unsatisfactory.

BENEFIT OF THE UNIVERSITY OF MINNESOTA CHEMICAL DEPENDENCY AWARENESS AND ASSISTANCE PROGRAMME

Derived benefits are as follows.

(1)   Improved work performance; a minimum of 50% increase in productivity.

(2)   Less absenteeism.

(3)   Better overall work results since others in the work unit do not have to pick up the slack caused by any individual's poor performance.

(4)   Better supervision through improved training and understanding of how to handle chemically dependent problems.

(5)   Improved employee's family relationships.

(6)   Improved service to faculty, staff and students with return of the chemically dependent employee to responsible productivity.

(7)   More return on the dollars invested in labour. Reduced requests for additional funds to cover up for poor performance.

(8)   Improved personal attitude on the part of the recovering dependent person.

CONCLUDING COMMENTS

Effective work performance is increasingly essential as University budgetary restrictions lessen the availability of funds for many departments. The ability to identify chemical dependency is essential and the chemically dependent employee's co-workers and supervisors must realize that sheltering the employee from disciplinary measures is no solution. But the programme outlined above does offer solutions: in terms of providing supervisory training for the identification of chemical dependency; and then in terms either of helping the employee reach a sustaining level of personal improvement and acceptable productivity, or of identifying the employee's inability to achieve these necessary levels.

Finally, the success of the programme argues that a strategy of confrontation with the chemically dependent employee is more effective than one which relies upon voluntarism.

32
Increasing awareness in young people of alcohol problems

D. ALLEN, J. C. GROVE and M. R. KEEN

An admirable booklet[1] published recently on alcohol misuse presents the issues of prevention and treatment in a lively but succinct manner. The authors hope to stimulate discussion and help people to clarify their minds about the proper aims of public policy and a sensible approach to individual behaviour.

Not in this discussion document nor in other weighty reports[2-5], nor in any other major policy statement on alcohol misuse is it proposed or implied that young people should be consulted about their views. With the exception of a report by one of us[6] we have not found an article on extensive consultations with young people about *their* views on alcohol and its place in society and in their personal lives.

Although realizing that our approach cannot be unique and that it is impossible to give an adequate description of a large scale empirical activity, we believe that a further report of our work will be of interest.

ORIGINS

Our Working Party of students, teachers, youth workers, health educators, probation officers and doctors came together in 1979. The aim of the group was to consult young people about community problems of alcohol and drug abuse. In particular we wanted their personal views, whether they regarded these abuses as problems, how they thought such problems as they identified could be avoided and in what way they could help.

We were stimulated to get together and start a widespread consultation with young people by the idea of holding an International Youth Forum within the meetings of the International Council on Alcohol and Addictions (ICAA) held in Cardiff in 1980. Behind this there was a growing concern at the failure of adult society, by precept, education or guidance, in preparing young people adequately for the complex, often unhealthy and sometimes bizarre and atrocious choices which lay ahead of them. With this concern there was a strong feeling that young people should have a voice and be involved at an early age in the determination of their own destiny. All members of our groups had extensive knowledge of today's young people with whom they were in almost daily contact. They had no doubt that properly confronted with facts and issues they would contribute opinions and ideas of their own on alcohol and drug problems. Whilst identifying their rights they would neither shirk responsibility for their own actions and choices nor disregard the wider social repercussions. Finally, our members predicted that young people would be keenly interested in what we proposed and that there would be no unwelcome side-effects.

These early judgements and opinions have been fully confirmed and it is noteworthy and encouraging that they have held true as the work is further extended in its third year to include disturbed and deprived groups.

THE TASKS

The population of Wales is just over 2.77 million. Our initial task is to promote discussion and ask the opinion of the 12—18-year-olds who amount to over 300 000 in total. In practice the target turned out to be about 189 000 in the 14—17 years' range. Probably a fifth and possibly more of the population was involved in discussion groups or small conferences within 2 years. This magnificent response was largely due to the immediate support of the Welsh Secondary Schools Association, which is the foremost Association of Heads in Wales. There are 14 440 teachers in the secondary schools and an ample proportion of them had the personality, skill and interest for group work.

A much larger cadre of 28 227 skilled youth workers are also available in the community. There are 165 employed fulltime in the Local Authority youth services, 386 are full- or part-time leaders and organizers in the Voluntary Youth Organizations in Wales and 27 666 are voluntary leaders and helpers (1978 figures). More recently, a large number of enthusiastic leaders are additionally employed in various schemes for unemployed school leavers under the Manpower Services Commission. If we take into account also school nurse counsellors, health visitors, health educators and therapists, it is evident that our objectives can be delegated to safe and sensitive hands.

Other primary aspects of our task include projecting the idea of genuine consultation to all participants, guidance on the reliable information necessary for informed discussion, categorizing the population so that discussions are extended to sections and groups which were initially missed out, seeking to ensure continuity in this mutual learning experiment and, finally, working out adequate feedback, evolution and reporting.

What might be termed secondary tasks claimed attention from the beginning. These were the need to collect, review and quite often devise techniques of initiating discussions and consultation. More disturbing were the large number of problems brought forward or brought to light which revealed unmet needs and anxieties in the community.

BACKGROUND STRESSES

According to recent research by the Schools Council, about 1 million children in England and Wales, or one in ten pupils, have marked emotional or behavioural problems. In addition to those developmental problems many are stressed by well-known social changes. These include latchkey children, family and marriage breakdowns, and street and school violence. Young people are increasingly aware of world-wide tragedies of environmental pollution and malnutrition. They are also worried by threats of nuclear wars and chemical warfare. In Britain, they are affected by unemployment, lower standards of living and urban riots. We have over 3 million unemployed and 4 million people eligible for supplementary benefit payments.

Professor David Donnison[7] opines that the real causes of urban violence are economic mismanagement and the social neglect and injustices rife in a society which stunts so many human hopes and talents. He believes that there are common features which link Derry's Bogside, Bristol's St Paul's, Liverpool's Toxteth, and Brixton's 'front line'. Riots, he argues, tend to occur where four conditions coincide: (1) an economic climate which predisposes people for trouble, (2) an urban setting which brings a lot of people together in potentially turbulent ways, (3) a community which enables them to react with rage to the humiliations they suffer and (4) an incident which ignites violence.

Of special interest are his comments on some neighbourhoods in which a lot of young unemployed people are concentrated. He points out that parental age groups have been moved out in recent years by slum clearance schemes or have migrated to more prosperous areas. This loss is serious because these are the people who bear the main responsibility for rearing the young, for helping youngsters to find jobs, for setting social standards and giving political leadership. Alternative less-balanced leaders move into the vacuum.

All these background stresses and conditions are relevant to our tasks, partly because social problems are causally linked and partly because in a consultative discussion young people will give opinions on and question all the issues which trouble or interest them.

INITIATIVES

A large variety of initiatives are needed for several reasons. We need to cater for differing social and educational categories and for special subgroups. Participation should be possible for a wide variety of statutory and voluntary personnel. Every effort should be made to introduce the subject and fortunately, as previously described[6] the opportunities are legion.

We found three aspects are of special importance.

Firstly, the organization and methods were left in the hands of those already in close contact with groups of children and adolescents. Local 'experts' such as community physicians, lecturers in social work or sociology, health educators, probation officers or senior policemen, were invited to make specific contributions on certain occasions only.

Secondly, only very general guidance was offered about sources of information, films and other teaching material about alcohol and drugs. Thus the teacher or youth leader sought out a teaching brief relevant to his own circumstance and favoured approach from a Health Education Unit or from a number of national organizations. Initially educational material was difficult to obtain but persistent and widespread demand led to improved supplies and stimulated several new studies.

It may be of interest to give our general impressions of the opinions expressed on this aspect of the work. Written material from the Teachers Advisory Council on Alcohol and Drug Education (TACADE) and the Health Education Council won the confidence of all concerned. Films, videotapes and slide—tape products were viewed with considerable disappointment and criticism. Clearly a great deal of thought and care is needed in order to produce special films and features for the consultative approach which we advocate. In the meantime, well-presented and reliable facts are readily available and much appreciated. Relevant topics and current issues can stimulate thought and discussion effectively.

Thirdly, we were surprised and concerned at the number and variety of problems disclosed during meetings with young people, especially those disadvantaged in any way. After considerable thought and discussion the Working Party members concluded that any expressions of anxiety and need should be accepted and an appropriate response made with care and without prevarication. Meetings should be of a kind that allow questions and challenges from young persons who are concerned by some disturbing and often urgent problem known to them personally.

DRAMA

Nowadays many young children, certainly from age nine upwards, are ready to protest when adults show that they are not really interested in their views or deal ineffectively with questions put to them. In such instances an able youth leader is willing to stand corrected. However, this is not always the case. It is a great pity if a meeting is a failure because a free consultation is not taking place. This is a matter of great concern to us and although it is a complex problem we suggest that better results are achieved by more active involvement of young persons in the preparation and planning of a consultation event.

Early involvement is unavoidable in drama and role-play groups. These activities are also commendable in that personal problems can be allowed reasonably safe and manageable expression. Illustrations from one initiative before the 1980 ICAA conference and another in 1981 are of interest in this regard and will be described briefly.

In the first case a teacher asked children aged 14 and 15 their views on alcohol and drugs. They were lower ability children but gave their views and opinions readily. These discussions took place during drama lessons. The majority of the children had experimented with alcohol and a wide range of drugs but mainly organic solvents ('glue'). As we would expect their reasons for this behaviour were much like those for smoking cigarettes. Most of them agreed that their behaviour was undesirable. Their teacher summed up their reasoning (which has a touching altruism) as follows: 'because it puts you in a situation where you don't know what you are doing and so are not responsible for your actions and as a result of this it is innocent people who suffer'. The value of these mini-consultations to each child will be evident to all. One serious case of drug taking was able to confide in the teacher (who had made the correct diagnosis almost immediately) after several weeks tactful guidance about her anxiety and depression. As a result she was able to part from older drug-taking friends and wean herself from heroin and other drugs.

In the second case the students were older and were the enthusiastic drama group of a Youth Arts Centre. The process of consultation with them started from the first approach. They were asked to present a dramatic portrayal of their views on key issues of intoxicant abuse. After discussions amongst themselves and with field workers and doctors, they produced a short drama which they presented at a National Conference of young people in 1981. On stage they telescoped the history of a young alcohol and drug dependent from the early group experiments to the last stages of apparently unhelpable isolation. The inadequacy of adult help for the young casualty was put across quite forcibly!

The audience which, as we shall describe later, was widely representative, watched and listened intently. Practically every aspect of the play stimulated considered comment and discussion. Drug users made technical comments and corrections somewhat reproachfully. Devotees of cannabis were discomfited and were probably prepared to launch a cannabis debate. Other youngsters defended 'society' and professionals who had come under criticism. There is no doubt that the drama production by these young actors had succeeded in raising a number of live issues which aroused serious interest.

1980 CONFERENCES

Several hundred young people attended the International Conferences in Cardiff in 1980. From previously-held regional conferences there emerged star speakers and debaters who (according to more than one experienced international delegate) outclassed most other contributors to the whole fortnight.

The points which emerged from the schools included a general opinion that the discussions and consultations should be taking place at earlier ages, and that more information was needed about alcohol and drugs. They could 'handle' the information and discussions and give their views and opinions without anxiety and were pleased to do so, and thought it was a good thing.

Less assertive and articulate young populations would be in agreement with these views but were, quite rightly, more concerned with other pressing issues. Disturbed or minor drug-taking groups were interested and co-operative. Nurses and college students were on the whole less open than the younger groups and tended to project what they thought would be views acceptable to their peers. It was reported that groups addicted to alcohol and drugs defended their actions vigorously and when challenged would fall back on vivid and enthusiastic descriptions of their alcohol and drug experiences. Even ex-addicts tend to follow this pattern. In view of our anxieties about contagion, addicts were not brought into the main stream of the exercise.

1981 CONFERENCE

The 1981 national conference was oversubscribed and too ambitious. Planning blemishes were thoroughly aired by all participants on the day and subsequently! The meeting was remarkably successful in bringing together young people of both sexes in the age range 14–18 from different backgrounds and educational status. We had heard during the preceding month of innovative, intuitive and caring work done with special groups including those emotionally and socially deprived or disturbed, unemployed school leavers, youngsters attending intermediate treatment centres or on probation, and these categories were well represented. The majority present were still at school or members of a variety of youth clubs and organizations. A large majority were cheerfully guilty of underage drinking, were probably tolerant of minor drug experiments and eager to have direct discussions with the minority present who were regular users of cannabis, solvents and other drugs. Tight organization of the group discussions and plenary discussions by reference to a questionnaire limited the risks of contagion to vulnerable youngsters. These arrangements were frustrating to many and would not have been accepted by them if they had been involved in planning the conference. On the other hand it is unlikely that the Working Party would again bring together such a diverse mixture of young persons without exhaustive preparation and consultation at every step.

Certain opinions emerged strongly and with little dissent. Great dissatisfaction was expressed about the lack of information of all kinds about alcohol and drugs and the problems caused by them. As expected there was more concern about drug problems than alcohol abuse. Use, abuse and ensuing difficulties for young people was of far greater interest than any aspects at a later age.

A wide range of views was evident on most issues. Preferred remedies for addiction problems among young people included greater parental responsibility, more and better leisure facilities, more information and at a younger age, making more use of the testimony of former addicts, better counselling services and stricter prescribing of drugs. They were sympathetic towards ethnic minorities which had certain cultural uses for substances illegal in this country. But the great majority were in favour of strict controls and suggested stronger measures to prevent underage drinking.

HEALTH EDUCATION VERSUS CONSULTATION

Health Education promotes good health individually and in the community. Within the general aim there are four important objectives.

First, is to give facts about their health and behaviour to persons individually or in groups. Second is to ensure that information is given in a way that can be understood and will influence behaviour. Third is helping people to understand that attitudes affect behaviour which is important to health. Fourth is listening to what people say about health and trying to understand the implications of their views for themselves, others and the health services.

The processes of consultation which we have been discussing can be included within the fourth objective suggested above. In relation to alcohol and drug use and abuse, it is a much neglected area. For children and young people it appears to be the method of choice and we shall argue the point more closely elsewhere. The need for such consultation has been amply demonstrated in our work. Due to lack of systematic knowledge about the theory and practice of consulting young persons innovative methods have been tailor-made for different ages, and group characteristics. Generally speaking the greater the emphasis on a true consultation and dialogue the higher is the regard and approval of the activity by all concerned. Two conditions have enabled us to proceed in a climate of interest and support bordering on enthusiasm. Firstly the field work is in the hands of those already involved with young people and by personality or training are sensitive and mature in their dealings with them. Secondly the prevention of accidents, illness and personal breakdown and the promoting of good mental, emotional and physical health are considered of prime importance by all concerned.

We seem to be along the right lines if youngsters are encouraged to think and express what is of interest and important to them and not necessarily to us. We have continually to guard against the urge to use the skills we have acquired to collect data for *us* to utilize. We have been trained to control our students, clients or patients in various ways for their supposed benefit and we have to avoid such temptations in this new style of work. Lastly we need to accept that we are subject to influences which affect later choices and have the right to be informed and consulted about important events and problems at a much earlier age than commonly supposed.

References

1 *Drinking Sensibly.* (1981). Department of Health and Social Services discussion document. (London: HMSO)

2 Department of Health and Social Services and Welsh Office (1978). Advisory Committee on Alcoholism, *Report on Prevention*. (London: HMSO)

3 House of Commons Expenditure Committee. (1977). *Report on Preventive Medicine*, Vols. 1–3. (London: HMSO)

4 Royal College of Psychiatrists (1979). *Alcohol and Alcoholism*. Report of a Special Committee on Alcohol and Alcoholism. (London: Tavistock Publications)

5 Office of Health Economics (1980). *Alcohol: Reducing the Harm*. (London: O.H.E.)

6 Grove, J. C. (1981). Consulting young people. Presented at the *27th International Institute on the Prevention and Treatment of Alcoholism*, Vienna

7 Donnison, D. (1982). The fire next time. *The Observer*, London, 14 March

Part 8:
ALCOHOLISM AND THE FAMILY

33
The need for 'recovery' of
the whole family

E. CUTLAND

GENERAL BACKGROUND

There seem to be two conflicting areas of thought in Britain about family therapy in the alcoholism field. One comes from the professionals who are concerned with arresting the disease but treat the alcoholic in isolation, sometimes excluding family members completely. The other point of view comes from family therapists who believe that if you help change the family dynamics, then the alcoholic will return to social drinking because the stress situation has been removed.

At Broadway Lodge, we believe that an individual has a predisposition to be alcoholic, that no stress situation causes the disease although it can give a reason to drink, that he/she is made able to go further into the alcoholism as a result of lack of knowledge and the various roles that people adopt within the family. As Gacic says: 'We believe that alcoholism is not an isolated individual problem, a personal problem or a private matter of the individual. It is a mutual problem of all those surrounding the alcoholic'[1]. Peter Nardi states: 'Viewing the family as a system of interacting roles which change as alcoholism becomes an issue, is a more realistic conception of the social situation. Each member in the family has a set of duties and rights they are expected to enact, based on their position in the system'[2].

Some treatment centres see the family as 'useful' as a tool of intervention, i.e. if you can persuade the family to toughen up and change its attitudes to the alcoholic, you have a better chance of getting the alcoholic into treatment and keeping him there. Then he is returned to the same groups of people who have been acting out the same protective roles for years, who are fused into viewing the patient as the problem and do not see the need for each of the individuals to look at themselves and change their behaviour. An appropriate simile is to describe the situation as similar to cleaning the wound but wrapping it up in the old, infected dressing. Swift and Williams[3] describe the steps that the family structure will undergo if the addict decides to stop using alcohol or drugs. 'The situation is similar to the one suggested in the example of the parents whose child leaves home, since having an addict in the family is sometimes like having another child. Certainly, this is a joyful time for everyone concerned, but we think that families often find this to be a confusing and bewildering time. For the family has lost one of its key members — the addict. In his place stands someone who looks the same but is, in truth, an essentially new person. Family members must begin to see themselves in new relationships to this changed person and this may not be easy. For when they lose the addict, they lose a familiar life style in which everyone knows what to expect from everyone else.'

Most of the relatives with whom I work during the treatment of the alcoholic, are not ready to look at themselves or their role in the alcoholic family. They are still obsessed with, or addicted to, the alcoholic and would much rather play the role of co-therapist than that of someone who needs help. It is only when the alcoholic returns home and continues to work on sobriety that the other people within that family network may come to terms with the fact that they need to change. This process can take years and sometimes family members are so rigidly 'locked' into the role of the enabler or victim, that it is impossible for them to change. A friend of mine described her feelings to me when her husband returned home from treatment. She said that he looked like the same man but he looked sober, more relaxed and happier. Part of her was delighted that he looked so well, the other part wanted to scream at him that he had no damned right to be so contented after all the pain that he inflicted on her and the children. She refused to get help. She saw the problem as his. He continued to stay sober but she continued to become more and more unforgiving and increasingly more angry. Eventually, after 2 years they started divorce proceedings.

At Broadway Lodge, we encourage family members to participate in our aftercare programme and in the last year have organized a number of couples' communication groups for people in early recovery. Again, not all spouses are ready to recognize the need for this and although they are usually happy for their alcoholic to receive aftercare, a small proportion decline help. In 1968, we started a residential programme for family members who were severely affected by the alcoholism and had not received enough help from our Sunday afternoon multi-family groups or Al-Anon. Since the origin of this programme, 46 people have been involved; 29 of those decided they needed help some time *after* the alcoholic had started to recover, i.e. three husbands, 13 wives, 11 daughters and two sons.

PROBLEM AREAS IN RECOVERY

Joan K. Jackson states, 'For the wife and husband facing a sober marriage after many years of an alcoholic marriage, the expectations of what marriage without alcoholism will be is unrealistically idealistic and the reality of marriage inevitably brings disillusionment'[4].

Communication

I believe that alcoholism is a disease of communication within the family. Everyone within that group has learned to deny most emotions, has ceased to share in a meaningful way and is therefore very unaware of what the other person is thinking or feeling. Often, there is a period of relief that the alcoholic is sober, but, even during this time, the family may continue to tread around him/her in eggshells and be frightened to say anything that will cause upset in case it provokes the alcoholic into drinking again. Recently, I worked with a family where the alcoholic had been sober for 5 years. Yet, although he lived with his wife and two teenage daughters, he was excluded from sharing in any family activity. The family was still adopting the same pattern as in the drinking days. Everyone was unhappy with the situation and each person wanted it to change but during the 20 years of alcoholic drinking, individuals had forgotten how to, or had never learned, to question or talk about uncomfortable feelings. In almost every case, families who come back for aftercare need help in learning skills on how to talk to each other.

Fear

Fear is one of the most difficult hurdles to overcome in early recovery for all members of the family; fear that the alcoholic might start drinking again, that if it happens, relatives might not be able to cope; fear of the new changing roles within the family, of letting the alcoholic function responsibly within that group. We teach our patients and their families that it is important that they recognize and deal with their feelings and that can be very frightening if one has been repressed or hiding in alcohol for many years. Most couples in early recovery have sexual problems. Very often this is due to fear of rejection, fear of not being able to make love sober, or fear of continued impotence. Again, because individuals have not learned to communicate this feeling, fear becomes augmented.

Anger

During the drinking days most relatives learn to present a facade of being a 'coper' to the rest of the world. Most are denying a great deal of repressed anger. This may be because they are guilty at feeling aggressive towards a sick person. Others disown their feelings because they are so intense and painful that the only way they know how to deal with them, is to push them down and try and forget them. Very often relatives do not recognize their wrath until well after the alcoholic is in recovery. Many continue through life playing the martyr and becoming more and more bitter. The majority of relatives need permission to express their anger. Why shouldn't he/she be angry? Why should anyone be expected to cope with the constant tension, the continual put-downs, the insensitivity to others' feelings, the aggression, the never knowing what to expect, the total self-centredness, the embarrassment, the lies, the deceit, the playing one family member off against another, all the worry and loneliness that comes from living with an alcoholic? How on earth can a person live in a situation like that and not be angry? Yet, the small number of relatives who have sought help before coming to Broadway Lodge, have been told by professionals and sometimes by Al-Anon members, to be grateful for the alcoholic's recovery and forget the past. Feelings of gratitude and the ability to forgive and forget are very difficult to find if anger is still being denied.

Low self-worth

Life with a drinking alcoholic can provide a terrible kind of security. There may be violence, abuse, blaming, disappearance for days or weeks at a time, but many family members remain in that situation because their remaining vestige of feeling a worthwhile person comes from believing he/she needs me. Unless family members get help in recognizing that the alcoholism is not their fault and that they are worthwhile people in their own right and not just a prop to the alcoholic, recovery of the addicted person will be very threatening. The other day, I had a long discussion with a man who was in a great deal of emotional pain. His wife, who had been sober for 2 years, was divorcing him 'after all he had put up with' during her drinking days. The basic problem was that he could not accept that she no longer had the same dependence on him and dealt with his insecurity by trying to control her and laying down rules which he expected her to adhere to. He was jealous of Alcoholics Anonymous because it had helped her get sober and more independent. She was devoting a lot of time to helping other people. This man and his wife had had a number of counselling sessions in the past but he continued to focus in on the areas he thought she needed to change and became very defensive when asked to look at himself and his need to be leant on.

CHILDREN IN THE RECOVERING FAMILY

During the drinking days, the most ignored people in the family are the children of the alcoholic. Like Claudia Black,[5] we find that many of the young people in the family slip through the net because on the surface they look so good. Like their non-alcoholic parent, the majority of children fall into the role of being the coper and take on a lot of responsibilities in the home. They learn not to question or 'rock the boat'. The rebellious child is very much in the minority.

Recovery of the alcoholic parent brings problems for the children in the family. The responsible child who has built up his/her self-esteem by encouraging everyone in the family to lean on him/her, often feels very alone and unloved when her alcoholic parent starts to recover. She no longer feels needed. Jealousy can result from the changing relationships in recovery. Sometimes, the non-alcoholic parent can develop a very dependent relationship with at least one of the children during the drinking days. When the alcoholic starts to work on being sober, the spouse can move rapidly towards building up the husband/wife relationship, unaware that the child is left feeling rejected and unable to express that emotion in a constructive way. That feeling of rejection may be augmented by the child's growing awareness that the parents are 'ganging up together' trying to instill some discipline in the home. This is very difficult to accept, especially as during the drinking days the children often took on the role of parent. Although some imposed structure may bring some relief to the children, it can also produce the conflicting feeling of resentment that the days of freedom are over.

Many people assume that if parents start to recover the children will automatically 'come right'. However, recovery from alcoholism is a long, slow process and the parents are quite often poor role models for a number of years. After all, the adults are just learning to communicate with each other. R. Margaret Cork[6] studied 115 children of alcoholics and states in her book *The Forgotten Children*, 'Many said that they did not want any other parents; they only wanted a chance to know and to be understood by the parents they had'.

CONCLUSION

Many family members are resentful that the drinking alcoholic is always the centre of attention in the family. Many object to the continued focus on that person in recovery. To treat an alcoholic in isolation is to be blind to the dynamics surrounding the person who has the disease. The family system needs to be looked at; each individual needs help in recognizing the role he/she plays and how change can be brought about. Treatment for the alcoholic is only the beginning in Britain. Much more work needs to be done supporting each person in the family until they learn to be comfortable with their own recovery and their new role in the family.

References

1. Gacic, B. (1981). Importance of the family and social network in the treatment of alcoholics. In *Proceedings of the 27th International Institute on the Prevention and Treatment of Alcoholism*, Vienna
2. Nardi, P. (1980). Children of alcoholics: a role theoretical perspective. Presented at the *Annual Meeting of the Society of Social Problems*, 24 August, New York City
3. Swift, H. A. and Williams, T. (1975). *Recovery for the Whole Family*. (Center City, MN: Hazelden Foundation)
4. Jackson, J. K. (1954). The adjustment of the family to the crisis of alcoholism. *Q. J. Stud. Alc.*, 562

5 Black, C. (1979). Children of Alcoholics. *Alcohol Health and Research World*, 23–27 (Fall, 1979)
6 Cork, R. M., (1969). *The Forgotten Children. A Study Children with Alcoholic Parents.* (Toronto: Alcoholism & Drug Addiction Research Foundation of Ontario)

34
Wives of alcoholics

S. RANGANATHAN

There is a tense, brittle air about that house. The children seem subdued, and move as if afraid to draw attention to themselves. The wife wears a fixed, determinedly cheerful expression on her face, while her eyes remain haunted, desperate . . . Another part of the city . . . In a tiny, dirty little hut, the rice-vessel is empty once again. The children are crying, shrinking against the flimsy walls while the shrill, bitter notes of their mother's voice clashes with the slurred, fumbling speech of their father. Their parents are engaged in yet another quarrel, because their father is drunk again. But here, the woman wears a hard, resigned look. This isn't anything new. Men come home drunk, they throw their pay after those bottles – it is the way of the world, and one must accept life as one finds it.

Two women – from different strata of society, with vast differences in terms of background, financial and social position, education – two women with one common bond – they are the wives of alcoholics. Suddenly, the gulf between them does not seem very wide after all!

From time immemorial, Man has used alcohol for its pleasurable and psychoactive effects. The history of alcohol dependence is no different in India. The Vedas, the oldest of India's religious texts, mention the existence and use of 'Sura', which was the equivalent of alcohol. Consumption of alcohol does not, however, appear to have been considered a virtue, and was, in fact, strongly condemned by the ancient rishies of India. In Manu's treatise, which is primarily an administrative code, drinking was considered to be one of the five sins, on a par with molestation of another man's wife, and infanticide. The treatise speaks of the negative effects of alcohol on the brain. It was believed that the only difference between Man and Animal lay in the existence of the human brain. Thus, when the brain was affected, men sank to the level of animals. Thiruvalluvar, an immortal poet of the pre-Christian era, devoted a full chapter with ten couplets to the consequences of drinking and alcohol abuse.

Religion plays an important role in the attitude of people towards drinking and alcohol abuse. In India, the major religions are Hinduism, Islam and Christianity. The Hindu religious texts abhor drinking. Islam condemns use of alcohol. However, Christianity, in general, is a little more tolerant towards drinking.

In India, alcoholism and related problems form an area in which very little research has been done to date. The data compiled by researchers so far, consist only of information on alcohol abuse pertaining to certain specific areas, such as students' attitude towards drinking and the study of some of the problems related to drinking.

Reliable data of prevalence rates for the entire country are difficult to find, although most of the existing studies[1-5] point out that alcohol is the second most widely abused drug in India. In the 40s only 5 % of students in university campus, on an average, drank alcohol. This has now increased to as much as 50 %. Increased drunken driving and accidents are being reported. Illicit liquor tragedies are steadily on the increase in every State. One such tragedy occurred in the City of Bangalore in the recent past, in which 226 persons died, out of whom 40 were women.

Very little research has been done so far on the impact of alcoholism on the family life of alcoholics in India. We do not have any single separate institution catering exclusively for the treatment and prevention of alcoholism. Except in marriage counselling, no importance has been attached to the families in the treatment plan of alcoholics.

The T.T. Ranganathan Clinical Research Foundation is therefore trying to involve the families of the alcoholics in the general treatment plan. We at the Foundation recognize the fact that alcoholism is not an illness that exists in isolation affecting the sufferer alone. The family of the alcoholic suffers along with the victim. They need help and counselling too. We also recognize the fact that if the alcoholic is to recover, it is important for his family to know and understand the facets of the disease. This is necessary because the alcoholic's family, through sympathy and understanding, can help reinstate the victim as a responsible member of society.

Over the past year, 70 alcoholics have been treated at the T.T. Ranganathan Clinical Research Foundation. The sample with which the present chapter deals is drawn from the wives of alcoholics who attended the outpatient department at the Foundation.

These observations have been made over the period when they were undergoing the active treatment as well as the follow-up programme. Since this chapter is concerned with the families of alcoholics, details regarding the alcoholics themselves have not been included. The findings have been summarized as follows.

SEX DISTRIBUTION OF SPOUSES*

From our observations we noted that out of a total number of 70 alcoholics treated last year, only one was a woman. In Indian society, the sight of a

* In the West, both men and women have been found to be alcoholics. Therefore the spouses of alcoholics are both males and females. But in India, alcoholics are usually males. Therefore the term 'spouses' refers exclusively to women.

woman drinking, particularly in public, is still not a very common one. However, it appears that the number of women who drink is on the increase, though very gradually. In the higher and sophisticated income levels, drinking in small amounts among women has become a fashion; in the very low income groups women are involved in the brewing and selling of illicit liquor and are found to drink too.

MARITAL STATUS

Out of the 70 cases, 64 were married and six were bachelors. Among the 64 married couples, no one was divorced. However, six wives had left their husbands because of alcoholism. We have the case of a professor of literature, who tried to give up alcohol but did not succeed. He lost his job and had his family walk out on him. His wife now lives separately with her children, and works and supports her family. The professor, unemployed and alone, is literally living on the streets. In another case, that of a merchant, his wife, having left him, is now living with her parents in her village. One fact that emerged was that in all the cases, women merely left their husbands. This is because divorces are not encouraged in India.

Of these married couples, 22 wives had been separated from their husbands at least for some time in their married life. Separation is one of the tactics used by the wives of alcoholics.

These findings have been corroborated by a study conducted by Bagadia, Shah, Pradhan and Mundra[6]. They have pointed out in their sample that a majority of alcoholics were married; very few divorces were noted.

These studies support the fact that divorces are not common among alcoholics — a greater number of alcoholics in India remain married as compared to Western countries.

SPOUSE OF THE ALCOHOLIC

There is no evidence that any particular relationship or marital problem causes alcoholism. A wife does not cause alcoholism, although she can aggravate it. However, studies have shown that in most cases wives of alcoholics share certain common characteristics. This could be because of the fact that they share a common problem.

In one study conducted by the T.T. Ranganathan Clinical Research Foundation on wives of alcoholics, the following characteristics were revealed. They were given both 16 PF and Beck Depressive Rating scales. On 16 PF they were found to be, in general, more outgoing, warm-hearted, of average intelligence, submissive, dependent and easily upset. At the time of testing they were found to be tense, frustrated and over-wrought. This may be due to staying with an alcoholic husband. They were not found to be psychiatrically disturbed. These findings have been confirmed by other recent studies[7].

Studies conducted in the West show that children of alcoholics, strangely enough, very often choose alcoholic spouses. A woman who divorces her husband on grounds of alcoholism chooses a new partner with the same problem. These situations, however, do not arise in India. There are reasons which explain why this is so. Most marriages in India are arranged, even today. There is really no question of anyone choosing an alcoholic partner. Parents scrutinise boys very carefully before giving their daughters in marriage to them. Even mild cigarette smoking sometimes results in certain young men being 'rejected'! Marriages are decided only after strict in-depth inquiries are carried out on both sides. Horoscopes have to match and play a very important role in decision making. Strangely, to the best of our knowledge, horoscopes do not appear to disclose whether the boy has a drinking problem or not! In spite of all this, however, some women do find themselves wedded to men with a drinking problem. It is a difficult situation from the very beginning, because most of our women are not aware of the properties, use and abuse of alcohol. They are for a large part intolerant of the husband having even one drink. This ignorance, intolerance and a strong tendency to over-react go a long way to make a tough situation worse. Women cannot be blamed entirely for this lack of exposure. Most homes do not store alcohol. A majority of women are not used to even the sight of liquor. Most men drink away from home. They also hide the smell of liquor on their breath by eating 'paan' (betal nut and leaves). Quite often the woman finds out about the husband's problem only after it reaches the stage of excessive drinking or when his health noticeably breaks down.

SEXUAL PROBLEMS

Through the ages, alcohol has been believed to be an aphrodisiac. In actual fact, it is a depressant and excessive use leads to impotence. Masters and Johnson in their work[8] mention that prolonged excessive use of alcohol is responsible for the onset of secondary impotence.

In our sample, we observed the following sexual problems between the couples. Women being intolerant of alcohol, severe conflicts arise between the couples. The wife shows her inability to respond to her husband's sexual advances; initially this occurs only while he is drunk and eventually whether he is drunk or sober. Another observation made was that some wives refuse to co-operate with their recovered alcoholic husbands. They have lost their sexual feelings because of forced sexual abstinence when their husbands were engaged in excessive drinking. According to Neil Kassel and Henry Walton[9], the alcoholic's sexual approach may repel the woman by his unfeeling attitudes and clumsiness. What was once of emotional importance is now only sordid and loathsome. She misses the companionship, the warmth and understanding which a husband should provide. Wife beating is also a cause for a further breakdown of marital relationships. In our sample, 27 cases admitted to physical abuse and battles. Since divorce is not encouraged in India, the amount of suffering the spouses underwent with their alcoholic husbands is enormous.

EFFECT ON FAMILY LIFE

Johnson in his book, *I'll Quit Tomorrow*[10], says that the entire family suffers the cruel and crippling consequences of having an alcoholic member in its midst. No proper research studies have been conducted to measure the extent of the impact of alcoholism on families. The nature and extent of impact of alcoholism can be described under three main headings – financial, social and emotional.

Financial impact

Alcoholism has the worst impact on the financial situation in the family. In our sample, the majority of which consisted of members from lower middle class and middle class, we found that the family finds it very difficult to make both ends meet. Patients who belong to the affluent classes did not exhibit many problems in this area. Eighty per cent of our cases had incurred debts. One of our patients has built up debts to the tune of one lakh (100 000) rupees, and has twice run away from home to avoid his creditors.

In India, when a woman gets married, she brings with her gold, silver, vessels, sometimes even furniture. This is her dowry. Her dowry is her social security, because most of our women do not work and are not financially independent. In many cases, the husband either pawns or sells his wife's dowry in order to pay for his liquor. The loss of her dowry is a traumatic experience for the average Indian woman, because she now has nothing of her own to fall back on. Many women in this position are forced to go out and seek work to help support the family.

Social impact

Alcoholism gradually, but invariably, leads to social isolation. It is not merely the alcoholic who finds himself isolated, but his family as well. As far as his family are concerned, the process of isolation begins due to a tendency on their part to avoid people. This is because the family members suffer from a sense of shame and embarrassment. The wife avoids accompanying the husband to parties and other social gatherings because she cannot bear the tension of never knowing when her husband will begin to misbehave due to drunkenness. She cannot face the pity and the comments. Gradually, people in turn begin to avoid them. The isolation gets worse. For example, no one is prepared to rent his house out to a known alcoholic. Society wishes to have nothing more to do with someone who is judged irresponsible and weak in every sense of the word.

However, the above facts are probably more applicable to the middle and higher income groups. At a lower income level, families do not suffer such rejection. Alcoholism is merely one more problem amongst the many they have learnt to live with.

Emotional impact

Alcoholism not only affects a family financially; it cripples them emotionally as well. The person who has to bear the brunt of it is the wife.

The intensity and the nature of the emotional impact depends on the depth of the drinking problem, the character and personality of the alcoholic and vulnerability to criticism from one's socioeconomic circles. The problems faced by the family members intensify as financial security lessens.

Indian wives do not cope with the problem in the same manner as their Western counterparts do. This is because there are certain factors characterizing their upbringing which tend to influence their attitudes and behaviour.

Indian wives are brought up to believe in the total sanctity of marriage. To an Indian woman, her 'mangal-sutra' is not merely a sign of marriage; it symbolises a relationship which has divine sanction, and which should never be broken. She reacts to her husband's alcoholism either by mutely accepting her 'fate'; or by throwing tantrums, sulking, losing her temper, or walking out on her husband for a brief while.

Very rarely does she decide to take the extreme step of divorcing her husband. A divorced woman, living on her own, bringing up her children, is not a very common occurrence in India.

Most Indian wives tend to hush up the fact of their husband's drinking problem. Once again, upbringing has a great deal to do with this. A woman is expected to put up a front and never disclose her husband's drinking to the outside world. Many wives try to hide their problem from others, even from their own parents for as long as possible. Pride very often prevents her from confiding in her parents, because it is considered undignified to run to her parents for help. In spite of the fact that her marriage was probably an arranged marriage, thus making the parents in a way responsible for the present situation, the wife very rarely blames them. She tries to battle with the situation alone, until it goes beyond her control, and she can no longer hide the fact that her husband is well on the road to alcoholism.

There is yet another factor that governs her attitudes. And that is, even today, most Indian girls grow up with the belief that to suffer for or because of the husband is a virtue. To bow her head down, and accept everything that her husband chooses to dole out to her, is considered the proper attitude for an Indian wife. It is almost as if she becomes a melodramatic heroine, even in her own eyes. In fact, many women actually appear to enjoy making martyrs of themselves in a masochistic way. Most wives tend to harbour guilt feelings about their husbands' drinking problem. They feel that it is some deep inadequacy in themselves that forces the husband to drink. Therefore, by making martyrs of themselves, they try to hold onto a melodramatic position in order to prevent their self-confidence from dwindling further.

Society is no help either. The wife is expected to 'do something' to 'prevent' her husband drinking. It is basic ignorance about the illness that leads to such ideas.

The wife has also to cope with the often hostile attitudes of the in-laws. Family ties being very strong in India, the husband's family also gets involved in the problem. If it is a joint-family set-up, the wife is under additional pressure. She tries to hide the fact of her husband's drinking from his family. She dare not voice her disapproval openly, because her in-laws will naturally support the man against her. She has to accept advice from them on how to behave, what to do, what to say in the present situation . . . all the advice being directed towards her, and not towards the person who is ill. The disease carries such a stigma with it, that most families do not wish to face up to the fact that their son has a drinking problem. They would much rather blame the wife, friends or other outside circumstances.

Most Indian women do not seek extramarital affairs. Although the possibility cannot be ruled out entirely, the wife's usual reaction is to cling to her children, lavish all her love and attention on them, throw herself into her housework and so on. Most women also believe in the beneficial effects of pujas — prayers offered to God — to save their husbands from drinking. Many women perform elaborate rituals and sometimes undergo many difficulties by observing certain vows all in the belief that they can save their husbands by the sheer strength of faith and prayer.

Even if a woman is willing to seek help, where can she go? There is no institution such as the Alanon here in India. Seeking psychiatric help, or even marriage counselling, is very rare in India.

The wife of an alcoholic really has very few choices open to her. She has to battle against ignorance, intolerance both within and without, the attitudes of her in-laws and society at large, her fears for her children and her home, and her desperate desire to keep up the illusion that her husband is a strong, dependable man, a husband straight out of her dreams as a young girl. She is thus caught in a web, and is dealt blow after emotional blow.

CONCLUSION

Alcoholism has not yet emerged as a study of interest to academicians, and has not made sufficient impact as a medical problem on doctors, as a social problem on society in general.

References

1 Deb, P. C. and Jindal, R. B. (1974). Drinking in rural areas: A study of selected villages of Punjab. (Ludhiana: Punjab Agricultural University)
2 Tacore, V. R., Saxena, R. C., and Kumar, R. (1951). Epidemiology of drug abuse in Lucknow with special reference to methaqualone. *Indian J. Pharmacol.*, **3**, 58

3 Mohan, D. and Arora, A. (1976). Prevalence and pattern of drug abuse among Delhi University College students. *J. Indian Med. Assoc.*, **66,** 28

4 Elnagar, M. N., Maitra, P., and Rao, M. N. (1971). Mental health in an Indian rural community. *Br. J. Psychiatry*, **118,** 499

5 Sing, G. and Lal, B. (1978). Drug abuse in the rural population. In *Drug Abuse in India.* (New Delhi: Ministry of Health and Family Welfare)

6 Bagadia, V. N., Shah, L. P., Pradhan, P. V. and Mundra, V. K. (1981). The management of chronic alcoholism. In Mohan, D. and Sethi, H. S. *Current Research in Drug Abuse in India,* p. 204

7 Edwards, P., Harvey, C. and Whitehead, P. (1973). Wives of alcoholics: A critical review and analysis. *Q. J. Alc. Stud.*, **34**

8 Masters, W. H. and Johnson, V. E. (1966). *Human Sexual Response.* (Boston: Little, Brown).

9 Kassel, N. and Walton, H. (1965).

10 Johnson, V. E. (1973). *I'll Quit Tomorrow: A Breakthrough Treatment for Alcoholism.* (New York: Harper & Row).

35
Children of alcoholics:
young – adolescent – adult

C. BLACK

Today, in the United States, there are an estimated 15 million children under the age of 18 living at home with at least one alcoholic parent. There are, inclusive of that number, 28–34 million people who are, or have been, raised in a home with at least one alcoholic parent. We know little about this special population of people. A review of the literature demonstrates an emphasis on genetic causation factors of alcoholism[1–8], Fetal Alcohol Syndrome[9–17], the relationships of alcoholism in a parent to asocial and problematic behaviours in the adolescent young[18–23], and the relationship of child abuse to alcohol abuse or alcoholism[24–33].

While research continues to explore the genetic causation factors of alcoholism and the Fetal Alcohol Syndrome, there is a great need for research on the emotional, social and psychological impact of children being raised in alcoholic homes. Research efforts have been based on children with noticeable social problems, thereby excluding children not displaying unacceptable behaviour or whose problems have not received professional attention. This research is dominated by those samples that were received from a population within agencies that have treated children with identified problems. The acceptably behaving children could be in the majority. Booz-Allen & Hamilton, Inc.[34], and El Guebly and Offord[21], Brown and Black[35, 36], and Black[35], lend support to the concept that children of alcoholics are not necessarily demonstrating problems in their youth. Black and Booz-Allen & Hamilton report that children of alcoholics often are 'overachievers'. While El Guebly and Offord suggest that all children of alcoholics are not victims, Black, Brown and Booz-Allen & Hamilton suggest that in spite of an appearance of 'survival', all are nonetheless affected.

While available data indicate children of alcoholics are at a higher risk to become alcoholic[37–42], than any other population group and have a higher tendency to marry an alcoholic[43,44], there is little information on the adult person once raised in the alcoholic home.

I wanted to understand better what variables might influence certain children to become alcoholic, to marry alcoholics, to do both, or to escape those possibilities.

The purpose of this chapter is to provide a better understanding of children raised in alcoholic homes and make pilot projects better known and to offer some of the initial data.

The survey method was a 12-page questionnaire, the sole way of retrieving information about respondent's past and present. Subjects were solicited via newspapers, magazine articles and public notices.

This study is representative of 405 respondents, all identifying themselves as having been raised in a home with parental alcoholism; 152 (37%) were males, 257 (62%) were females; 236 (58%) had a father alcoholic, 52 (13%) mother alcoholic and 110 (27%) both parents alcoholic. Respondents were 28 years and older, this age range being chosen for the purposes of their having more time to develop into their own alcoholism, and related marriage or other emotional problems, making it possible to see the long-range effects.

This sample is geographically representative of all parts of the United States, and represents all educational and socioeconomic levels.

At this time those respondents that were of a racial minority, or influenced by the death of a parent in childhood, or single parenting were eliminated from this first analysis.

Typically, parents and professionals do not acknowledge the need for bringing children into a treatment programme, except to treat a behavioural or disciplinary problem or to assist in a confrontation among family members. The tendency is to focus on a problem child who is often stereotyped as a potential future alcoholic; one who exhibits the defined high-risk characteristics of (1) having a low self-concept, (2) being more likely to perform poorly in school, (3) being more easily frustrated and (4) having adjustment problems in adolescence and early adulthood[45]. I believe, however, that the child with behavioural problems in the alcoholic home is in the minority. Although he or she may receive attention by drawing notice to him or herself, I believe that all children in alcoholic homes have a high risk of becoming alcoholic and that the majority of the children, those who appear to have adjusted and so are not focussed on in the research, are easily overlooked.

ROLE PATTERNS

Three role patterns which seem to allow children to survive in alcoholic homes appear regularly. The dynamics discussed here are not revolutionary in psychology, but rather are similar to Adler's birth order and the more recent family systems approaches. However, I do not believe these concepts have been generally related in practice to the children of the alcoholic.

I have labelled these role patterns as (1) The Responsible One, (2) The

Adjuster and (3) The Placater. A child may adopt one role or any combination of the three. As will be illustrated, these roles create strengths which in turn hide the scars that develop from living in an alcoholic family system. It is important to recognize the deficits in such roles in order to believe in and support the need to address all children of alcoholics. Family system theorists view the family as an operational system and believe that 'change in the functioning of one family member is automatically followed by a compensatory change in another family member'[46]. To each action there is an equal and positive opposite reaction in the family. The roles these children play are compensatory changes or reactions to parental alcoholism, allowing the children to maintain a sense of balance or homeostasis to survive.

The Responsible One

The role most typical for an only child, or the eldest child in a family, is one of being responsible, not only for him or herself, but for other siblings and/or parents. This child typically provides structure and stability for him or herself and others in an often inconsistent home setting. An example is the 10-year-old daughter who took it upon herself without telling anyone to complete the household chores daily and to oversee the other two children. Aware of the plans of every member, she attempted to organize the family. She felt this role was necessary because the mother was working 7 days a week, 10–14-hour days, and the alcoholic father was not working and was not responsible to anyone in the home for his whereabouts. In this situation where the child assumed the responsible role, one that provided order for her, she carried this sense of responsibility to other areas of her life. She excelled in school, for she learned to structure good study habits. She learned to manipulate others about her to get done what was necessary, thereby developing leadership qualities. She became goal-oriented on a daily basis. She learned not to project ahead, knowing her alcoholic father could interfere, so her goals became realistic. A self-worth developed as she accomplished these goals.

The Adjuster

Another role that may be combined with the previous responsible role, or adopted separately, is that of the adjuster. This child easily follows directions, not feeling the great responsibility the elder child feels or to whatever is called for on a particular day. For example, a 28-year-old man, the son of a male alcoholic, describes his childhood as 'bouncing from one extreme to the other'. He said he fluctuated physically and emotionally never knowing what to expect from either parent. One day his mother was leaving his father and the next day she was behaving as if the thought of separation could never enter her head. For weeks at a time, the child would sit outside a bar in the car, waiting while his father drank for hours. Other weeks, his dad would not drink at all. Another example, a young woman, said she too learned to be flexible in her alcoholic family — she felt she had little choice but to adjust. In the most extreme situation, she could not follow through with her plans because her parents would move without notice. And these were major moves – from the north-eastern states to Florida, to California. Adults who were 'adjuster' children say that, as a result, they see themselves as flexible and able to adapt to a variety of social situations.

The Placater

The placating child greatly needs to smooth over conflicts. This child, often very sociable, develops the admired quality of helping others adjust and feel comfortable. This child often adopts his role to alleviate a sense of guilt that he caused the alcohol problem. An example is the 22-year-old daughter of a male alcoholic who talked of being aware since the age of six of tension in her family, especially of great sadness in both parents. So she spent years trying to help both parents feel good. Everytime her dad said, 'Hey, let's go for a ride', she'd go, now reflecting that the ride always resulted in a series of stops at local taverns. She combined the placating and responsible roles, additionally doing a great amount of housework to please the mother who worked because dad did not work. For hours at a time, she would wait on and listen to dad's buddies as they drank and talked. She said she did not understand what was happening in the home, but she knew people hurt, and she would do whatever she could to please them, thinking it would take away the pain. Strengths developed out of this role. She felt she was popular and got many strokes for helping others, being sensitive to their feelings and listening well.

Survival is key

I have found that children in alcoholic homes are busy surviving. We admire the way they assume the role(s) that make(s) the most sense to them – roles that will help bring peace to the chaotic, denying family in which they live. Displaying behavioural problems is not a role that helps attain peace. We do see some – but not most – children from alcoholic homes in the acting-out role.

Unfortunately, it is easy to overlook the children who are responsible, adapting sociable, and bright. But they are possibly being set up to be 50–60% of society's future alcoholics. Whatever the role these children adopted in the family, there will be some negative consequences for them.

As these children reach their late teens and early twenties, they are often busy leaving the primary family. They make decisions on education, employment, marriage and childbirth. Focussing on their futures, these children usually are unaware of the negative effects of their alcoholic upbringing. They often recognize their strengths because they have been rewarded for being so healthy. As adults, they say they often heard from others and/or told themselves, 'You've really done well in spite of your home life'. Again the scars are unseen even by those who are close.

But these children whose roles have allowed them to survive do not change roles just because they leave the alcoholic environment; these roles become patterns carried into adulthood. It is after the children have begun to lead settled lives as adults that they begin to realize that old methods of coping are no longer working to provide a sense of meaningfulness to live. It is at this time the effects of living in the alcoholic home begin to show. These adults often find themselves depressed, and they do not understand why; life seems to lack meaning. They feel a loneliness, though many are not alone. Many find great difficulty in maintaining intimate relationships. And many become alcoholic and/or marry alcoholics.

In addition to the strengths developed through adopting these roles, there are some equally powerful deficits. Many of these children learned it was not all right to experience certain feelings like anger or sadness. It did not help to feel. When they showed their sadness, their fear, no one was there to comfort them. When they became angry, they found themselves punished. Or when they wanted to talk about anything important, they simply found themselves ignored. It did not take long for these children to learn first, not to express their feelings, and second, not to feel.

Children who ascribed to the responsible role often found their leadership and self-reliance led them to being 'too alone', unable to depend on another person, to trust that another person would be there for them when they needed someone. This can carry over to adulthood.

Many of these 'responsible' children have talked about their 'need to be in control' which has led to difficulty in relationships at work and socially. These children, too, end up often working alone and not having meaningful relationships.

A classic example was the 31-year-old daughter of a male alcoholic. She was bright and a successful lawyer. But she worked alone, had no close friends. Her marriage was failing. I definitely believe her fear of trusting others as well as her fear of her own feelings, which she learned in her alcoholic family, were responsible for her confusing, lonely life.

'Adjuster' children became 'adjuster' adults, unless there has been some direct intervention as a result of their own insight for a need to change. They continue to allow themselves to be manipulated by others, thereby losing self-esteem and power over their own lives. Their option is to invite someone into their lives, often an alcoholic, who has problems or creates problems. This allows them to continue their reacting role. Adult placaters will try to continue the childhood habit of taking care of and trying to please others. Both adjusters and placaters will often not respond to or even be aware of their own failings and desires. As one woman said, 'After I raised my kids and only had my husband to please, it seemed life had little meaning, and before long, I was here in the hospital for alcoholism'.

The examples given have been those of adults who were raised in alcoholic families. I used adult examples because most of the children still at home appear to be doing well; not until adulthood are negative consequences apparent. I see these young children learning to find the role that helps them feel better, either taking care of others and the environment (being

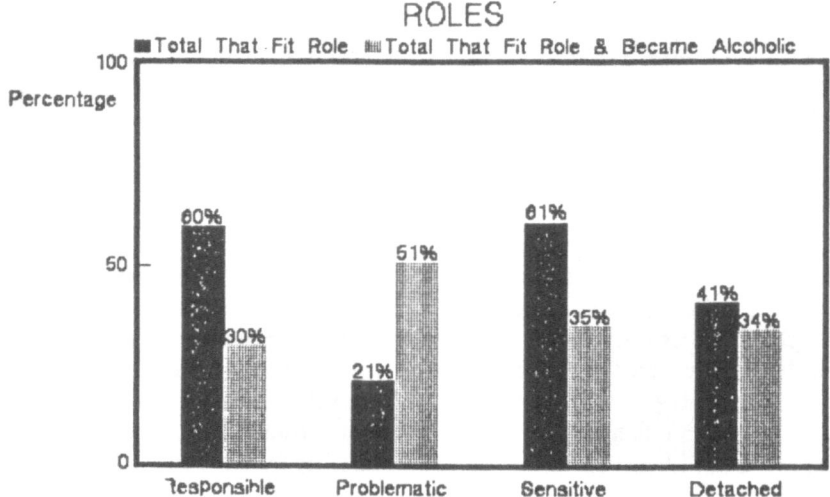

Figure 35.1 While 60 % of the sample identified themselves as responsible, 30 % became alcoholic. 21 % identified themselves as problematic. 61 % of that sample became alcoholic. 61 % identified themselves as sensitive (placaters), 35 % became alcoholic. 41 % of those identified as detached (adjusters), 34 % became alcoholic. Adjusting and problematic qualities are role adoptions most conclusive to becoming alcoholic, while the greatest number of respondents identify with the other 2 roles

'responsible'), adjusting, not questioning, or busy trying to please others and trying to take away others' hurt.

DON'T TALK

The Family Law: *Don't talk about the real issues.* The real issues are: Mom is drinking again. Dad didn't come home last night. Dad was drunk at the ballgame. I had to walk home from school because Mom had passed out at home and forgot to come and get me.

Some say it is a rule; I believe, for most alcoholic families, it has become law. As one 9-year-old daughter of an alcoholic said, 'When you have a rule in your house for so long, to not talk about dad's drinking, it's r-e-a-l-l-y hard to talk now (even when he is sober)'.

In the earlier stages of alcoholism, when someone's drinking seems to become a more noticeable problem, family members usually attempt to rationalize the behaviour. They begin to invent excuses: 'Well, your dad has been working hard these past few months', or, 'Your mom has been lonely since her best friend moved away'. As the drinking increases, the drinking and the irrational rationalizations become a 'normal' way of life. Family members focus on the problems drinking causes, but have difficulty associating drinking with those problems.

It is easier to invent reasons, other than alcoholism, for crazy behaviour. If the drinking takes place outside of the home, and dad doesn't act falling-down drunk when he comes home, or if they don't see him when he comes home, the children may more readily accept what the other parent tells them — drinking is not the problem.

If children do not understand alcoholism, it is difficult for them to identify their parent as alcoholic. Children are like adults in that they too will believe all alcoholics are old men on Skid Row, without jobs or families. Such fragmented information is typical of childrens' lack of knowledge concerning the disease of alcoholism.

Another way which helps family members rationalize the alcoholic's behaviour is for them to not discuss or, in any manner, talk about what's really happening at home. Thirteen-year-old Steve said, 'I thought *I* was going crazy. I thought *I* was the only one in my house who knew dad was an alcoholic. I didn't know anyone else knew'. I asked him why he believed this to be true. He answered, 'because no one else ever said anything'. Steve described an incident which occurred when his father, in a semiconscious state from drunkenness, was on the floor, had thrown-up, had hit his head on the coffee table and was bleeding. Steve's mother and sisters had returned home within moments after his dad had hit his head. They just picked dad up and carried him off to the bedroom. No one spoke to anyone else. Steve said again he thought, 'maybe this is all in my head'. I asked the two older sisters and Steve's mother why they had not talked about this incident with Steve. They responded, 'because he hadn't said anything, and we hoped he hadn't noticed'. I believe helplessness, despair and hopelessness cause family members to believe that *if you just ignore it, maybe it will not hurt; if you just ignore it, it may just go away.*

Many adult children have told me they were instructed not to talk about things which would upset mom or dad; or they simply learned by themselves that things went a lot easier when they did nothing to 'rock the boat'. One young man said, 'dinner was pretty quiet. Anything we said rocked the boat. And then, if we were too quiet, *that* rocked the boat!' These children not only don't talk about boat rocking issues, but they don't talk about, or share, their fears, worries or hurts with anyone.

Children will share the same bedroom with a sibling for years, both hearing the arguing taking place between mom and dad. Or, they hear mom crying night after night. But they only hear, they never speak to one another about it, although they may each cry — silently and alone. In one family, the six children were between the ages of 12 and 21 when dad sought treatment for his alcoholism. Three to four months prior to seeking help, the father would return home late at night after having been drinking for several hours. Not having seen his children all day, he'd make his nightly rounds, passing from one room to another, until he'd seen each of his children. He would scream, shout and harass each child until moving on the next room. All of the children were awake as he went from room to room, but they never spoke to each other about these nightly episodes. The family simply acted as though nothing out of the ordinary was happening.

In another family, young Billy told me how he was taking the air out of the car tires so dad wouldn't drive when he was drinking. His youngest sister, Ann, was putting water in dad's vodka bottle; his oldest sister, Lisa, was putting apple cider in dad's whiskey. Each was unaware of the other's actions concerning dad's drinking because they were unable to talk about the *real* issue — their father's alcoholism.

Well-adjusted children who experience daily childhood problems would, most likely, talk about these problems with other family members. Because of the *denial* of the *alcoholism* in an alcoholic family, seldom are any of the children's problems recognized, and the family problem — alcoholism — is never discussed. These children (accurately or inaccurately) do not perceive others, inside or outside of the family, to be available to them for help. Many adult children of alcoholics have questioned where their aunts and uncles were when they needed them. Many wondered why grandpa and grandma weren't more concerned for them. Nora, another adult child, told me if she had told anybody what her home life was like, she couldn't possibly have been believed. 'They wouldn't believe me, because if it was so bad, I couldn't be looking so good. They never saw my mother getting drunk every day, they never saw her raving like a maniac, passed out upstairs. They never saw her bottles all over the house. They just never saw.'

While many children fear not being believed, they may also experience guilt talking about the problems of their parents. They feel a sense of betrayal in talking about such delicate problems. Children find the family situation so complex and confusing, they feel inadequate in attempting to verbalize the problems — they just don't know how to tell others. Children feel very loyal to their parents, and invariably, they end up defending their parents, rationalizing that it isn't really all that bad, and continuing in what has now become a denial process.

It is most despairing to be a child in an alcoholic family, to feel totally alone, and to believe talking to someone will not help. (Figure 35.2.)

FAMILY VIOLENCE

In retrospect, most adult children who were raised in alcoholic homes remember the frequent arguing which took place in the home. Some children say the arguing was about 'money' or the kids, most say the arguing was about 'anything and everything'. The children and the non-alcoholic parent experience a significant amount of verbal harassment, no matter what the disagreements. The impressions and feelings caused by this type of harassment remain with those children, and are carried into adulthood. In some instances, the harassment escalates and suddenly erupts into violence, and in physical or sexual assault. While the direct relationship between alcoholism and physical

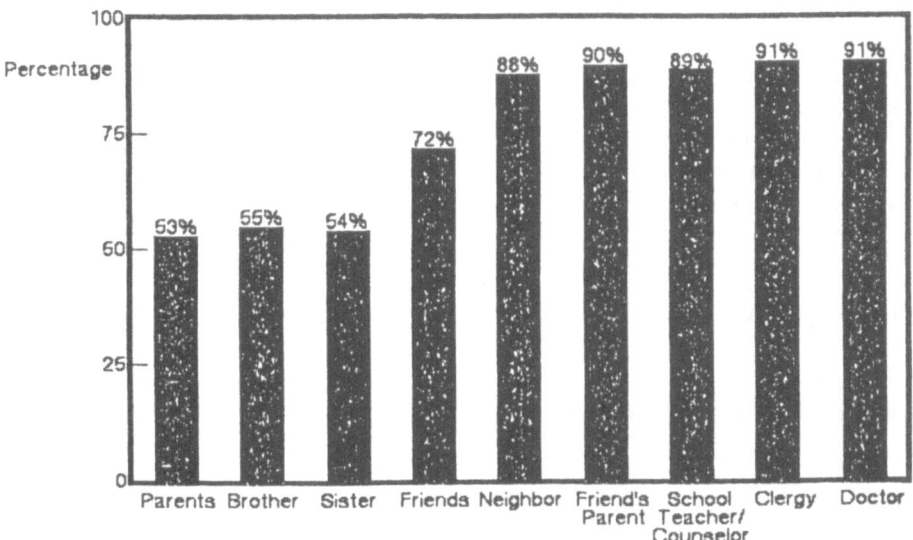

Figure 35.2 In asking this population who they spoke to as a child within the home, it was clear most children didn't talk about what was happening at home. The figure shows that 53 % of this population say they never *once* spoke to the other parent. 55 % never once spoke to a brother. 54 % never once spoke to a sister. If children did talk they spoke at home because 72 % never spoke to a friend. 90 % never spoke to friends and parent. 88 % never once utilized a neighbour, 89 % never once utilized a teacher or school counsellor, 91 % never utilized clergy, or a doctor. All are potential resources, most not utilized

or sexual abuse has not been clearly delineated, a strong association between those problems is consistently identified.

'While dad's drinking increased, mom became more erratic. She was playful and fun one moment, and full of rage the next. She would pick up anything (whip, vacuum cleaner hose, spoon) and hit and hit and hit, and would never apologize. Even when we were bleeding, somehow it was still our fault'. (Candy, age 34)

My own research indicates 66 % of children raised in alcoholic families have been physically abused, or have witnessed abuse on another family member. In more than one third of these families, such abuse occurs on a regular basis.

Consequences for children

Research about domestic violence indicates that witnessing violence may be just as detrimental to the emotional and psychological development of a child, as of the child actually being abused. Just as children who are abused tend to be abusers themselves in adulthood, children who witness assault on parents or siblings, also tend to be abusers and/or abused victims in adulthood. Many children of alcoholics become alcoholic and marry alcoholics; many children of batterers become batterers and marry batterers; many children of both, do both.

My research indicates 26% of daughters in alcoholic homes have been incest victims. Five per cent of sons were incest victims; for sons who were violated it was evident both parents were alcoholics and both parents sexually abused.

CONCERNS

This group was asked to identify in order of priority their concerns as they felt them within the alcoholic home. (Table 35.1.)

PROBLEMATIC AREAS

As adults, this group was asked to identify whether or not they saw these areas to be a major problem in their adult life (Figure 35.3a,b,c).

Greatest problematic areas for this sample group were:

74% have difficulty letting others know what they need.
65% have difficulty with expression of feelings.
65% have difficulty putting themselves first.
62% have difficulty with intimacy.
60% have difficulty with trust.
57% have difficulty with identification of feelings.
52% have difficulty with dependency issues.
46% have difficulty with general confusion.
45% have difficulty with depression.
27% have difficulty in problem solving.
24% have difficulty in taking responsibility for self.
20% have difficulty in working with others.

CONCLUSION

This paper is an enticement, hoping it will engage the reader to be aware of the severity of the impact alcoholism has on children. My hope is that it (1) allows you an awareness of children that look good, and their need for assistance, (2) impacts you with the isolation that is imposed regarding this ability to let others be available to them, via the use of potential support systems, (3) makes you more aware that violence is a part of such family systems, (4) demonstrates that children's concerns are more than the drinking and (5) shows that, as adult children, this specific population identifies continuing problematic areas.

Table 35.1 Concerns

Total		Married alcoholic		Male alcoholic		Female alcoholic	
Quarrelling	56%	Unhappiness	50%	Unhappiness	52%	Unhappiness	52%
Drinking	53%	Drinking	49%	Quarrelling	48%	Quarrelling	48%
Unhappiness	47%	Quarrelling	45%	Drinking	46%	Alcoholic parent's lack of interest	47%
Alcoholic parent's lack of interest	39%	Alcoholic parent's lack of interest	28%	Alcoholic parent's lack of interest	46%	Drinking	43%
Non-alcoholic parent's lack of interest	23%	Non-alcoholic parent's lack of interest	22%	Non-alcoholic parent's lack of interest	22%	Non-alcoholic parent's lack of interest	31%

Drinking was never identified as the child's number 1 concern, unhappiness and quarrelling being identified as the main concerns
For those that became alcoholic the alcoholic parent's lack of interest in them was a significantly greater concern than for those who did not become alcoholic

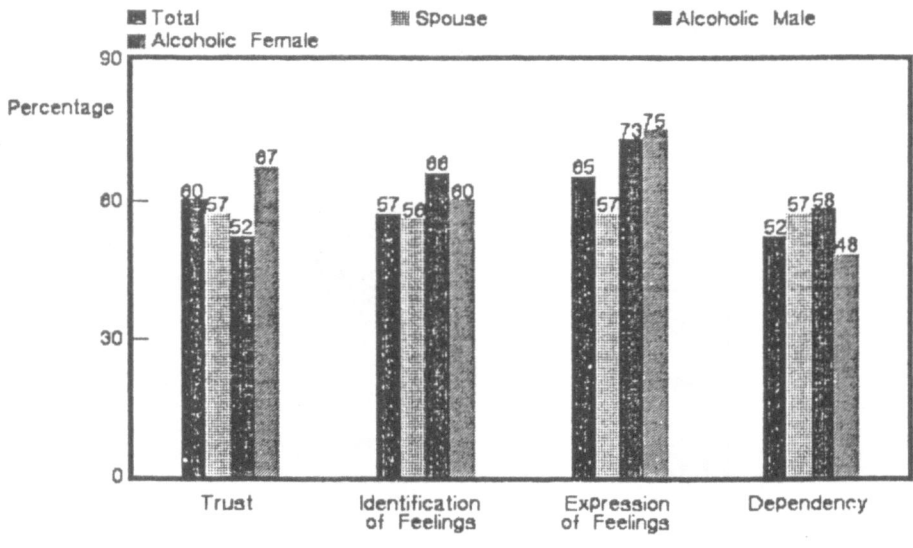

Figure 35.3a

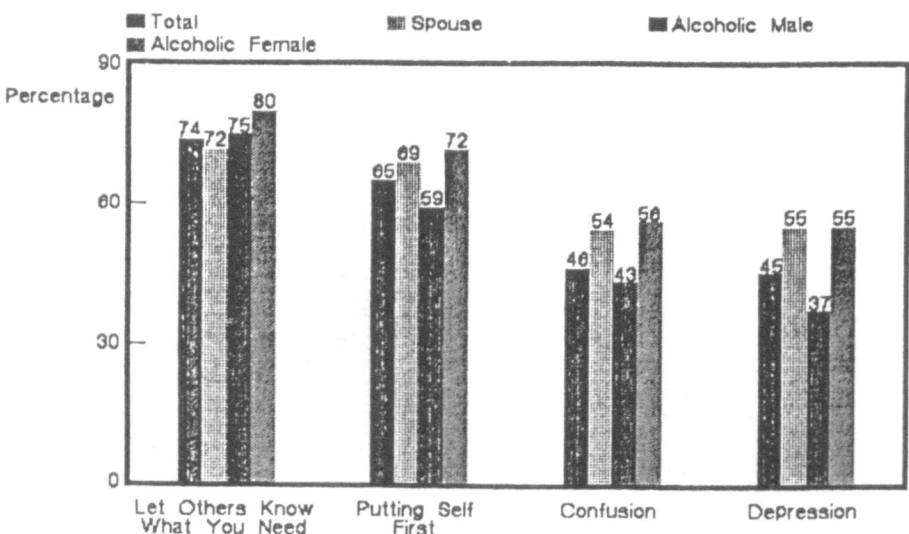

Figure 35.3b

As indicated earlier these data are only initial frequency data of a major study. I am not yet making conclusions from the data. This is a pilot study of which there will be multiple regression analysis to identify predictors of those who will become alcoholic and/or marry alcoholics, as well, a control group data base.

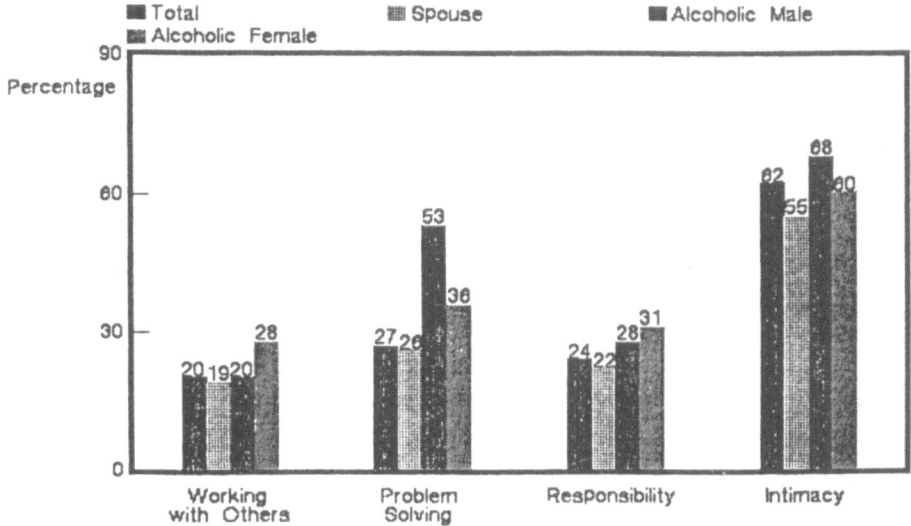

Figure 35.3c

I will be looking at variables such as (1) sex of child, (2) sex of alcoholic parent and (3) drinking style of alcoholic parent, birth order, role adoption, support systems utilized, perceptual concerns. Hopefully, these data will not only provide information about this specific population group but also indicate possible prevention and treatment strategies.

References

1 Goodwin, D. W. *et al.* (1973). Alcohol problems in adoptees raised from alcoholic biological parents. *Arch. Gen. Psychiatry*, **28,** 238
2 Goodwin, D. W., Schulsinger, F., Moeller, N. *et al.* (1974). Drinking problems in adopted and non-adopted sons of alcoholics. *Arch. Gen. Psychiatry*, **31,** 164
3 Kaij, L. (1960). *Alcoholism in Twins.* (Stockholm: Almquist & Wiksell)
4 Partanen, J., Bruun, K. and Markhanen, T. (1966). Inheritance of drinking behavior. (New Brunswick, NJ: Rutgers Center for Alcohol Studies)
5 Roe, A. and Burks, E., (1945). The adult adjustment of children of alcoholic parents raised in foster homes. *Q. J. Stud. Alc.*, **5,** 378
6 Schuckit, M., Goodwin D. and Winokur, G., (1972). A study of alcoholism in half siblings. *Am. J. Psychiatry*, **128,** 1132
7 Seldin, N. E. The family of the addict: a review of the literature. *Int. J. Addict.*
8 Westermeyer, J. and Bearman, J. (1973). A proposed social indicator system for alcohol-related problems. *Prev. Med.*, **2,** 438
9 Jones, K. L. and Smith, D. W. (1973). Recognition of the Fetal Alcohol Syndrome in early infancy. *Lancet*, **2,** 999
10 Jones, K. L., Smith, D. W., Ulleland, C. N., *et al.* (1973). Pattern of malformation in offspring of alcoholic mothers. *Lancet*, **1,** 1267
11 Landesman-Dwyers, K. L. S. (1977). Naturalistic observations of high and low risk

newborns. Presented at the *Meeting of the Society for Research in Child Development*, March, New Orleans

12 National Institute on Alcohol Abuse and Alcoholism. (1977). *Critical Review of the Fetal Alcohol Syndrome*, pp. 1–58. (Rockville, MD: NIAAA)

13 Quellette, E. M., Rosett, H. L., Rosman, N. P. *et al.* (1977). Adverse effects on offspring of maternal alcohol abuse during pregnancy. *N. Engl. J. Med.*, **297**, 528

14 Streissguth, A. P., Martin, J. D., Martin, D. C. (1977). Research design and assessment of alcohol consumption during pregnancy. Presented at the *Meeting of the Society for Research in Child Development*, March, New Orleans

15 Streissguth, A. P., Barr, H. C. (1977). Brazelton Assessment of neonatal offspring of moderate and light drinkers. Presented at the *Meeting of the Society for Research in Child Development*, March, New Orleans

16 Ulleland, C. N. (1972). The offspring of alcoholic mothers. *Ann. NY Acad. Sci.*, **197**, 167

17 Winokur, G., Reich, T., Rimmer, J. *et al.* (1970). Alcoholism III: diagnosis and family psychiatric illness in 259 alcoholic probands. *Arch. Gen. Psychiatry*, **23**, 104

18 Alltop, L. B. *et al.* (1980). Do children seen in mental health clinics come from 'problem drinking' households? *Inventory*, **19**, (4)

19 Chaftez, M., Blane, H. and Hill, M. (1971). Children of alcoholics: observations in a child guidance clinic. *Q. J. Stud. Alc.*, **32**, 678

20 Conference Report (1974). Runaway and alcohol conference. *National Institute on Alcohol Abuse and Alcoholism*, 8–10 April

21 El-Guebly, N. and Offord, D. (1977). The offspring of alcoholics: a critical review. *Am. J. Psychiatry*, **134**, 357

22 MacKay, J. R. (1961). Clinical observation on adolescent problem drinkers. *Q. J. Stud. Alc.*, **22**, 124

23 Schuckit, M. (1972). Family history and half-sibling research in alcoholism. *Ann. NY Acad. Sci.*, **197**, 121

24 Arentzen, W. P. (1978). Impact of alcohol misuses on family life. *Alc. Clin. Exp. Res.*, **2**, 349

25 Behling, D. (1979). Alcohol abuse as encountered in 51 instances of reported child abuse. *Clin. Pediatr.*, **18**, 87

26 Blumberg, M. L. (1974). Psychopathology of the abusing parent. *Am. J. Psychother.* **28**, 21

27 Fontana, V. J. and Besharov, D. J. (1977). *The Maltreated Child; The Maltreatment Syndrome in Children — A Medical, Legal and Social Guide*. (Springfield: Thomas)

28 Gil, D. (1970). *Violence Against Children: Physical Child Abuse in the United States*. (Cambridge, Mass.: Harvard UP)

29 Helfer, R. E. and Kempe, C. H. (eds.) (1974). *The Battered Child*. 2nd edn. (Chicago; University of Chicago Press)

30 Hindman, M. (1975–6). Children of alcoholic parents. *Alc. Health Res. World*, Winter 1975/6, 2

31 Hindman, M. (1979). Family Violence. *Alc. Health Res. World*, **4**, (1), 2

32 Kempe, R. S. and Kempe, C. H. (1978). *Child Abuse*. (Cambridge; Mass.: Harvard UP)

34 Booz-Allen & Hamilton, Inc. (1974). *An Assessment of the Needs of and Resources for Children of Alcoholic Parents*. (Springfield, VA: National Technical Information Service)

35 Black, C. (1979). Children of alcoholics. *Alc. Health Res. World*, **4**, 23

36 Brown, S. and Cermar, T. (1980). Group therapy with the adult children of alcoholics. *Newsletter*, California Society For Treatment of Alcoholism And Other Drug Dependencies, **7**, (1), January

37 Chaftez, M. (1979). Children of Alcoholics, *NY Univ. Educ. Q.*, **10** (3), 23

38 Kearney, T. R. and Taylor, C. (1969). Emotionally disturbed adolescents with alcoholic parents. *Acta Paedopsychiatr. (Basel)*, **36**, 215

39 Miketic, B. (1972). The influence of parental alcoholism in the development of the mental disturbances of children. *Alcoholism*, **8**, 135

40 Nylander, I. (1963). Children of alcoholic fathers. *Q. J. Stud. Alc.*, **49,**
41 Rosenberg, C. M. (1969). Determinants of psychiatric illness in young people. *Br. J. Psychiatry*, **115,**
42 Stott, D. H. (1971). The child's hazards in utero. *Mod. Perspect. Int. Child Psychiatry*, 19
43 Bailey, M., Hoberman, P. and Sheinberg, T. (1965). *Distinctive Characteristics of the Alcoholic Family.* Report of the Health Council of the City of New York. (New York: National Council on Alcoholism)
44 Clifford, B. (1960). A study of the wives of rehabilitated and unrehabilitated alcoholics. *Soc. Casework*, **41,** 457
45 Bosma, W. (1975). Alcoholism and teenagers, *Maryland State Med. J.* **24** (6), 62
46 Bowen, M. (1973). Alcohol and the family system. *The Family*, **1** (1), 20

36
Experiences of the counselling unit for families with alcohol related problems

M. MINIEVIC

A family represents a small primary group that has direct and intimate relationships. The family unit implies almost complete consistence of interests and a firm, continuous relationship among the family members. It is also a unique community because of its importance in the life of each individual, both in all the periods of life and in nearly all fields of functioning. This represents one of the main factors in the gaining and maintaining of psychosocial stability and emotional balance in its members.

It is well known that alcohol related problems are most dominantly reflected in the family unit in the sense of disturbed and misconducted relationships, as well as the fact of their influence on individual and interpersonal functioning. It should be underlined that these disorders, by definition, come first, before the other social and health symptoms of alcoholism. All investigations in this field point to the importance of factors tending to keep alcoholism confined within the family system. Although family problems play an important role among the reasons for accepting treatment, what often happens is that 10 years could pass before the patient and his family come to seek help. This point most frequently represents the moment when all individual, family and extra-family social problems come to a head.

The early recognition of the family problems related to alcoholic drinking contributes very much to the successful treatment and rehabilitation, i.e. it contributes to the prevention of health disorders and bad professional functioning, as well as to the prevention of mental and other disturbances among the other members of a family.

Our intention is not to deal with all of the various problems related to alcoholism. Our aim is to find out the methods and approaches in giving help to the family in the early phase of alcoholism, before their alcoholic member 'goes to the bottom'.

During our work with alcoholism significant groups of problems are noticed:

(1)   The ignorance that alcoholism is an illness until serious health and social complications make their appearance.

(2)   Partial acceptance connecting the family problems to alcoholism and alcoholic behaviour.

(3)   Denial of any possibility for changes within the family system until the alcoholic himself makes a decision to go to treatment or to give up drinking.

All these important points have an influence on the environment because of their similar attitudes, and the tendency to enormous tolerance and adaptation to the drinking behaviour as a socially acceptable and favoured manner of behaviour.

Taking into account all the observations and impressions as well as many years of experience in work with alcoholics, and under the constant pressure and demands of families, the Institute for Mental Health in Belgrade founded in 1978 the Counselling Unit for families with alcohol related problems.

The basic idea of this initiative has been an attempt to offer qualified help to a family in identifying the problem and finding out the possibilities for its solution. The essence of this work lies in the motivation and preparation of the family, and the alcoholic himself, for complete family treatment. The Counselling Unit has been organized by the Centre for Family Therapy of Alcoholism in Belgrade, and represents the first service of this kind in our country. Counselling is performed by a team of experts – a psychologist, social worker, defectologist, and, periodically, a psychiatrist. The financial support has been provided by means of the preventive programmes for mental health protection, which ensures a service free of charge and administrative procedures. Our clients can contact the staff directly or by writing (if they do not live in Belgrade) and by phone – by so-called 'hot line'.

PRINCIPLES AND METHODS

In the Counselling Unit the accent is laid on the individual treatment of each client and each family. This approach involves the complete analysis of specific problems of every member and his family as a group in its natural environment, and all these elements help to create a special plan for every case and each family.

All impressions, observations and information, as well as the mode of behaviour in the Counselling Unit, indicate the disintegrated attitudes of the family members in their efforts to find an adequate solution for the problem drinking.

The communications are generally aimed at the effort to find out who is responsible for the actual situation and reasons for drinking. The attitudes of all family members toward drinking and alcoholic behaviour are chiefly moralistic. The actual dependence on alcohol is not fully recognized and all expectations are aimed at the alcoholic himself and his goodwill to give up drinking. The reason for not coming earlier to the treatment, according to the family members' explanation, is lack of information about the Counselling Unit and methods of treatment. At the same time it became obvious that action directed only towards the cognitive components of a person's attitude, through education, does not represent a sufficient condition for changing the behaviour and habits. Some clients, under the impression of new information, become certain that they can find the right way to bring the patient to treatment, but later they completely fail. On the other hand, there are persons who believe that the newly received information cannot bring any changes, for they have already tried all they could. To them the only solution is to wait until the patient is hospitalized.

The collected data require a continuous and extensive approach to the family with alcohol related problems. Our experiences reveal the importance and necessity for including key persons, relatives, friends, in order to obtain a more complete observation of the factors which keep alcoholism within the family. Despite the tendency for an independent family life (growth of nuclear families), in our environment there still exist the firm traditional connections and a great influence of parents and relatives on the young married couples. As an example, the wife who recognizes her own contribution to alcoholism in her husband might decide to change her behaviour. Instead of quarrelling and warning him of the dangers every day, she gives up taking care of his personal hygiene and dressing (cleaning shoes, ironing etc). But after a while she will soon become faced with reproaches of being a bad housewife, who neglects her husband. She is then forced to continue suffering and taking responsibility for the formal functioning of her family. Only a few persons realize that she is overburdened, nervous, scared, while the children live in constant insecurity without real parental care and love. This influence is especially expressed when the wife, after innumerable warnings, makes a decision to leave her husband in order to bring both of them into a situation of choice — either to dissolve their marriage or to begin with the treatment and a new life.

These influences from the environment can be very important in holding up a therapeutic change, assuming that her decision will be met with criticism. These are the reasons why we expand the scope of our work and influence on the wider family circle and key persons from the social environment.

The basic approach is education combined with other psychosocial methods; i.e. informing of the characteristics of alcholism in a context of family interactions.

In our practice we apply:

(1)   Lectures
(2)   Written material (brochures)
(3)   Sessions consisting of conversations in a family group when the roles of all present are defined.

Special sessions with the family members clear up the particular relationship problems, and make possible an approach to the emotional relationships which are usually disturbed and poor. The family members train in a new manner of communication (clear, direct and defined). From this they can find the best solution to their problem. The special role of the expert is to point to the tendencies to look for the guilty person or the position 'who is right'.

The process of preparation and motivation of the family is long and slow, especially at the beginning. It must be done step by step (sometimes for several months), with permanent testing of the capabilities of the family. The instructing is done by presenting tasks corresponding to the data about the specific difficulties. At the same time the main aim of the staff is to dispel the prejudices that the patient has when he realizes that he needs help. Until they are dispelled, nothing can be achieved.

The recognition of the mechanism of defence (minimization, denial, rationalization and projection) is very important for all the involved persons because it is, in some way, present in all of them.

The collective work, recorded at least once a week (with some or all members), will progressively give a family more security in the realization that the problem can be solved, provided it is accepted as a common one. Everyone becomes aware of his new role, is constantly encouraged, and this contributes very much to the increase of self-confidence.

During the period of intensive work with so-called healthy members, important changes are happening within the family circle. The alcoholic knows that his family visits the Counselling Unit and he relates all modifications in his life to this fact. He is now very rarely in a position to quarrel and to charge somebody with bad intentions. Now his threatenings and orders are without their usual effects. This, of course, can intensify his anger, tension and aggressive behaviour or can be the reason for his absence from home. Some of the patients may succeed at abstinence, and, after a period of not drinking, believe that no further treatment is necessary. However, the family accepts this state of abstinence in a different way. Since they are aware of the temporary character of this state, it now represents a good chance for an open conversation about their visit to the Counselling Unit, especially for those who only gave numerous promises but did not participate.

The consistent behaviour in reference to the real needs of the family and its members is the best warning for the alcoholic himself that he must come face-to-face with a decision about future life. When the patient joins his family and visits the Counselling Unit, the staff, in collaboration with the family members, can start with the plan of treatment.

The patient and his family can also come to a decision to get divorced. In this case the staff of the Centre for Social Work and other institutions will become involved. During the process of divorce the decisions can be altered and this represents a new chance to save the marriage. When divorce is the only solution, the Counselling Unit still helps the family to solve various difficulties and supports them in a new state of adaptation and accommodation to changed life conditions, especially in their emotional crisis which follows every divorce. In these situations the so-called 'therapy of divorce' is put into effect.

OUR RESULTS

When the information about the establishment of the Counselling Unit was given to the newspapers at the end of 1978, the first visitors came immediately seeking help for their family members and relatives. Some of them called us up and asked for more detailed information or fixed an appointment. We also received letters with various questions and requests for advice for some efficient medication. Two thirds of the total number were wives of alcoholics.

Many people are afraid of their visit to the Counselling Unit being discovered by the drinker, as they feel it will worsen the family relationships. Only a small number of these visitors were alcoholics themselves asking for help and trying to find solutions for their difficulties and their alcoholism.

Up to the end of 1981 we had registered 428 families with problems related to the drinking of one person, but sometimes two or even three persons in the family (husband, wife, son, etc).

The population of alcoholics was very heterogenous – from the individuals who have already been clinically observed and seriously treated, to those in the earlier phases of alcoholism and mostly with family difficulties and problems.

The work with alcoholics and their families is continued until we establish a solid contact with the alcoholic and are able to attain a mutual agreement about the plan of treatment. Through motivation in the Counselling Unit, 226 alcoholics have been included in the programme of family therapy, or 62%. We are quite sure that we did not fulfil all the expectations of some clients, or, perhaps, the tasks we set for them were too difficult.

DISCUSSION AND CONCLUSIONS

Our experiences in this specific field and our approach to the family of alcoholics, over the other key persons, can be estimated as a modest one. The staff of the Centre for Family Therapy with its therapeutical and other activities has not been in a position to satisfy all the requirements of the people who have been asking for help at the Counselling Unit. We did not enter their homes and persuade the alcoholic by argument of the necessity to be treated; instead we have aimed at helping the families and friends of alcoholics to recognize the problems of alcoholism in their real extent. We have tried to support them in their better personal functioning and so increase their self-respect and ability to make decisions — either to remain as a family or to separate.

Our impressions and experiences we present in the following conclusions:

(1) The Counselling Unit for help to the families with alcohol related problems has been justified from the professional and social points of view as a necessary institution.

(2) It is also necessary to develop co-operation with other responsible institutions that have their own place and position in withstanding alcoholism and its consequences on other people, e.g. centres for social work, educational institutions, industries (enterprises) etc.

(3) The unity of prevention and treatment as a continuous activity has been confirmed in the practice of the Counselling Unit. Many problems in individual and interpersonal functioning are often affected and even disguised by alcohol.

(4) This method occupies a significant and important place in the social-psychiatric approach to the other categories of psychiatric disorders, and (but) especially in the demystification of psychiatry.

37
Sexuality and the alcoholic family:
effects of chemical dependence and co-dependence upon individual family members

E. COLEMAN

In alcoholic and chemically dependent families, we have found a significant correlation with intimacy dysfunction. Intimacy dysfunction is defined as an inability to express feelings (both positive and negative) in a meaningful and constructive manner, which is mutually acceptable and respectful, and leads to the psychological well-being of the individuals involved. In order to engage in intimate behaviour or to be involved in an intimate relationship, one must be able to communicate feelings and thoughts. The purpose of this communication is to define the boundaries of the relationship and to express feelings of caring, concern, commitment. It is to negotiate roles and rules of the relationship and to resolve conflicts. Intimacy dysfunction is also an attitudinal dysfunction which prevents the individual from having meaningful relationships.

Intimate relationships can be of different durations and intensity and are certainly not limited to the parental unit. Sexual activity which is sometimes viewed as the apex of intimacy is only a part of intimacy and one way of expressing it. In addition, sexual activity can occur without an intention of intimacy expression. In so far as we are all sexual beings and express our sexuality (sex roles, physical attractions and repulsions, needs for warmth, tenderness and touch) in all that we do, our sexuality is always a part of our intimacy or sexual activity. Figure 37.1 illustrates the relationship between intimacy expression and sexual activity as a part of sexuality.

Examples or symptoms of intimacy dysfunction might include: physical abuse of children, emotional neglect of children, sexual abuse of children, relationship discord, violence in relationships, rape, and sexual dysfunction.

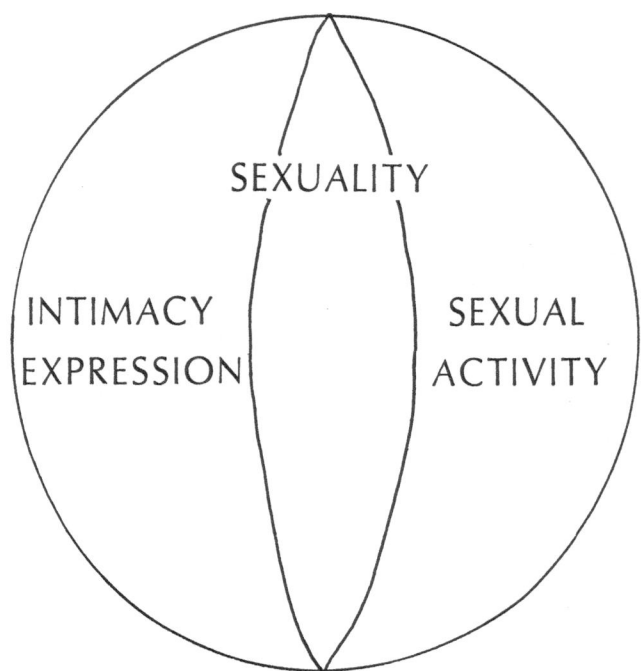

Figure 37.1   Relationship between intimacy expression and sexual activity

These intimacy dysfunctions are correlated with alcoholism, chemical dependency and co-dependency[1]. These are often correlated with other addictions or abusive patterns such as food addiction, work addiction, or sex addiction.

While these are only correlations, questions are often raised whether chemical dependency causes intimacy dysfunction or whether intimacy dysfunction leads to chemical dependency. This is a 'chicken or egg' type of question and is answered using the following integrated model (see Figure 37.2). The cycle can begin at any point; the starting point is often irrelevant because of the longstanding pattern which is passed on from generation to generation. Disturbed family dynamics and individual intimacy dysfunctions are an inevitable consequence of chemical dependency and co-dependency. This leads to intimacy dysfunction in the family. As a coping mechanism and to retain family stability, there is an increased need for alcohol or chemical abuse and co-dependent behaviour patterns. With unhealthy expressions of intimacy in the family, sexual attitudes are developed in the children which are based upon unhealthy parental role models. As the chemical dependency and co-dependency patterns progress there is damage to the self-esteem of family members. With a lack of healthy sexual and intimacy attitudes, a lack of healthy role models and a lowered self-esteem, the child tries to develop

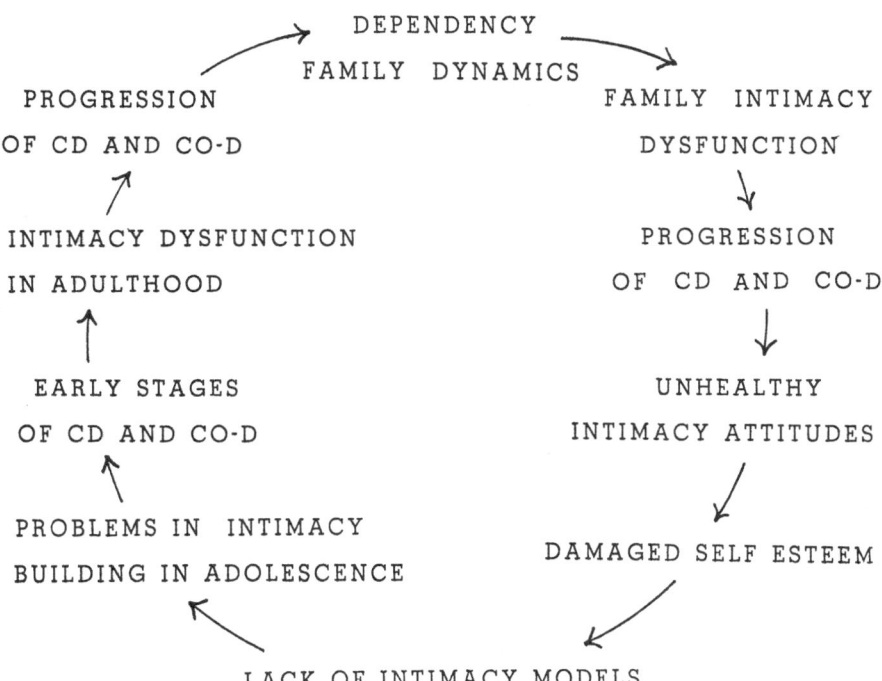

Figure 37.2 Integration model of the CD-Intimacy Connection

intimate and sexual relationships in adolescence and adulthood. With these handicaps and developmental deficiencies it is no wonder the adolescent would have difficulty. The adolescent turns to alcohol, drugs or co-dependent behaviour patterns to cope with existing pressures and to cope with the chronic pain of the family intimacy dysfunction. Excessive use of alcohol, drugs, sex, food, work, enabling or co-dependent behaviour can all be methods to anaesthetize the family pain. All these methods are used to feel better about oneself. However, this positive feeling is artificial and temporary. In fact, as the dependency and co-dependency patterns develop, they begin to cause further damage to intimacy patterns and self-esteem. This adolescent enters adulthood with further problems of intimacy. There is, then, greater need for coping mechanisms and this feeds the progression of dependency and co-dependency. This dependency leads to the continued dependency family dynamics and begins the process again, handing down this family pattern from generation to generation.

Now that the model of intimacy dysfunction has been described, some particular effects of this family pattern on the individual family members will be described. The following areas, while not exhaustive, are the most common areas affected by life in an alcoholic or chemically dependent family.

LACK OF BOUNDARIES

Marilyn Mason has described how the element of boundary ambiguity is found in most chemically dependent families. This ambiguity causes 'one person not knowing where he/she and another begins' (reference 2, p. 309). A person suffering from boundary ambiguity will not know how to set boundaries or will not be able to respect other's boundaries. Nor will the individual understand clear boundaries and appropriate family roles, (e.g., a mother, father, grandparent, child etc.). Often these roles are confused and interchanged among family members.

Confusion in boundaries is often a result of physical or sexual invasion of boundaries. We know that physical violence between family members is not uncommon in chemically dependent families[3]. We have clinical evidence which also suggests psychological damage occurs to all family members who witness this abuse, not necessarily to those physically victimized. We also have clinical evidence which suggests that the physical violence can increase after treatment of chemical dependency.

Incest is also not uncommon in chemically dependent families[4]. Estimates have been made that 40-80% of female alcoholics have been incest victims. Little is known about male alcoholics and their incidence of incest because these questions have not been asked.

Lack of personal boundaries, overly rigid boundaries, or lack of respect for other's boundaries are ingredients for intimacy dysfunction. Skills at boundary setting form an essential ingredient in developing and maintaining healthy, intimate and sexual relationships.

INTIMACY AND SEXUAL ATTITUDES AND VALUES

It is no wonder that, with boundary ambiguity and being exposed to unhealthy intimate and sexual attitudes and values, offspring develop similar unhealthy attitudes and values. Attitudes about intimacy which are common among chemically dependent family members:

"Intimacy doesn't exist"
"Intimacy is something you only have when chemicals are involved"
"Intimacy is something that you take; it is never given freely"
"You can only be intimate if there is sex involved"
"Sex can never be associated with intimacy"
"Sex is dirty"
"Seductive behaviour gets you what you want"
"Sex will give you power"
"Sex will make you feel powerless"

These are just a few examples. They give an idea of how these attitudes serve as barriers to healthy intimacy and sexual expression.

SHAME

One predominant attitude which is often found in chemically dependent individuals and their family members is shame about their sexuality. Shame is a feeling of unworthiness, sinfulness or feeling unwanted. Shame inhibits an individual from feeling worthy of an intimate relationship. Feelings of shame are a result of family intimacy dysfunction. Having been unloved, neglected or abused, individuals will feel bad or sinful about every aspect of their personhood.

Sex is also a common source of shame. Alcohol or other drugs are used to overcome shame in order to be sexual. Adolescents begin using alcohol or other drugs at the same time they are learning to be sexual with others. Individuals with shame-based personalities need alcohol or other drugs to be sexual. When the use of alcohol or drugs stops, the coping mechanism for shame is removed. The individual becomes inundated with feelings of shame regarding sexuality. The individual needs to find some other coping mechanism. Some stop having sex and others develop sexual dysfunctions. Ironically then, chemical dependency treatment often causes an individual to experience sexual difficulties.

SEXUAL DYSFUNCTION

Lack of desire, premature ejaculation, retarded ejaculation, female orgasmic dysfunctions, erectile and lubrication difficulty are common dysfunctions among alcoholic, chemically dependent and co-dependent individuals. These dysfunctions are often a result of discomfort and anxiety about sexuality. These dysfunctions can also develop as a result of the disruption of the association of drugs and sexual functioning. When an individual has always relied on drugs in order to be sexual, the removal of this 'crutch' leaves the individual a 'sexual cripple'. The individual needs to learn 'how to walk again without the crutch' and deal with the source of shameful feelings about sexuality.

Sexual dysfunctions can also be a result of physiological damage caused by alcohol or other drug abuse. Liver disease and alcoholic hepatitis are particularly responsible for this type of damage. Since the liver is involved in the metabolization of sexual hormones, liver disease will result in altered hormone levels and secondarily cause sexual difficulties. Pancreas damage due to alcohol abuse will result in diabetes. Diabetes in turn can cause erectile dysfunction and vaginal lubrication problems. Circulatory problems may be responsible for this or peripheral neuropathy.

Organic brain damage is another way that alcohol damages the brain and secondarily impairs sexual functioning. Fortunately, we are treating alcoholism and chemical dependency in early stages so this kind of cortical damage is avoided or minimized.

Examination for physical causes of sexual dysfunction is always important in working with alcoholic and chemically dependent individuals. The psychogenic aetiologies are often present with organic aetiologies, and they very often interact to produce the sexual dysfunction.

SEX ROLES

Feeling good about one's masculinity and femininity is a feeling that eludes most chemically dependent and co-dependent individuals. Research has indicated that people drink or use chemicals to deal with the disparity between one's ideal sex role image and one's actual sex role image. Men who feel inadequate as males often drink to feel more masculine. Other males who feel restricted by male sex role stereotypes will use drugs or alcohol to engage in behaviours which are stereotypically feminine (e.g., expressing feelings, crying, embracing a friend).

Women will turn to alcohol or drugs to feel more powerful and masculine. Others who have taken on many traditional male roles in society may use alcohol or other drugs to permit them to engage in stereotypical feminine behaviour.

Research has not documented the link between sex roles and co-dependent behaviour patterns. However, we see from a clinical perspective that many co-dependent individuals are struggling with these same sex role issues. Out of the insecurities of sex role identities, many chemically dependent and co-dependent individuals hold on to rigid sex role behaviours. They are afraid to express a mixture of masculine and feminine behaviour for fear they will be less of a man or woman.

The pressures created by sex role standards or the confusion created by changing sex role standards are a definite part of the aetiology or the damage created by chemical dependency or co-dependency. While drinking or drug use may make an individual feel better about his or her sex role identity, when the individual loses control of use of alcohol or drugs or develops serious co-dependency patterns, his masculinity or her femininity is questioned. An alcoholic or an addict feels less of a man or less of a woman and no longer can that individual fulfil the roles they or society would like him or her to fulfil.

SEXUAL PREFERENCE

Chemically dependent and co-dependent individuals are almost universally concerned about sexual preference. Whether because of insecurity about sex roles, incidental homosexual encounters, or mixed or predominant homosexual arousal patterns, these can be a source of anxiety, shame and discomfort. For some, fears of being or becoming homosexual are an ongoing concern or unconscious fear. Closeness to same-sex individuals can lead to confusion about these feelings. Thoughts of past homosexual activity can cause confusion, discomfort, guilt and shame. Even an awareness of a same-sex fantasy or dream is enough to generate stress.

There are also those with predominant same-sex attractions who have hidden from these feelings through alcohol, drug abuse, or co-dependent behaviour patterns. They have denied these feelings and used these behaviour patterns to help them forget. Others have acted on these feelings, felt shame about them, and used alcohol, drugs or co-dependent behaviour patterns to mask the shame. Many individuals going through treatment for chemical dependency or co-dependency and who identified themselves as homosexual prior to treatment, will invariably feel the guilt and shame about their homosexuality once alcohol, drugs or co-dependent behaviours are removed.

The problem of alcohol and drug abuse among homosexuals is enormous[6]. Oppression, alienation and shame all contribute to self-abusive patterns and naturally lead to alcohol and drug abuse. To be sober and homosexual means the individual is faced with the task of embracing his/her homosexuality, developing self-acceptance, and skills to function in intimate relationships in a society which is predominantly heterosexual and oppressive towards homosexual.

SEXUAL ADDICTIONS

Sex can also become a coping mechanism or an anaesthetic to the psychological pain caused by intimacy dysfunction. Like a quick 'fix', sex becomes a way of shoring up damaged self-esteem or creating a false sense of intimacy. In fact, sex may have the same physiological effect as alcohol and other drugs and thus there is a potential for dependency. Chemically dependent or co-dependent individuals can develop patterns of sexual addiction before treatment or as a replacement to chemicals or co-dependent behaviours in recovery. Examples of sexual addiction include sexual acting-out, compulsive sexual activity, certain fetishistic behaviours, and compulsive masturbation. Just as chemicals and co-dependent behaviour has formed an intimacy barrier and caused further intimacy dysfunction, sexual addiction can do the same.

TREATMENT CONSIDERATIONS

In order to treat alcoholism, chemical dependency and co-dependency, therapists must address the intimacy dysfunctions of the individuals involved. As a preventative measure, these issues need to be addressed in order to break the vicious cycle of family intimacy dysfunction. Treatment of all individuals in the family is necessary to break the cycle. Removing alcohol, chemicals or co-dependent behaviours from a family system leaves all family members insecure and lacking the healthy tools to express intimacy. Treatment of intimacy issues will be a key in preventing recidivism and creating sobriety in all family members.

References

1 Coleman, E. (1982). Family intimacy and chemical abuse: The connection. *J. Psychoact. Drugs*, **14**, 153

2 Mason, M. (1983). Sexuality and fear of intimacy as barriers for recovery for drug dependent women. In Reed, B., Beshner, C. and Mondanaro, J. (eds.) *Treatment Services for Drug Dependent Women*, Vol. II. (Washington, DC: US Govt Printing Office, for US Dept of Health and Human Services)

3 Kempe, C. H., Silverman, F. N., Steele, B. F., Droegemulle, W. and Silver, H. K. (1962). The battered child syndrome. *J. Am. Med. Assoc.*, **181**, 17

4 Benward, J. and Densen-Gerber, J. (1975). Incest as a causative factor in anti-social behaviour: An exploratory study. *Contemp. Drug Probl.*, **4**, 323

5 Wilsniak, S. C. (1976). The impact of sex roles on women's alcohol use and abuse. In Greenblatt, M. and Schuckit, M. A. (eds.) *Alcoholism Problems in Women and Children*. (New York: Grune & Stratton)

6 Fifield, L. (1975). *On My Way to Nowhere: Alienated, Isolated, Drunk.* (Los Angeles: Gay Community Services Center)

38
Women's sexuality and alcoholism

M. STERNE, S. SCHAEFER and S. EVANS

This paper represents an encapsulated version of the results of a research project undertaken at a women's chemical dependency treatment programme located in the Midwest of the United States of America. Before discussing the results, a description of the context out of which the research began will be given.

In the Fall of 1977, Chrysalis, a Center for Women in Minneapolis, Minnesota (the agency from which the research was gathered) became one of the original 13 women's treatment programmes awarded grants by the National Institute on Alcohol Abuse and Alcoholism (NIAAA). From the onset of the programme, sexuality was viewed by the staff (of which the authors were a part) as an essential component of the treatment programme.

Within the first year of operation the staff at Chrysalis conducted a needs assessment of the clientele, asking the women to prioritize issues they saw as most critical to their recovery. Ten major areas of recovery were questioned, including (1) chemical use, (2) personal awareness, (3) health, (4) family, (5) social, (6) legal, (7) occupational, (8) economic, (9) sexuality and (10) other – clients could list an additional untapped area.

Of these ten categories surveyed, sexuality was rated in importance second only to the category called 'personal awareness', which consisted of items related to self-esteem, assertiveness and independence.

The area of sexuality was rated even higher than the 'chemical use' category. Many of the women seen at Chrysalis had been through multiple prior treatments and seemingly had a working knowledge of alcoholism; yet many discovered even with this knowledge something critical to a quality sobriety was missing. For many women this involved unresolved sexuality issues. For some women, fear of sex sober compelled them to begin using alcohol again. For others, coming to grips with the pain of past sexual assault or incestuous experiences led to self-medicating with alcohol or pills. For still others, attempting to work through sexual identity issues served to promote the seeking of psychological refuge with a chemical high.

To explore further the relationship between women's sexuality and recovery from alcoholism, an extensive sexuality questionnaire was developed. The questionnaire consisted of a ten-page self-report inventory tapping nearly 800 bits of information, from which the present research was derived.

The questionnaire was distributed to clients who had completed primary treatment (Phase I) and were considered relatively stable in their sobriety (for demographics see Appendix to this chapter). These clients were in the second phase of the treatment programme, where they were working on issues related to their sobriety, including relationship dependency, parenting skills, assertiveness, sexuality and feelings group.

The sexuality questionnaire included a two-page glossary of terms so that all subjects would be operating from similar working definitions. In addition to closed-ended questions, (Yes-no and scaled attitudinal questions), a number of open-ended questions were included. The open-ended questions provided a rich source of material, though more difficult to quantify. When possible, objective criteria were formulated within which to place subjective comments to aid in the interpretation of information.

The information provided today represents the results of analysing 75 questionnaires. Major areas surveyed include: childhood sexuality, incest and sexual assault, sexual identity, celibacy, level of sexual satisfaction, medical and gynaecological concerns, prostitution, the use of alcohol and/or other drugs in conjunction with sexual activity, and general areas of sexual conflict.

The following is a summary of results reported from the questions surveyed.

(1)   Sexual preference:
    (a)   heterosexual, 61%
    (b)   lesbian, 29%
    (c)   bisexual, 3%
    (d)   Uncertain, 7%.

(2)   Sexual partners over past 5 years:
    (a)   Males only, 55%
    (b)   Females only, 15%
    (c)   Both, 30%.

(3)   First sexual (genital) experience:
    (a)   Sex of partner: female, 15%; male, 85%
    (b)   Age: range 5−31:
        (i)   14 or less, 24%
        (ii)   15−17, 35%
        (iii)   18−20, 29%

    (iv) 21 +, 11 %
    (v) N/A, 1 %
(c) Positive or negative experience:
    (i) Positive or reasonably so, 18 %
    (ii) Negative, 82 %.

(4) Voluntary periods of celibacy: yes, 79 %; no, 21 %.

(5) Use of alcohol and/or other drugs in conjunction with sexual activity:
  (a) Always or frequently, 71 %
  (b) None or rarely, 29 %.

(6) Satisfaction with pattern of sexual behaviour over the past 2 years:
  (a) Satisfied, 33 %
  (b) Dissatisfied, 67 %.

(7) Number of sexual partners over past 5 years (average per year):
  (a) One, 51 %
  (b) Two, 17 %
  (c) Three, 4 %
  (d) Four, 4 %
  (e) More than four, 12 %.

(8) Pregnancy, abortions, miscarriage:
  (a) Experienced pregnancy, 57 %
  (b) Experienced abortion(s), 44 %
  (c) Experienced miscarriage, 23 %.

(9) Gynaecological Concerns: Greater than 80 % reported having experienced one or more gynaecological concerns (most frequently ranked categories):
  (a) Yeast infections, 57 %
  (b) Irregular menstrual periods, 33 %
  (c) Crabs, 31 %
  (d) Gonorrhoea, 17 %.

(10) History of prostitution: 8 %.

(11) Incest/sexual abuse:
  (a) Proportion victimized: 53 %
  (b) Sex of perpetrator: male, 87 %; female, 13 %
  (c) Category of perpetrator (according to most frequently ranked):
    (i) Father
    (ii) Neighbour
    (iii) Brother
    (iv) Mother
  (d) Age of onset:
    (i) One third before or during age 6
    (ii) One third between the ages 7−13
    (iii) One third age 14 or older

    (e)   Frequency:
          (i)   Single incident, 31%
          (ii)   Multiple, 33%
          (iii) Chronic (one or more times a month for a year or more),
                 36%
    (f)   Exposed incident:
          (i)   Two thirds did not report incident.
          (ii)   One third reported incident to an adult.

(12) Admitted to the victimization of a minor themselves:
    (a)   Physically abused, 21%
    (b)   Sexually abused, 13%.

(13) Reported the following had become sexual with them:
    (a)   Doctors, 9%
    (b)   Lawyers, 7%
    (c)   Clergy, 7%
    (d)   Professor, 9%
    (e)   Boss or Supervisor, 31%
    (f)   Therapist, 5%
    51% reported one or more of the above categories of professionals had
    become sexual with them.

(14) Major areas of sexual conflict:
    (a)   Having sex when partner wants it, she doesn't, 93%
    (b)   Fear of unattractiveness, 92%
    (c)   Inability to reach orgasm, 92%
    (d)   Fear of intimacy, 86%
    (e)   Doubts about performance, 85%

(15) Sexuality issues most wanted to address in treatment:
    (a)   Learn how to develop intimacy
    (b)   Learn to be more direct in communicating sexual needs (setting
          boundaries, being assertive, communicating what pleasures
          them)
    (c)   Learn more about sex
    (d)   Explore sexual identity
    (e)   Become more comfortable with own body
    (f)   Regain power, take back control of sexuality and assume
          ownership.

    The data gathered corroborate clinical observations and offer information
to alcoholism professionals in designing women's treatment programmes or
in formulating individual treatment plans for women clients. Women often
report their difficulty in broaching the topic of sexuality with their
counsellors. One obvious treatment implication is the necessity of counsellors
asking questions related to sexuality directly – either verbally or through
questionnaires. The direct asking of questions serves a permission-giving
function and thereby begins to facilitate the therapeutic process.

APPENDIX

Characteristics of Chrysalis' outpatient clients (1979–1980) were as follows.

(1) *Mean Age*: 29.2 years.

(2) *Ethnicity*:
White, 93 %
Black, 2 %
American Indian, 5 %.

(3) *Marital status*:
Never married, 53 %
Married, 18 %
Separated/divorced, 29 %.

(4) *Mean Years of Education*: 13.4.

(5) *Percentage employed of those in labour force*: 74.5 %.

(6) *Occupation*:
Professional/manager, 16 %
Sales/clerical, 20 %
Crafts, 7.5 %
Labour, 1 %
Service, 20 %
Student, 5.5 %
Homemaker, 9 %
None, 20 %.

(7) *Mean Income*: $8276 (annual household).

Part 9:
ALCOHOLISM AND INDUSTRY

39
The history, the philosophy and the essential components of employee assistance programmes

D. A. MASI and L. A. TEEMS

PHILOSOPHY

Employee assistance programmes (EAP) have emerged as a method for effectively dealing with employees whose alcohol, drug and mental health problems are eroding job performance. An EAP is a combination of assessment and referral services designed to restore these employees to full productivity. They are viewed as particularly effective in combating job deterioration due to alcohol abuse. In fact, the highest rates of recovery from alcohol problems occur in EAPs, not in hospitals and other treatment facilities[1]. The reasons for the success of the EAPs lie in their philosophy.

Job performance is the pivot of employee assistance programming. The workplace constitutes a unique setting in that there is a contractual relationship between the employer and employee which allows the employer to intervene if work production deteriorates. Such deterioration must, of course, be carefully documented by supervisors or managers and must meet the standards that are established in agreements between employers and employees[2]. If a worker is not performing according to these agreements, the employer then has a justification to take action. But their action does not have to be adverse; an EAP offers a humane method of intervention.

This intervention can occur at the worksite with a great deal of leverage. Jobs are very important to people. By using the threat of job loss, EAPs have the potential for breaking through the alibis, the denial and the excuses that people in trouble with personal problems, particularly alcoholism, often exhibit. Usually, they will not seek help voluntarily. When the facts of deteriorating job performance can be documented, the stage is set for a rather unique form of intervention — confrontation. Confrontation, coupled with job leverage, provides a strong motivation for individuals to do something about their problems before dismissal results.

Another basic supposition of an EAP is that of early referral by supervisors and managers. Except for an employee's family and friends, the supervisor is perhaps the person most affected by a personal problem. Because of the stigma and denial often evidenced in family and friends, the supervisor can more easily identify the early warning signs of a problem employee. An integral component of any EAP is the training of managers to determine the facts about an employee's performance, *not* the nature of his or her personal problem. Their role is to be alert to performance changes, document these changes, and with the advice of an EAP staff member, refer the employee to the programme.

SIZE OF PROBLEM

Every business, no matter how well managed or what size, has employees with such troubles as alcoholism and drug abuse. Studies in the USA indicate that at any given time, 18 % of a workforce consists of troubled employees whose job performance has deteriorated by 25 %[3]. The National Institute on Alcohol Abuse and Alcoholism (NIAAA) estimates that over half of these, or 10 % are employees in the middle stages of alcoholism[4]. Another 2 % of the employees have problems due to drug abuse[5] and 6 % are suffering from other emotional problems such as depression[6].

Employee problems affect job performance in a number of ways: increased absenteeism, tardiness, increased sick leave, on-the-job absenteeism, poor judgement, lowered morale, resentment from co-workers, erratic behaviour, on and off the job accidents, wasted supervisory time, damaged public relations, excessive spoilage, missed deadlines, overtime costs, grievance costs, and training costs.

The traditional way to deal with a troubled employee has been to adopt a 'hands-off-policy'. Often, these employees were fired, transferred, hidden etc. But the effects of these problems on work performance are of vital concern to businesses. From an economic perspective, profit-minded and productivity-minded corporations can no longer afford to close their eyes or ignore the costly alcohol, drug and mental health problems which directly affect an employee's performance as already stated. In the USA alone, the cost to industry is estimated at $25 billion[7].

HISTORY OF EAPS IN THE USA

The idea of programmes to assist employees with personal problems is relatively new. Formal counselling and referral programmes did not emerge until the early 1940s. At that time, occupational alcoholism programmes began to evolve in a handful of major industrial firms such as Dupont, Kemper Insurance and Eastman Kodak (see reference 8, p. 5). Their outgrowth was the result of efforts by recovered alcoholics who were perceptive enough to realize the importance of a job in the life of an alcoholic. These crusaders pursued their programmatic ideas with their employers who sanctioned the initiation of these early programmes.

Despite their demonstrated effectiveness, EAPs did not proliferate for the next 20 years. The early achievements were attained only through enormous efforts by a few strong advocates. Apathy and stigma were often the barriers to the growth of industrial programmes (see reference 8, p. 7).

In the 1960s, industrial alcoholism programmes began to show some accelerated growth. A study done by the National Council on Alcoholism in 1964 indicated that 203 work organizations reported having some formal programme[9]. Hughes Aircraft and Standard Oil were among the major corporations in this group.

The passage of the Hughes Act by the US Congress in 1970[10] was perhaps the greatest impetus to the development of occupational alcoholism programmes. Senator Harold Hughes is a recovered alcoholic and had the courage to speak out in the halls of the Senate on behalf of separate alcohol legislation. This law established the National Institute on Alcohol Abuse and Alcoholism in the US Department of Health and Human Services. Within the Institute, the Occupational Branch was established which granted money for special demonstration contracts as well as for two occupational programme consultants in each state.

The Hughes Act also mandated the development and maintenance of prevention, treatment and rehabilitation programmes for federal employees with alcohol problems. The Department of Health and Human Services programme has been mandated the model for the federal government. Both authors work in this programme. Similarly, the US Department of Defense initiated such programmes for their military and civilian employees.

Other changes were taking place for occupational programmes in the 1970s. Research was beginning to find that programmes focussing on all types of employee behavioural problems tended to avoid the liability difficulties and ambiguous supervisory feelings that had hampered the effectiveness of most alcoholism programmes[11]. Due to these developments, the late 1970s saw expansion of alcoholism programmes into broader-based employee assistance programmes. They began to reflect services for an extensive range of behavioural/medical problems. Today, there are over 5000 EAPs in the USA[12] including over 50% in the *Fortune 500* Corporations[13].

PROGRAMME COMPONENTS

When developing an EAP, there are essential components which must be addressed to ensure an effective, smoothly-operating system. They are:

Development of programme support

It is vital to the programme's existence to have support of the organization's key personnel. This will include those persons who make direct decisions about the EAP, those persons who can operate as political allies to the EAP, and those persons who make indirect decisions that may affect the EAP. Top level support for the programme must be ensured *before* its actual start. This includes placement of the EAP at a sufficiently high level in the organization in order to demonstrate top level endorsement. Financial support along with staff positions must also be considered. The company must be willing and able to fund the EAP at an adequate level. This component is essential for assessing the company's commitment. For every 3500 employees, one professional full-time staff member is needed. Companies sometimes will give lip services to a programme and it is important in the beginning that this be flushed out.

Development of a programme plan

It is critical that a plan for the programme's development be written initially. A 5-year projected plan as well as incremental annual plans are important. The plan will delineate the goals and assumptions as well as the strategies and remedies for achieving the goals. The process for the plan should include:

(1) Visiting the organization's various sites or plants.

(2) Studying the organization's existing systems to learn the potential interface with EAPs. For example, this will include the personnel system, procedures for performance management appraisal, the equal employment opportunity office, the health facilities as well as the disciplinary procedures.

(3) A demographic study of the employee population should also be conducted to include sex and level in organization.

(4) Interviews with the company's key personnel for input.

Development of a policy statement

One of the early concerns of any programme's formulation is the development of a written policy statement. It is most beneficial to complete the policy after the EAP has been operating for a period of time. This will ensure a full understanding of the organization and how each system in the organization will affect the EAP. Persons of critical importance to the programme must be involved in the policy's design. This should include unions (where they exist). The policy must state:

(1) The purpose and authority of the policy, which includes the organization's recognition that employees who demonstrate problems with work performance may potentially be suffering from an alcohol, drug abuse or mental health problem as well as their recognition that

these problems are treatable. This policy should also include any organizational mandates for such a programme.

(2) The eligibility of employees for the programme's services.

(3) The integration of the programme into the overall management system of the organization.

(4) The roles and responsibilities of the various personnel in the organization.

(5) A delineation of the procedures for the programme's use.

(6) The record-keeping procedures which must stress confidentiality.

(7) The criteria for professionally staffing the programme.

(8) The importance of and procedures for supervisory training.

(9) Provisions for an evaluation of the programme.

(10) That an employee's participation in the EAP will not jeopardize his/her future opportunities.

It is imperative that the policy be signed by the industry's top management and where appropriate, should be signed jointly with the unions.

Staffing

When deciding about staff, it is important to consider a balance between administrative staff and counselling staff. It would be a serious mistake to place heavy emphasis on the counselling aspect of the programme. In the developmental stages of a programme, a disproportionate amount of staff time will be spent on administrative and coordinating functions such as policy development, training, employee education etc. When considering staff for these functions, a professional with strong administrative skills, who has an understanding of business and systems analysis, would be most appropriate. Counsellors must have demonstrated ability to work in an industrial arena and to advise/assist supervisors, managers and unions. They must possess excellent counselling and assessment skills, particularly in alcoholism, and must have a thorough knowledge of the treatment resources in the community. All staff must exhibit professionalism or the respect of the organization will be lost.

Establish a confidential record-keeping system

Every EAP must develop procedures for compiling records. All individual case files must be confidential and must be located in a manner that ensures maximum security. All files should be locked and as much as possible should not identify the employee or make reference to names and diagnostic information. Only the minimal amount of data should be maintained for a counsellor to work with an employee. Procedures for accessing the files should be made perfectly clear. Only EAP staff should ever have access to the employee files. Reports and statistical information should never contain identifying information on employees. Finally, procedures must be established for destroying closed files.

Supervisory/union training

Supervisors, managers and union stewards (where appropriate) are the personnel in any organization vested with the responsibility of identifying and documenting deteriorating job performance, confronting the staff member and making referrals to the EAP. Consequently, they must be properly trained to do so. The objectives of the training should be to define the EAP and its philosophy, to define the EAP's target population in terms of work performance, absenteeism etc. and the related symptoms, to demonstrate that the EAP provides an alternative to the previous mishandling of employees with personal problems, and to provide the guidelines for supervisory/union action and use of the EAP (see reference 8, pp. 209–10). Training should be designed to discourage the tendency of managers to act as diagnosticians and counsellors, which is not their area of expertise. They must be made aware of focussing on obvious job performance and work-related problems. The regulations and policies on confidentiality and their reasons must also be explained (see reference 8, p. 209).

Location of EAP

The location of the EAP must be considered at two levels: (1) its location organizationally and (2) its location physically. Organizationally, it is vital that the EAP be located under the personnel functions. This follows from the basic premise that EAPs are based on job performance, which is clearly the concern of personnel. Some companies place their programmes in the medical units. In most instances, however, the medical units are still encompassed under the company's personnel functions.

It is also critical to consider the physical location of the EAP. First of all, every employee should have access to it. This will mean making provisions for handicapped personnel. Secondly, the programme should be located in such a manner that confidentiality is maximized. In other words, it should be placed inconspicuously so that employees will not be identified as going to the EAP.

Employee education and outreach strategies

It is equally important to educate and reach the employees of a company, because 'supervisory referral is not the only avenue of case finding. Promotion of self-referrals and other referral sources can be aided by a well-planned use of employee health education' (see reference 8, p. 210). In addition, outreach and education keep the EAP highly visible.

No one brochure, pamphlet, etc. is equally effective in an organization. An

EAP must explore a variety of strategies such as posters, news releases, home mailouts etc. and discern which methods are effective with which group of employees. Presentations, alcohol awareness weeks etc. are also useful in educating the employee population. The objectives of educational strategies are to introduce the EAP, familiarize employees with the EAP staff and the programme's procedures and, finally, to raise their consciousness about the emotional problems which may be affecting them.

Develop a referral network

It is critical that any EAP develops a network of community treatment resources to use in referring employees. It is the responsibility of the EAP staff to evaluate the available agencies on their quality and adequacy of services. When evaluating a treatment facility, consideration must be given to their location, their fees and their agency philosophy. The EAP should establish a liaison with the key staff at each agency to ensure smooth coordination of referrals and to coordinate follow-up activities.

Programme evaluation

EAPs should be set up initially to include specific evaluation plans. Any EAP must be evaluated for its cost-effectiveness and efficiency. Evaluation and dissemination of the results are critical for the survival of the programme. Case records and office records should be designed to facilitate data retrieval. Evaluation instruments must be developed and implemented as the programme begins. The evaluation should gather data in relation to work performance and should contain control groups.

A number of cost-effective studies have been done which bear out the financial savings in these programmes.

One of the most widely publicized studies is the Kennecott Copper evaluation of its "INSIGHT" programme. Their programme dates back to the 1950s, but it was not until 1973 that a randomly selected sample of 150 men who had used the programme was evaluated on a before and after basis. The study calculated their absenteeism rates, weekly indemnity costs; and hospital, medical and surgical costs over a 6-month period before their involvement with the programme and compared this with a 6-month period immediately following their programme involvement. After an average of 12.7 months in the programme, the 150 men had improved their attendance by 52%, decreased their weekly indemnity costs by 74.6% and decreased their hospital, medical and surgical costs by 55.4%[14].

Another interesting study published in 1981 by Comp-Care Corporation reported on their summary of 68 separate corporate and government programmes. The study found that the employees that used the programmes had reduced their absenteeism rates, reduced their utilization of hospital, medical and surgical services, and there was a significant improvement in their production rates. In addition, all of the companies involved in the study reported lower insurance premiums since establishing the counselling programmes.

Several other studies have reported similar results. General Motors reported a return of $5 for every dollar invested in their programme. They have had over 10 000 employees go through their programme and the study found that they were saving $3700 a year for each employee or a total saving of $37 million a year[15]. Northrup Corporation reported a saving of $19 800 a year saved on each of the employees that went through their programme. United Airlines has recently reported a return of $16.95 for every dollar invested in their programme[16]. Other programmes at Kelsey-Hayes, Dupont, IBM, EXXON and Bell Telephone have documented and reported similar positive results. In the public sector the HHS Region III ECS programme has documented a $13.32 return for each dollar invested in their programme during 1981[17]. The US Postal Service and the US Navy have also reported a high cost-benefits ratio for their programmes.

The Department of Health and Human Services evaluation plan will study six personnel items including absenteeism and sick leave as well as health insurance claims. This will be measured against a control group matched to job level in the workplace and sex.

CONCLUSION

In conclusion, it is becoming increasingly evident that a partnership between business and alcoholism can be most fruitful. Not only can money be saved but more important, alcohol abusers as well as alcoholics can be reached before they lose their positions.

References

1 Masi, D. (1981). *Human Services in Industry*, p. 70. (Lexington: Lexington Books)
2 Roman, Paul (1976). The promise and problems of employee alcoholism and assistance programs in higher education. Presented at *University of Missouri, Conference on Employee Assistance Programs*, Columbia, p. 2
3 *Prevalence Study of Alcoholism in Industry.* (1968). (New York: National Council on Alcoholism)
4 *Fourth Special Report to the U.S. Congress on Alcohol and Health.* U.S. Department of Health and Human Services, NIAAA. Publications No. (ADM) 81–1080. (Washington, D.C.: U.S. Government Printing Office)
5 Gibbons, R. et. al. (1975). *Research Advances in Alcohol and Drug Problems.* Vol. 2. (New York: Wiley)
6 Rosen, B. et. al. (1973). Identifying emotional disturbance in persons seen in industrial dispensaries. In Noland, R. (ed.) *Industrial Mental Health and Employee Counseling*, p. 57. (New York: Behavioral Publications)
7 *Costs to Society of Alcohol Abuse, Drug Abuse and Mental Illness.* (1981). Report by the Research Triangle Institute for the U.S. Department of Health and Human Services (Alcohol, Drug Abuse and Mental Health Administration), Rockville, Maryland
8 Presnall, L., (1981). *Occupational Counseling and Referral Systems.* (Salt Lake City: Alcoholism Foundation)

9 *Survey on Industrial Action Regarding Alcoholism.* (1964). (New York: National Council on Alcoholism)

10 Public Law 91–616 (42 U.S.C. 4582) *Comprehensive Alcohol Abuse and Alcoholism Prevention, Treatment, and Rehabilitation Act of 1970,* 31 December 1970

11 Trice, H. M. and Roman, Paul (1978). *Spirits and Demons at Work: Alcohol and Other Drugs on the Job.* 2nd Edn pp. 152–168. (Ithaca, NY: Cornell University)

12 Opening Remarks by Thomas Delaney, Executive Director, Association of Labor-Management Administrators and Consultants on Alcoholism (ALMACA), *10th Annual ALMACA Conference,* November, 1981, San Diego, CA

13 Roman, P. (1981). Executive Caravan Survey Results. In *Labor-Management Alcoholism Journal,* November–December. (New York: National Council on Alcoholism)

14 Schramm, C. J. (ed.) (1977). *Alcoholism and Its Treatment in Industry,* p. 80 (Baltimore: Johns Hopkins University Press)

15 Lanier, D. (1981). Presentation at *Department of Agriculture, Association of Labor-Management Administrators and Consultants on Alcoholism (ALMACA),* Spring, 1981

16 *Alcoholism.* **1,** (4), 46 (March–April 1981)

17 Sullivan, D. W. (1981). Department of Health and Human Services, Region III, Employee Counseling Services Annual Report. (Unpublished document, Philadelphia, PA)

40

A contemporary view of employee assistance

W. MALONEY

We know that alcoholism has plagued employers since the dawning of the industrial revolution. It's even a safe bet that addiction frustrated the general contractor who put up the Parthenon. Over the centuries, employers have watched helplessly as skilled and valued employees gradually degenerated until termination was unavoidable. There was no remedy. Threats, discipline, promises were all useless.

In the USA, the response by industry ranged from vigorous witch hunts to blatant denial. At one extreme were the nation's railroads, who decreed that any employee seen entering a saloon was subject to immediate discharge. But then there were other employers who provided beer breaks, a practice that still exists in some breweries.

Of course, industry wasn't alone in being baffled by alcoholism. Clergy, the health care system and educators were all impotent in the face of this disease.

Eventually industry did begin to find answers, and in this paper we will touch briefly on the history of these efforts. We will then examine a contemporary model that is in ascendancy. This is a model that has been employed by Hazelden for several years, so we can next give you the results of our evaluations. Finally, we will give you some of the 'how to' as seen by Hazelden.

THUMBNAIL HISTORY

Starting now with a bit of history, it was only when alcoholics banded together to help themselves that any signs of hope emerged. Alcoholics Anonymous became a wellspring of miracles that transformed alcoholics into productive members of society. This new phenomenon was noted by enlightened members of American industry. Here and there, employers established AA-related alcoholism programmes. But by 1970 the employer with a programme was still very much the exception, and for a good reason: except in situations where the employer had limitless faith and gave continued strong support for many years, industrial alcoholism programmes just didn't yield dazzling results.

The need was there, and the practitioners were dedicated. But those who instituted programmes were disappointed when very few alcoholic employees knocked on the counsellor's door; we know now, of course, that such volunteerism would be quite inconsistent with the nature of this disease. Persistent employers tried a predictable management solution. They demanded diagnosis by the supervisor, who then had to force employees to see the counsellor.

Alcoholism stigma being what it is, the supervisor doesn't look upon this as diagnosis – but as prosecution. He is the accuser, and the employee is the alleged perpetrator. We shouldn't be surprised that there is a low level of supervisory participation! Supervisors, like family members, will tend to hide the problem, thus enabling progression of the disease.

What we are seeing, of course, are manifestations of our old friend *denial* – denial by the employee and denial by his or her supervisor. The industrial alcoholism programme is structured to combat denial head-on, to work harder and harder to shake the alcoholic out of the woodwork. This approach can be successful, but most employers just aren't willing to allocate the resources that it takes for such an all-out war.

Then, in the 1970s, we saw the emergence of comprehensive *employee assistance programming*. We know that we risk being labelled as evangelists, but many of us who have grown with employee assistance see it equal in significance to the emergence of alcoholism treatment in the fifties and sixties.

The literature distribution branch of Hazelden gives us indicators of the employee assistance explosion. We provide a series of pamphlets that seemingly have no application, other than as supplementary material for comprehensive employee assistance programmes; they certainly would not fit into traditional industrial alcoholism programmes. Our sales of these pamphlets exceeded 400 000 copies over the last 4 years. We also provide a handbook for employee assistance programme managers; 30 000 of these have been purchased. These data reflect the escalating growth of employee assistance in the USA.

THE EMPLOYEE ASSISTANCE MODEL

Why has it caught on? Because it meets industry's bottom line standard: it works. And employee assistance programming succeeds because it does an end-run around denial.

These comprehensive efforts are not called 'alcoholism programs'; and if they do employ alcoholism counsellors, that is not their job title. The programmes are not set forth as an answer to alcoholism. Rather, in all respects, the programme is designed and promoted as a vehicle for helping employees and dependents with *any personal problems*. There are bountiful side-effects from this approach that I will touch upon; but for now, let's look at the effects on addicted people in the work force.

First, we see voluntary referrals. Now there are employees knocking on the counsellor's door. After all, it's not all that shameful to ask for help with financial problems, or for marriage counselling, or to get the name of a good attorney.

Most alcoholics encounter personal problems. These problems may be legal, marital or emotional. Most alcoholics do not associate these problems with their alcohol use. Therefore, they will seek help for these problems so long as the focus is on their 'problem' and not on their alcoholism.

This is the key to how comprehensive employee assistance programmes bring help to more alcoholics than do the alcoholism specific programmes. Consistently, there is a large variance between the number of employees who present alcoholism as their problem and the number who are actually diagnosed alcoholic.

For example, Mr K. is a stockbroker in a midwestern US city who was finding it impossible to cope with his depression, a sick child and a complaining wife. As a last ditch alternative to suicide, he called our employee assistance counsellor. He told the counsellor he didn't know how to unwind, that he wondered whether he could ever do his job well again, and that he was depressed about family income.

After a half-hour phone interview the telephone counsellor acted quickly to initiate crisis counselling and further assessment. Three diagnostic interviews involving both Mr K. and his wife resulted in a decision that radically changed Mr K.'s life. He decided that his other problems could be resolved if he did something about his drinking first.

Mr K. completed a treatment programme and returned to work with the full support of his manager. He reports that his life has become progressively better, particularly his ability to do his job. He never knew his problem was alcohol, but with the help of his family and the counsellors he now has begun the process of recovery from alcoholism.

Mr K. is a typical example of the way comprehensive programmes facilitate self-referral by alcoholic employees. The frosting on this cake is that this self-referral can and often does occur at a relatively early stage in progression. Our case files include many employees who had to ask for time off for treatment, where existence of the disease came as a complete surprise to the supervisor.

Speaking of supervisors, let's look at their role in the comprehensive employee assistance programme. No longer are they diagnosticians – indeed, in our supervisory training programmes we emphasize that diagnosis is a highly *improper* role for them. Their contribution is in the area where they are proficient and feel comfortable – that is, in the evaluation of job performance. When they see performance falling off and there is no apparent job-related reason, they can conclude that there may be some personal problem – *some unspecified personal problem* – underlying the behavioural change. They then refer the employee to the personal problems counsellor. How much easier than saying, 'I think you're a drunk and I want you to see the alcoholism counsellor'.

I noted earlier that there are spin-off benefits. The alcoholic does not have a monopoly on the world's problems. There are a host of non-alcohol-related syndromes that undercut serenity and productivity on the job. In our experience, with well trained counsellors about 40 % of the case load will be chemicals-related. It's not difficult to justify the cost of the programme on the basis of the recoveries that generate from this 40 %. But the other 60 % are getting help, too. These are employees who are hurting, and who are not leaving their problems in the parking lot when they come to work. Research by US governmental agencies, by Hazelden and by other private organiz-ations indicates that at least 10 % of the work force are functioning at depressed levels of productivity due to interference from personal problems. These problems include financial hardship, depression, sexuality difficulties, probate entanglements − the entire spectrum of human travail. The skilled employee assistance counsellor helps all these people *find the resource in the community that offers the right help at the best price*. Note that the employee assistance counsellor does not provide direct assistance to the client. The counsellor's role, after helping the client define the problem, is to achieve referral to the least expensive appropriate resource.

EARLY EVALUATION FINDINGS

Hazelden is currently providing employee assistance counselling for em-ployers with a total employee population in excess of 25 000. Representative data from some of these programmes will illustrate the benefits that we consistently see in employee assistance programmes.

Our approach is to maximize self-referral. We want the benefits of earlier intervention, and we want to make the supervisor's job easier. With effective communications and counsellor behaviour that builds trust, self-referral can be accomplished, as shown in Table 40.1.

The 'self-referral' percentages need clarification in later research. They include some undefined proportion of *informal* management referrals. The 7−9 % 'supervisory referrals' are those instances where the superior was very directive.

Table 40.1   Sources of Hazelden employee assistance caseload (1981)

Organization	Number of employees	Utilization rate (%)	Supervisory referral (%)	Self-referral (%)
County government	6500	4.9	7	93
Utility	5329	6.1	7	93
Brokerage Co.	868	9.1	9	91

Now let's check on the benefits of self-referral. We followed through on a random sample of 109 cases from the county government unit included in Table 40.1. The follow-through is shown in Table 40.2.

Table 40.2 Job changes within 4 months after programme contact

Referral type	Transferred	Promoted	Terminated	No change	Total Number
Self	6	4	5 (5%)	85	100
Supervisor	1	0	5 (56%)	3	9

We have to cross-validate these findings with a larger sample, but the degree of the difference here is extreme. These data suggest that self-referral facilitates problem identification and resolution before work performance has degenerated to a level demanding disciplinary action.

To us, one major justification for employee assistance is facilitation of alcoholism identification. We maintain that alcoholics will come to the counsellors for help with less threatening problems, without admitting or even knowing that the underlying difficulty is related to chemicals. Our position was supported by an analysis of the problems brought to us by one sample of 325 clients from a single employer (Table 40.3).

Table 40.3 Before and after: presented vs. assessed problems

Problem type	Presented by client	Assessed by counsellor	Assessed/ presented
Financial/legal	54	52	0.96
Occupational/educational	73	70	0.96
Family	125	138	1.10
Health	20	23	1.15
Personal/emotional	101	123	1.21
Alcohol/drug	62	134	2.16

We see other advantages to employee assistance programming that, so far at least, are supported by our evaluation.

(1) Family members are urged to utilize employee assistance, on the assumption that a personal problem anywhere in the household will affect an employee's productivity. It is easy for family members to access the service, and they do. For instance, we looked at 204 clients who came to us in one 6-month period from one of the companies we serve. Twenty-one per cent of the 204 cases were other family members. This is representative of most of our contracts.

(2)   Most recovering alcoholics have other life problems to resolve; leaving them unsolved indefinitely is not healthy *vis-à-vis* continued recovery. Employee assistance counsellors are trained to identify all client problems and, over time, to guide the person to help for all problems. Looking at the 1981 Hazelden caseload, clients assessed as alcoholic had 3.2 problems each, on the average. Other clients averaged 2.2 problems.

(3)   Usually it is difficult to obtain access to personnel files and to management staff in order to measure cost effectiveness of employee assistance programmes. In one instance, though, we had full co-operation. We evaluated pre- and post-data for a sample of 109 clients from an organization with 6000 employees. In this sample, absenteeism dropped 75% during the 4 months after first contact with the programme.

(4)   Of course there is another way to measure cost effectiveness. In one of our more mature programmes for several thousand employees, our charges to the employer work out to $176 per client seen. If we choose to allocate all programme costs to the caseload where alcoholism was the assessed problem, we are still at a figure of only $409 per case. That's almost infinitesmal, given the costs that are incurred by addicted employees.

HAZELDEN APPLICATION OF THE MODEL

Hazelden has always worked closely with employers. We have known for a long time that employers' programmes have unique virtues. Looking at admissions to treatment at Hazelden, referrals from industry are 1.8 years younger, and have been in serious collateral difficulty 2.1 years less, than the total admitted patient population. We have known for some time that employer programmes are achieving earlier intervention.

With this favourable inclination, we moved into the employee assistance field ourselves in 1975, establishing hundreds of programmes in our home state of Minnesota. In 1978 a major petroleum company asked us to establish a national programme for their employees. After designing a model that would meet the demands of their dispersed population, we accepted their invitation. We are now in the third year of a successful programme for them, and in 1981 we began adding other national employers to the service. As of this writing (1982), our counselling service is available to 25 000 employees and their families in 600 communities scattered across 32 of the 50 states.

The model we developed gives the employer reasonable assurance of consistency across the organization, even though there might be staff in several parts of the country. All employees are encouraged to call our Minnesota counselling staff on a toll-free number, any time day or night. We use the telephone to introduce them to the service, and for crisis intervention. Then, our counsellors arrange for the caller to meet with a local agency who is contracted to us. In-person counselling is taken over by that agency.

Our model is dependent, of course, on the local agencies' dedication and proficiency. We select agencies with experience in referral counselling, since that is the thrust of employee assistance. They must have staff with proven capability to identify the presence of addiction. The agency must be willing to use the diagnostic tools we have developed, and must be willing to conform to the requirements of our information system. This is a computerized information system that provides measures of agency effectiveness, and also facilitates Hazelden monitoring of agency case handling.

Entering 1982 we had 33 agencies under contract to Hazelden. New agencies are added most months, as new contracts require the addition of agencies in new locations.

Some of these agencies are already providing employee assistance in their local communities. Others are mental health clinics or social agencies of various types who want to become employee assistance providers. As they are serving Hazelden they are using our technology and training to facilitate their entry to this expanding health care delivery function.

The Hazelden model of employee assistance relies heavily on approval from management and employees. Beginning at the upper levels of the organization, Hazelden briefs executives on the topics that are to be covered in supervisory training and employee orientation. Without executive commitment, the best designed employee assistance programme will have minimal success. Executives must provide support and encouragement to obtain the support of those under them.

Training is then provided to supervisors. They have the most difficult role in the programme while at the same time playing the most important role. Because supervisors themselves are supervised, they have conflicting roles that may inhibit their enthusiasm for the employee assistance programme. They are provided with the necessary understanding and skills that will help them work through these situations.

As I noted earlier, our definition of the employee assistance model does not include total dependence on supervisory referrals. This does not mean that we exclude this means of access; we're only saying that self referrals are advantageous and possible within the employee assistance model. Supervisory referral is still essential in many cases. In this model, though, the referral is usually less stressful for supervisor and employee, since the referral is related only to job performance − not to addiction.

Supervisors are therefore trained to document job performance. Then, supervisors are oriented to the broad scope of human difficulties which affect employee performance − including marital and family problems, emotional and mental health problems, financial and legal problems, alcohol and drug problems and physical health problems. Supervisors are also trained to meet the requirements of confidentiality and privacy.

Group employee orientations are often conducted, though in dispersed organizations written communications have to suffice. In either case the objectives are to describe the scope of the problems for which assistance is available, to describe programme policies and procedures, to stress the confidentiality of the programme, to examine attitudes about reaching out for help, and to explain to employees how they may access the programme.

These front-end communications are followed by quarterly mailings to employees' homes. Because these mailings are addressed to the home, families are kept informed of the availability of assistance. Hazelden has developed an extensive series of pamphlets that are used for these mailings.

Typically the counsellors will be voluntarily contacted by troubled employees, shortly after the front-end orientation. Job performance based referrals can also come in early, but may be slow until management develops trust in the programme staff. Family members and fellow workers are also sources of referral. Labour unions, the judicial system and health care practitioners are also referral sources as they learn about the programme.

Employees who realize the need for help and take action on a voluntary basis are provided direct and confidential services. The employee or the family member receives immediate problem assessment. Counsellors welcome referrals from all appropriate sources. Clients who call on the telephone are encouraged to make in-person appointments as soon as possible. Walk-in clients are assisted immediately or by scheduled appointments.

Because our programmes are nation-wide, we are serving employees in isolated locations, nowhere near any agency that could provide in-person counselling. Our counsellors are, therefore, trained to perform referral service over the telephone. It's not the preferred way, of course, but it is surprisingly successful and it's the only answer for people in remote rural locations.

The basic purpose of the assessment process is to identify the primary problem as well as any related problems underlying job performance deficits and client concerns. Experience indicates that there is often a discrepancy between the presented problems and the problems later identified by the counsellor through the assessment process. The desired outcome from assessment is to achieve agreement between the client and the counsellor as to the actual primary problem or problems requiring further assistance.

Problem evaluation and intervention usually involve several stages with the counsellor utilizing a variety of skills. These levels of involvement with the client include the following: (1) developing rapport, (2) structured interviewing, (3) collateral interviews, (4) intervention steps and (5) assessment recommendations.

After listening to the client's statements about the reasons for referral, the counsellor will gather information about the client's functioning in all major life areas. This attention to the whole person helps to identify possible problem areas not immediately offered by the client. It also helps to place the client's functioning in perspective by identifying areas of strength as well as liabilities. A thorough assessment facilitates identification of the primary problem as well as the ability to prioritize other problems requiring action.

Finally, after the assessment process has been completed, the counsellor makes recommendations to the client and/or family regarding a preliminary diagnosis of primary and relevant secondary problems. The counsellor's assessment is based on many factors including the number of life areas disrupted, the client's feelings, the availability of support systems, the client's history of involvement with helping systems and the client's willingness to act for change.

The next step is referral to a community resource. At this point the counsellor explains that additional assistance must be at the employee's expense; only the initial assessment and the referral recommendations are covered under the employee assistance programme. However, the counsellor knows the employer's benefit package, and will inform the client of possible health insurance or health benefit plans that may be utilized to cover the follow-on work.

After the client has accepted the referral, the counsellor will monitor the client's progress and co-operation with the recommended treatment resource. Careful documentation of the case is important. The counsellor, by staying in touch with the community resource, will be able to ascertain whether the referral was appropriate. The counsellor will also be able to confirm the client's attendance at the recommended treatment programme.

The Hazelden model also provides for a complete and detailed report to management concerning the utilization of the programme. We accomplish this through our computerized information system.

Another element of Hazelden employee assistance is our evaluation of the quality of our service. As one measure, employee surveys are conducted to measure awareness of the programme and attitudes toward its value.

But the truly unique elements of the Hazelden model are the toll-free national telephone line and the network of local agencies. These two strategies have been developed to enable employers with multiple locations to deliver consistent, high quality employee assistance care to their entire population.

So this is how we look at employee assistance. We forecast continued growth, noting that we are renewing all of our old contracts and steadily adding new programmes, despite the current recession. We conclude that the employer is seeing economic benefit. Adding that to the enhanced recovery of addicted people and the resolution of other difficulties for employees and family members, we are inclined to call employee assistance the 'Everybody Wins' programme.

41

Alcohol problems at the work-place in the Federal Republic of Germany

H. ZIEGLER

INTRODUCTION

Since 1978 the alcohol problem at the place of work is being increasingly discussed in the FRG. The problem is more and more recognized as a management task, and is thus regarded as a subject of equal importance amongst a series of other problems. Apart from those firms which are directly engaged with solving the problems with alcohol-addicted employees, the head organizations of employers' associations and of employees' associations are now dealing with this problem.

THE EMPLOYEES' ATTITUDE TOWARDS ALCOHOLIC BEVERAGES

Society and its attitude towards alcoholic beverages is reflected in business life. In general, alcoholic beverages are regarded as 'drinks of choice' with high symbolic values. With an alcoholic drink, contact-making is easier (e.g. at a 'warming-up' party given by a new staff member), it loosens the atmosphere and brings about a feeling of 'fellowship' (e.g. at a company's party given for the staff).

Within a firm the drinking pattern, the drinking occasions and the drinking standards differ from one department to another. The attitude towards alcohol also varies considerably in the different professional categories.

The kind of profession and the environment of work can restrain but also amplify the consumption of alcohol. The availability of alcoholic beverages at the place of work, the tolerated or the actually practised consumption of alcohol during working hours, and the extent to which it is invited, are factors of an amplifying or restraining effect.

THE COLLEAGUES' ATTITUDE TOWARDS AN ALCOHOLIC AMONG THEM

In spite of the rather positive opinion of alcoholic beverages, the opinion about alcohol-addicted colleagues is rather negative. The alcoholic is always regarded as a burden and he is seen in a very negative light when, on account of his illness, he can no longer control his drinking capacity and when his consumption of alcohol constantly oversteps the drinking standard of his group of fellow workers. For this reason the alcoholics will try to hide their illness from their colleagues as long as possible, and for some considerable time they believe they are 'normal drinkers' although in actual fact they are already alcohol-addicted. They are constantly admonished by their colleagues, their friends, their family. Quite often they try to live up to the urge to do better, try to control the alcohol consumption. Yet they cannot solve this problem on their own.

The complexity of relations and the different possibilities of attitudes towards each other, are shown in Figure 41.1.

WHO IS AN ALCOHOLIC?

Again and again the question arises at the workplace as to who among the employees should be classified as alcoholic in need of treatment. First of all, it has to be realized that each alcoholic has once started as a normal consumer. The transitions from use to abuse and to addiction are fluent. This means that the alcoholic often only recognizes after a long time that he has become addicted. Clear lines between these phases cannot be drawn. Missing such a marking point leads thus to uncertainty and to special questions. Experience has shown, however, that often it is not so important to set such marking points but that such definitions are only wanted to take action against an

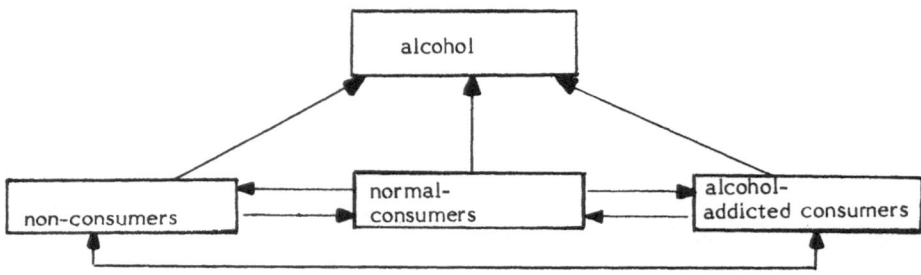

Figure 41.1 Alcohol and consumer groups: the relations and attitudes are predominantly emotionally based

employee with more supporting certainty. The definitions 'abuse' of alcohol and 'endangered' by alcohol often mar the view and result in an omission of help[1]. Valid criteria for the working field are therefore:

(1) if alcohol creates problems, then alcohol is the problem
(2) whoever does himself psychical, physical and social harm through alcohol, is an alcoholic.

EVALUATION OF THE INDIVIDUAL SYMPTOMS OF ALCOHOL ADDICTION

A standard question to an alcoholic is what quantity he drinks. Here it is essential to be aware that problematic drinking conduct will always be played down, be minimized. The alcoholic will always name very much smaller quantities in order to remain inconspicuous. The named quantity, however, is often accepted as the true quantity, that is, one fails to ascertain or to put the right questions. Already in the initial phase of alcoholism social strains are experienced in the family, in the work team and in the circle of friends.

In this phase, however, the burdens and strains will still be shouldered and shared by his social ambient field because he is still regarded as a likeable, nice person. A typical characteristic of alcoholism is the 'conspicuous inconspicuousness'[2]. This means that to a great extent alcoholics adapt themselves to their social environment and that they try to hide their addiction as long as possible before their colleagues and superiors. The alcoholic is usually swathed in the odour of peppermint or mouthwash, trying to overlay the smell of alcohol. He takes great care in his outer appearance (and also his wife will ensure that he goes to work cleanly dressed) – all for not becoming conspicuous. The many days of absence are carefully spread over the week.

A most important characteristic of addiction is trying the do-it-yourself treatment: intermittent phases of abstaining. The alcoholic stays off alcoholic drinks for these periods in order to prove to himself and to others that he is still and at any time able to drink in a controlled manner. Erroneously such attempts at self-treatment are mostly taken as a symptom of improvement, but they are in fact a very significant index for addiction, for alcoholism.

The initial, minor social problems at work and in the family now become increasingly more grave. Now come the first reprimands for drinking alcohol at the place of work. Now come the first differences and difficulties with the fellow workers who are exasperated by the many hours of absence. And finally come the first cracks in the comradeship of the fellow workers because the attempts to help and save have failed.

WEAK POINTS IN DEALING WITH ALCOHOLICS

Appropriate and early help for the alcoholic is hindered by emotionally determined attitudes, by strong emotions towards the alcoholic. Whenever an attempt is made to solve the alcohol problem, the attempt is made on a rational basis. This procedure does not always lead to success as the emotional barriers were not removed. Many negative sorts of reactions in connection with the alcoholic employee, can, however, only be clarified on an emotional basis (see Figure 41.1). A very grave problem in dealing with an alcoholic fellow worker is the tendency to minimize, which happens at all levels of the firm's structure. When remarks are made such as, 'in any case, he is still doing his work', or 'as long as he doesn't drink, he is one of the best' or 'even drunk, he hands in better reports than Mr X does sober', and the like, then it is quite certain that there is an alcohol problem among the employees. Out of fear that when the alcohol problem becomes officially known, the management has no alternative but to dismiss the person concerned, out of this fear the problem will be kept secret until the problems with the alcoholic become greater than the anxiety over the resulting consequences.

So far, the employing firm has responded to alcoholism among their staff by resorting to disciplinary measures, hoping that these disciplinary actions will bring improvement in the alcoholic's conduct.

Usually an escalating series of disciplinary measures is employed, going from verbal reprimands and severe warnings to cuts in wages, transfer to another department (or lesser qualified work), up to instant dismissal. The reprimands often contain the demand that the alcoholic must change his attitude towards alcohol and change his drinking habits. Such a demand, however, is a very high imposition for the alcoholic, as a change in attitude and behaviour can only be learned during the course of lengthy therapy. The demand made in such a reprimand cannot be obeyed, and consequently further steps will be taken. Depending on position and grade of qualification either the 'strong method' or the 'soft method' will be applied in dealing with the alcoholic employee[3].

With the 'strong method', the attempt is made by certain compulsory measures (sanctions) to bring the potential alcoholic back on the 'right track'. If this doesn't succeed, endeavours are made to get rid of him by the quickest means. Further actions mostly only serve the purpose of making a dismissal watertight in the legal sense.

When the 'soft method' is used, the attempt is made to give sympathetic help, to create for the alcoholic a 'trouble-free' area within the firm. When this procedure does not lead to the anticipated success, the trust and understanding often turn into severe disappointment which then results in a harder approach and finally the desire to dismiss this employee.

It is not infrequently the case that demand for dismissal was not voiced from a superior level but came from among the group of fellow workers who for years have tried to improve the situation. The wish to have someone dismissed is in most cases accompanied by negative stored-up emotions and the helplessness of the superior.

A particular problem, and one of great significance among the weak points in dealing with alcoholics, is that of the talks held with the sick person at different levels. If and when the initial restraint is overcome, a good contact with him can be established. The alcoholic sets the signal that he is at ease in this conversation, that he is being treated with understanding, and thus shows his superior that he appreciates him as an interlocutor. If, however, the superior accepts this hidden praise, he is — for the purpose of any further proceedings — 'disarmed'[2]. Such a conversation mostly ends with the promise that from now on, the man will change his conduct. Such promises cannot, as experience has shown, be kept. If he has a lapse, the alcoholic will try, with grave self-reproach and self-accusation, to 'disarm' his speaking partner again. Time and again the alcoholic is so successful that in such talks he is not the subject — the conversation turns around the boss, the wife, the colleagues. In this manner he diverts attention from himself and is in the clear. But the aim of such a talk must be to keep and demarcate the social distance in order that the superior keeps his freedom of action.

WORKPLACE AND MOTIVATION FOR THERAPY

Several studies have shown that the place of work has a high index for successful therapy and an alcohol-free life[4]. Being out of work is regarded by alcoholics as a far greater strain than, for instance, the missing of social ties after a divorce. By keeping an alcoholic on the payroll, a firm therefore has a good chance of motivating the person to undergo therapy. It can be presumed here, that an alcoholic will always try to evade the step of giving up — of his own free will — his 'problem-solver'. He will always find new ways and means to be nearby his 'stuff'. If through bad conduct, however, his job is in danger, indirect motivation for taking up therapy may show success. It is therefore of the utmost importance that in all talks the threat of possible severe disciplinary action should be accompanied by an offer of help. It is therefore of great significance to offer to the alcoholic understanding and help but at the same time to confront him with the realistic difficulties. In such way a positive-acting 'constructive pressure' may form[5], which curtails the development of the illness. In talks with his superior the alcoholic must therefore unmistakably be informed in what way his conduct gives reason for complaint, what consequent disciplinary measure may result, and which possibilities of help exist. The superior should furthermore outline quite clearly the full problem, as for a long time the alcoholic has only gone by intimations, assumptions, vague threatenings or indistinct promises.

ESTABLISHING A LINE OF ACTION REGARDING ALCOHOL-ADDICTED EMPLOYEES

Besides the tasks for the individual superiors, lines of action are important for the whole firm.

All members of staff who come in contact with the alcohol problems should first of all form a working group to clarify the following.

(1)   How great is the alcohol problem in the firm?

(2)   Which preventative and therapeutical measures can be offered personnel-wise?

(3)   How, and by which steps, is action to be taken in the individual case of an alcoholic fellow worker?

(4)   Which external possibilities of help exist (self-help groups, advisory and information offices, special therapeutical clinics)?

(5)   How could treated alcoholic be reintegrated in the firm?

(6)   What kind of structural measures could be taken (e.g. removing beer-machines, changing delivery contracts, arranging alcohol-free parties, prohibiting in general the consumption of alcoholic beverages at the workplace)?

(7)   Which public effective measures should be undertaken by the firm (e.g. informative actions, posters, leaflets, articles in the works news-paper, instruction of leading personnel)?

Such a working group can consist of members of the personnel department, of the social services, of the works medical department, of the workers' council, but also of 'ex-alcoholics'. The duties of the individual members should be laid down in written guidelines, and the individual steps for equal treatment of all alcohol-addicted employees should be fixed.

FURTHER MEASURES

The members of the working group have to establish contacts with the external self-help groups and advisory offices so that they themselves get a better know-how and can cut down their own reservations through mutual information. If an alcoholic member of staff undergoes treatment in a special therapeutical clinic, then this time and occasion should also be used for establishing contacts with such institutions. This may favourably influence the success of therapy, and in urgent cases may help in obtaining a therapy place. In addition, the full programme of possibilities of help should be made generally known in the firm, which may contribute to an early recognition and early treatment of so far undetected alcoholics. In many firms the experience has been that open information, about such programmes of help, encourages superiors as well as colleagues to start the first rather delicate talk. For making these programmes known as widely as possible, given informa-tion channels should be made use of. The working group should further give thought to the questions of how drinking occasions can be reduced or alternatively be held with non-alcoholic beverages, with soft drinks. Such discussions, especially, very often lead to an opinion forming about the 'alcohol problem' which is shared by all members equally. Within the range of discussion of the working group, the question of general prohibition of alcohol in the firm will most surely arise, unless prohibition is already in force. Prohibiting alcohol in general can be very helpful, especially when preventative measures are carried through. But it should not be regarded as the solving factor for the problems with alcohol-addicted employees. Very often the situation of an alcoholic will become worse if alcohol is officially forbidden. As an addict he is forced to drink, but each time he must drink he consequently at the same time violates the working rules.

CONCLUSION

Past experience with therapy concepts and preventative measures shows that effective measures for helping the alcoholic in the occupational sphere can be developed when the problems are regarded free of emotions and with a cool analysis of costs and gains. The series of escalating disciplinary measures against alcoholic employees, the hushing-up out of fear of a possible dismissal – these should belong to the past and should be substituted by adequate treatment projects and by preventative measures. The alcohol-sick employees should not only be regarded from the purely economic point of view but stronger consideration should be given to the social aspects which lie within the social welfare obligations of the employer. It is very often the case that when the appropriate therapeutical efforts have been made, an employer keeps an employee who has worked for him many a year, who knows his job and the firm, and who will – after coming through therapeutical treatment – serve the firm with his full working capacity without requiring any time for vocational adjustment. It is therefore a demand on all responsible in personnel management that measures for help and preventative considerations become an integrated part of modern personnel policy.

References

1 Gerchow, J. and Schrappe, O. (1980). *Alkoholismus – eine information für Ärzte* (Alcoholism – Information for Physicians). A DHS publication. (Cologne: Arzte Verlag)
2 Dörner, K. and Plog, U. (1978). *Irren ist menschlich oder Lehrbuch der Psychiatrie: Psychotherapie* (To err is Human, or a Text-book on Psychiatry/Psychotherapy). (Wunstorf: Psychiatrie-Verlag)
3 Aßfalg, J. (1980). Der konstruktive Druck, unveröffentlichtes Manuskript (The constructive pressure, an unpublished manuscript). DHS-Fachausschuß 'Alkohol und Beruf' (Alcohol and Profession)
4 John, U. (1979). Zum Stellenwert der Arbeit im Therapieerfolg bei Alkoholkranken (The index of work in the successful therapy of alcoholics). *Suchtgefahren*, **25**, 145
5 Ziegler, H. (1979). Therapieprogramme in den USA. (Therapy programmes in the USA.). In a DHS publication: *Suchterkrankung am Arbeits-platz* (Addiction at the place of work). (Hamm: Hoheneck-Verlag)

42
Employee alcoholism programmes in Ireland

M. QUINLAN

INTRODUCTION

Irish industry is now in the tenth year of its operation of employee alcoholism programmes.

The introduction of EAPs was brought about by a resolution passed by the Irish Congress of Trade Unions at their Annual Conference in 1972. The unions were concerned about the overall effects of alcoholism on their members and mentioned job-performance as one of the key areas for concern. As a result of this resolution a subcommittee was set up to examine the whole area of alcoholism in the workplace and to make recommendations.

FURTHER DEVELOPMENTS

The next major development took place in 1974.

In that year the Electricity Supply Board (E.S.B.), which is the national power company, introduced their first employee alcoholism programme. The E.S.B. had conducted a survey of restricted staff and one of the areas that they identified as a problem area was alcoholism. The company then appointed 16 Staff Services Officers to look after the welfare of their staff with particular reference to problems caused by alcoholism.

The development of the E.S.B's employee alcoholism programme was relatively slow but had the advantage of trade union and management backing.

In 1978 the Irish Congress of Trade Unions subcommittee released its findings. Its report concluded that there was a '200 % increase in the incidence of alcoholism in the past 5 years', that 'alcoholism is Ireland's predominant drug problem' and '95 % of alcoholics are at work'. The recommendations were not acted upon by any employer organization.

A NEW DECADE

It should be mentioned at this stage that 1980 was a very significant year in the development of employee alcoholism programmes.

In that year the Alcoholic Rehabilitation Centre (ARC) was set up from funds provided by the trade unions. This strong trade union sponsored initiative was funded by deductions from the pay-packets of trade union members. Its purpose is to set up a treatment centre in Dublin from the monies raised.

There was also an increased awareness of the levels of absenteeism in Irish industry. Absence rates of up to 25 % had been recorded in some industries and there was growing concern at the amount of money lost due to absenteeism.

In 1980 the Economic and Social Research Institute in its report on *Drinking in Ireland* indicated that Irish industry was losing at least £30 million annually due to the problems caused by alcoholism. In that same year the Federated Union of Employers in its report on absenteeism issued strong recommendations for procedures on alcoholism in industry.

The Confederation of Irish Industry conducted a study and released a *Newsletter* quoting some Irish companies as having found that alcoholism and alcohol-related problems had been responsible for 10−25 % of all absenteeism. The study proved to be very effective as a means of motivating Irish employers to develop employee alcoholism programmes.

This employer initiative was based on an urgent need to counter the growth of absenteeism which was quickly putting some Irish industries out of business.

By *1981* 32 Irish companies had developed procedures for assisting employees who develop alcoholism during the course of their employment. This number included many public bodies as well as private sector industries and the approach was as varied as the range of industries would indicate.

There is no doubt that the employee alcoholism programme run by the Electricity Supply Board is the most progressive. Not only was it the first programme to be introduced in Ireland but it has been constantly updated and now consists of:

(1) general education on the problem of alcoholism at induction of staff,
(2) intervention where considered necessary,
(3) aftercare programme which insists on membership of Alcoholics Anonymous.

CONCLUSION

The current position in Ireland is that there are many programmes working very effectively to assist the alcoholic.

The Employer Labour Conference has convened a Working Party on Alcoholism and the trade union sponsored Alcoholic Rehabilitation Centre now has 11 000 subscribers.

All these factors, no doubt, set the pace for the future development and growth of the employee alcoholism programme in Ireland.

43

Employee assistance programmes and the treatment network: building an effective relationship

J. C. CLARNO

Too frequently employee assistance programmes (EAPs) and alcoholism treatment programmes are discussed as separate and isolated activities. However, it is more appropriate to discuss these two aspects of the alcoholism network as a continuum in regard to occupational alcoholism and employee assistance programming. Most traditional EAPs are structured as so-called 'broad brush' models which encompass other behavioural/medical problems beyond alcoholism. Some EAPs also include legal and financial counselling. It is now likely that some EAPs will include pre-retirement and/or vocational guidance. But the wisdom of broadening EAP models too wide at the expense of the life-threatening and most prevalent problem, alcoholism, is questionable. An alcoholism focus is essential, as it is a serious and fatal illness. Employee assistance programmes should be considered as pre-treatment activity, unless the employee assistance programmes are specifically designed to provide direct in-house primary treatment. Certainly, most EAPs provide some counselling but in a conceptual sense the predominant EAP models are considered pre-treatment.

To foster EAPs and to build a good relationship between EAPs and treatment, two objectives must be met. First, how does the treatment network develop in response to the evolving EAP movement? Second, what are the expectations of both parties in the EAP–treatment relationship?

If a treatment network is to be developed to respond to EAP referrals it is necessary to undertake an active effort to heighten the awareness of the entire community toward alcoholism and its consequences. Most people agree that the problems of alcoholism comprise 50–70 % of the potential EAP referrals. Unless the community – the employers – admits the existence of the problem of alcoholism, little will be accomplished in dealing with it. This single fact is *very* important for encouraging the support of local alcoholism councils or community volunteer groups. Many resources exist that will spark community interest to develop a continuum or helping network for the illness of alcoholism. If this task is accomplished, the broader service network for the treatment of 'other problems' identified through an EAP will also naturally evolve. Some of the sources for achieving support to develop a treatment network include contacts within:

(1)   business and industrial leadership
(2)   pastoral or ministerial associations
(3)   medical, hospital, or community health groups
(4)   existing alcoholism treatment services, including local alcoholism councils
(5)   government
(6)   individuals and volunteers with a personal interest, including recovering persons, AA, Al-Anon members.

Employee Assistance Programming and treatment will develop from the combined activities of representatives from the above groups. The evolution of an area-wide or regional continuum of care can then result from the growth of both employee assistance and individual treatment programmes. But the development of this treatment continuum must be built on two principles, cost consciousness and quality. A delicate balance between these two factors will provide an optimum in patient care.

In regard to quality, time will not allow for a full discussion of all levels of care in alcoholism treatment (e.g. hospital based, outpatient), but some relatively simple criteria for the assessment of non-hospital, free-standing treatment programmes can be identified. But these criteria are also valid for other levels of care. They are as follows:

(1)   Is the treatment programme under medical management and how is it provided? The physician providing the medical management should have an in-depth knowledge and understanding of the disease process of alcoholism and other chemical dependencies.

(2)   Are all other members of the staff trained and knowledgeable in the disease concept of alcoholism and other dependencies?

(3)   Does the treatment programme maintain a relationship with other EAPs in the community and, if so, what is the quality of the relationship?

(4)   If the programme does not provide outpatient aftercare services, does the programme have a good working relationship with other community outpatient programmes?

(5)   Does the treatment programme philosophy incorporate the recovery principles of Alcoholics Anonymous? For example:

(a)   Is the non-alcoholic professional staff knowledgeable and accepting of the principles of Alcoholics Anonymous as a means of recovery?

(b)   Does the clinical staff include recovering alcoholic persons who are currently active in the fellowship of Alcoholics Anonymous?

(c)   Does the treatment programme provide scheduled educational sessions to include a presentation and discussion of the Alcoholics Anonymous Twelve Steps of recovery and its Traditions and philosophy?

(6)   Does the treatment programme provide for planned interviews with the family (when appropriate) and with the appropriate company representative?

(7)   Is the human dignity of the patient enhanced throughout the treatment environment?

(8)   Is there an informal, personal, and open communication with the patients indicating positive staff attitudes toward patient care?

(9)   Does the programme concentrate on the detoxification and rehabilitation of the employed alcoholic, chemically dependent person, or are admissions primarily chronic and indigent alcoholic patients?

(10) In those facilities where treatment programmes for illnesses or medical problems other than alcoholism and chemical dependencies are provided (e.g. mental illness, acute or chronic physical illnesses) are the components of the alcoholism programme effectively isolated from the other services?

(11) Does an evaluation system exist to measure treatment outcomes?

When this series of basic questions is answered, one must then ask if clinical evidence supports the responses. Some of the criteria may be met in full, but frequently some criteria are partially met. Ultimately the overall programme evaluation is usually a matter of assessment and judgement by the purchaser of the care. These criteria are not comprehensive enough to completely evaluate a programme, but are merely suggestions that an EAP specialist may wish to incorporate in a survey of treatment programmes.

An effective relationship is built on understanding mutual needs. A good relationship between an EAP and the treatment sector must be based on this principle and one of the key ingredients in this process is good communications. It is a fact that all patients do not require the same level of care for alcoholism. In building an effective relationship between the treatment sector and the EAP, it is essential to have a full understanding of the triage responsibilities regarding referrals. Prior to admission for treatment a careful triage of patients will eliminate needless time and effort. Once into treatment it is also natural to expect that additional patient assessment might indicate a need for an alternative level of care. Physical or emotional problems might be identified requiring a level of care which demands psychiatric or acute medical management. An EAP specialist may not have the ability to identify this need prior to the referral.

In regard to alcoholism and other chemical dependencies some of the considerations that will assist the EAP specialist in the triage process are as follows:

(1) How chronic is the illness?
(2) What is the history or pattern of recent excessive alcohol or drug use and the potential for withdrawal?
(3) What is the overall type and pattern of alcohol and drug usage?
(4) What social and familial supports exist?
      What is the chronology and degree of marital discord?
      Are there children living at home?
      What is the quality of employer support?
(5) Is there a history of medical or emotional problems, including suicidal threats or attempts?
(6) Is there a history of previous hospital admissions?
(7) What is the employee's level of motivation to accept help?
(8) Does the employee have a good potential for life style change?
(9) What is the degree of denial?
(10) What is the geographic location of residence?

An EAP specialist who has some clinical skills and experience can utilize the above criteria in making a more accurate referral judgement. It is important that the EAP−treatment relationship be built on developing the treatment to meet the patient's needs. Too frequently the reverse occurs.

Treatment programmes also need to know, as early as possible, the work history and job behaviours of the employee who is entering the treatment programme. Additionally, any acute medical problems that should be immediately known by the treating staff must be conveyed with proper releases. This is also true in the case of the job performance history. The treatment programme should also expect assistance from the EAP in getting the family involved in the treatment process when appropriate.

The company's interest in the employee's treatment can make a significant contribution to the treatment outcome. An 'employer interview' or meeting is arranged during the treatment experience to include the primary counsellor, the appropriate company representative and the employee. Sometimes it is appropriate to include a family member. These meetings are of course, coordinated with a prior understanding and agreement with the patient. Without a prior approval the trust relationship between all parties could be jeopardized. There are also the legal considerations if a proper release is not completed.

An effective EAP−treatment relationship also continues beyond the point of the employee's discharge from primary care. Again, with proper releases, ongoing communication between the EAP and treatment will provide the employee with support throughout the recovery process.

The EAP specialist should maintain close contact with the employee to monitor his or her commitment to the aftercare plan. Job performance is also measured to determine treatment outcome. Beyond job measures, many other factors can be used to determine successful outcomes. Some are determined by the aftercare staff and some by the EAP specialist, for example, physical health, emotional growth and family stability. The proper flow of this information, with consideration given to confidentiality, will also strengthen the EAP—treatment relationship.

CONCLUSION

An attempt has been made to describe the strengthening of the relationship between an EAP and the treatment sector. Though some of these constructive principles might appear to be somewhat simplistic, a tendency exists to complicate matters. It is essential to frequently return to basics if the employee assistance and alcoholism movement is to grow and survive.

44
Unemployment and alcohol abuse

K. FRUENSGAARD and T. ARNGRIM

It is well known that there is a significant association between alcohol abuse and occupational malfunction, sick leave and dismissal.

In particular with regard to alcoholics treated in public institutions (hospitals, treatment homes, alcohol clinics etc.), it has been found that there is a considerable predominance of clients belonging to the lower social strata or who have experienced social disaster including unemployment. This seems surprising as alcohol consumption – at least in Denmark – tends to be relatively high among the upper classes[1]. However, this inconsistency may be due to the better opportunity for concealment of abuse open to persons of high social status, and because treatment of the abuse frequently is more 'discreet' (access to private consultations, admission to somatic departments etc.).

These points can be illustrated by data from an investigation carried out in a Danish treatment home for alcoholics ('Ringgaarden'), where the principles of treatment are close to those of Broadway Lodge – that is to say, modified Alcoholics Anonymous principles[2, 3]. The material is composed of 347 ex-patients, approximately 85 % of whom came from the working class, almost all had experienced social collapse and only one sixth had not previously had one or another form for treatment of alcoholism. Of those available to the labour market only 15 % were employed at the time of admission. At the time of discharge, after on average a period of 3 months, this frequency had reached 37 % and at the follow-up investigation, 1–5 years later, this frequency was 56 %. A shift between the groups of those available and those not available to the labour market took place, but this only affected the mentioned percentages to a minor degree. A distinctly significant correlation was found between the pattern for alcohol consumption after discharge and the work situation.

467

A current investigation from the same treatment home[4] shows that at the time of admission only 4 % of those available to the labour market were employed. This trend towards a lower frequency of employed among those admitted may be a reflection of the general rise in unemployment in the period 1973–1977 to 1981.

In the following study the problem complex related to alcohol abuse and unemployment will be elucidated from a somewhat different angle, as the starting point is an investigation of unemployed patients who were admitted to a psychiatric emergency department[5]. Particular focus is placed on circumstances that appear to be pertinent in the stable re-establishment of the unemployed alcoholic in the labour market.

INVESTIGATION OF CONSECUTIVE GROUP OF UNEMPLOYED PERSONS ADMITTED TO PSYCHIATRIC EMERGENCY DEPARTMENT

The investigation covers a consecutively admitted group of unemployed persons who in the first 5 months of 1979 had to be admitted to the psychiatric department at Odense University Hospital. In all, 70 persons − 47 men and 23 women − were involved. There was a predominance of persons between the ages of 25 and 49 (two thirds), the great majority were single (four fifths), approximately two thirds were unskilled workers and up to half were not members of a trade union.

Habitual personality was assessed partly through a semistructured psychiatric interview, partly via Eysenck Personality Inventory. The majority of those who were not psychotic or borderline psychotic could be characterized as easily tired, sensitive and inhibited. On the slightest provocation they felt themselves criticized or belittled and in such situations had difficulty in expressing irritation or anger. Under the influence of alcohol, however, this inhibited behaviour often changed radically. Almost half of the persons involved had a constant or periodic alcohol abuse (average consumption seven or more drinks daily) and one quarter had an abuse of benzodiazepines. In fact only three were registered who, prior to actual unemployment period, had not required treatment for a psychiatric disorder and/or abuse problems.

A follow-up investigation was carried out both 6 months and 1 year after admission.

At the 1-year follow-up investigation, of the 70 persons seen 17 were assessed to be occupationally well situated, that is they had steady work or were judged to have a good chance of quickly resuming work again. In addition one person was judged to be well settled as a student.

The group of 18 persons just described (group I) was compared with the remaining persons who coped less successfully with regard to occupation (group II).

On the whole the persons in group I were found to be relatively 'strong' individuals because, in comparison to the persons in group II, they had a significantly lower frequency of earlier admissions to psychiatric departments, 22 % as against 69 %, ($p < 0.1$ %, χ^2-test) and sick leave prior to dismissal, 50 % vs. 76 %, ($p < 5$ %, χ^2-test). Further, in significantly fewer instances the actual unemployment period was > 3 months, 33 % as against 65 %, ($p < 2.5$ %, χ^2-test) and therefore was probably less stressful. In group I significantly more were admitted for more than 4 weeks, 56 % as against 24 %, ($p < 2.5$ %, χ^2-test). It can be assumed that on the part of both the patient and the therapist there was a relatively high degree of motivation for initiation of a more prolonged and relatively intensive treatment. Because of the pressure of work in a psychiatric emergency department, situations cannot be avoided in which the therapists are faced with the necessity of deciding how to use the scanty resources available most effectively.

CONNECTION BETWEEN THE COURSE ON THE VARIOUS LEVELS

The course on the occupational level was compared to the course on a number of other levels. It was found that a positive occupational course was significantly connected with a positive development in alcohol consumption (see below). This also applied to improvement in the general mental condition, 83 % as against 24 %, ($p < 0.5$ %, χ^2-test), and to improvement of relations with family, friends and acquaintances, 61 % as against 16 %, ($p < 0.05$ %, χ^2-test).

DEVELOPMENT WITH REGARD TO ALCOHOL CONSUMPTION

The average alcohol consumption per day prior to dismissal for both group I and group II is indicated in Table 44.1. It can be seen that there is a tendency towards a greater number of abusers in group I than in group II. This tendency increases during unemployment (see Table 44.2), in which period there is a great increase in consumption generally.

At the time of the 1-year follow-up investigation the picture had however

Table 44.1 Average daily alcohol consumption prior to unemployment

	Drinks (10−12 g)				
	0−1	2−6	7−10	11−20	> 20
Group I ($n = 18$)	8 44 %	2 11 %	2 11 %	3 17 %	3 17 %
Group II ($n = 52$)	30 58 %	8 15 %	5 10 %	3 6 %	6 12 %

Table 44.2 Average daily alcohol consumption during unemployment

	Drinks (10−12 g)				
	0−1	2−6	7−10	11−20	>20
Group I (n = 18)	5	1	1	4	7
	28%	6%	6%	22%	39%
Group II (n = 52)	22	8	2	5	15
	42%	15%	4%	10%	29%

changed (Table 44.3), as it can be seen that at that point only one patient in group I consumed from seven to ten drinks daily, while in group II there were five with a consumption of seven to ten drinks daily and five who consumed over 20 drinks daily. On comparison of the alcohol consumption prior to dismissal with that at the 1-year follow-up investigation, a significant preponderance of instances of reduction as against increase in consumption for group I can be demonstrated, nine as against one ($p = 5\%$, sign-test) while this is not the case in group II (13 as against six).

Thirteen of the 18 patients in group I had alcohol problems prior to admission. The situation for these 13 patients at the 1-year follow-up investigation was as follows: five were abstinent with the help of constant or periodic use of disulfiram (Antabus) − a couple of these patients used disulfiram only when they felt particularly stressed by external factors. Three patients had a minimal alcohol consumption without the help of disulfiram. Four patients managed day-to-day control of their alcohol intake, in that they took at the most only a few drinks daily, but now and then at week-ends indulged in what could be termed as 'time off'.

A single patient still had a constant alcohol abuse, though moderate, (seven to ten drinks daily) but in spite of this abuse maintained steady employment following discharge.

Table 44.3 Average daily alcohol consumption at 1-year follow-up investigation

	Drinks (10−12 g)				
	0−1	2−6	7−10	11−20	>20
Group I (n = 18)	13	4	1	0	0
	72%	22%	6%		
Group II (n = 47)	29	8	5	0	5
	62%	17%	11%		11%

OTHER FACTORS OF SIGNIFICANCE FOR A POSITIVE COURSE OCCUPATIONALLY

Interaction between the significantly associated parameters in the follow-up period, positive occupational course, sanification of the alcohol abuse, improvement of general mental condition and improvement in relations with family, friends and acquaintances could be complicated but often sanification of the actual abuse was the primary factor.

On closer examination of the single case histories a number of other factors were earmarked which could be of significance for a positive subsequent course. Stabilization in new employment – apart from sanification of the abuse if any, was particularly dependent on the following factors:

(1) experiencing the job as relevant work
(2) feeling of responsibility for the work done and towards fellow workers
(3) a general feeling of good relationship with fellow workers.

A significant number, i.e. two thirds, of the persons in group I had contact with one or several 'in-between stations' following hospitalization in the psychiatric department and before re-establishment in the labour market. In this respect the difference between group I and group II was statistically significant, 67% as against 29% ($p < 1\%$, χ^2-test).

In group I, the 'in-between station' in six cases was a psychiatric day centre, in three cases high school sojourn (see below), in three cases rehabilitation via rehabilitation workshops/apprenticeship.

It should be briefly mentioned that at the psychiatric day centre, attached to the department of psychiatry in Odense, activities include group therapy directed at personal insight, diverse practical activities such as workshop crafts, cookery and finally various outgoing activities (e.g. visiting exhibitions and home visits to clients). The high schools – colleges of a type peculiar to Denmark – have a wide range of educational subjects to offer, and further great weight is laid on sociability. The courses most often cover a period of some months. The salaries of patients obtaining placement in rehabilitation workshops or apprenticeships are paid in part or full by the public authorities.

Case histories

It is felt relevant to give a brief summary of some of the case histories.

Case 1

A 20-year-old man in childhood and adolescence presented behavioural disorders and had been involved in criminality. He had been addicted to alcohol for several years and periods of employment as an unskilled worker had been of short duration. He was admitted because of alcoholism and nervousness, and after discharge was admitted to a treatment home for alcoholics ('Ringgaarden'). Following this he was hired on a coaster where he continues to work. He finds his work responsible and interesting, saying: 'It makes demands on me, and that is what matters. I have become more mature. We are seven or eight men on board and I can't let them down, and am not permitted to, either'.

Case 2

A 20-year-old man had had various forms of unskilled work. When he went to sea 7 years earlier he developed an overriding taste for alcohol and since had difficulty in coping with his work. He was admitted because he swallowed a handful of sleeping tablets on being rejected by his girlfriend. During his short period of admission he appeared depressed, somewhat immature and lacking in self-confidence. He was then referred to an ambulatorium for alcoholics but soon neglected coming there. He started working $3\frac{1}{2}$ months after discharge. Through a friend he heard of work available in the railway company and after an interview he obtained the job. He grew to like his work, not least because of the comradeship it offered and through it he started to cultivate various forms of sport, something new to him. At the 1-year follow-up his condition was found to be completely satisfactory, his daily consumption of alcohol modest, and family relations were described as 'first rate'.

Case 3

A 24-year-old man earlier had been apprenticed to a printer for 3 years. He was last employed 2 years earlier when he had casual seasonal work. He had a tendency to alcoholism since adolescence. His alcoholism was massive, particularly in periods of adversity. He tended to tire of his work and had contact difficulties in relations with the opposite sex. He was admitted as an emergency because of drunkenness and suicidal threats following rejection by his girlfriend. During hospitalization, arrangements were made for him to resume his apprenticeship with the opportunity of completing his training, but within a few months of its completion, anxiety symptoms set in, and his alcohol abuse started once more. It turned out that he had never been really interested in his trade. At the 1-year follow-up he had started working as a helper for pensioners in a project 'Youth in Work', and currently considered that work as 'more than relevant'.

Conclusion

When an unemployed psychiatric patient needs to be re-established firmly in the labour market, it is considered of great importance that sufficient time is used to determine the patient's actual competence, probable abilities, and wishes and expectations regarding future occupation etc. It is important, not least when dealing with young unemployed patients attached to work projects, apprenticeships and the like, that a form for contract is drawn up of the conditions agreed upon for future co-operation. At regular intervals joint evaluation should be made of the extent to which these conditions are satisfied by both parties. If this is not done, there is a great risk that months will pass by before it becomes clear that the educational or occupational efforts instituted are merely waste of time and money.

References

1 Vilstrup, H. and Nielsen, P. E. (1981). Alkoholforbrugets fordeling i den danske befolkning i 1979. *Ugeskr. Læg.*, **143**, 1047
2 Fruensgaard, K., Larsen, I., Schmidt, H. and Vaag, U. H. (1980). *'Ringgaarden' undersøgelsen. En efterundersøgelse af institutionsbehandlede alkoholmisbrugere*. (Odense: Fyns Stiftsbogtrykkeri)
3 Fruensgaard, K. (1982). Psychotic conditions occurring in patients while in a treatment home for alcoholics. In Golding, P. (ed.) *Alcoholism: A Modern Perspective*, pp. 383–388 (Lancaster: MTP)
4 Arngrim, T. (1983). Psychosocial analysis of patients admitted to a treatment home for alcoholics (In preparation)
5 Fruensgaard, K., Benjaminsen, S., Joensen, S. and Helstrup, K. (1983). Psychosocial characteristics of a group of unemployed persons consecutively admitted to a psychiatric emergency department. *Soc. Psychiatry* (In press)

Part 10:
ALCOHOLISM – SOME RECENT RESEARCH

45
Alcohol research and its implications for prevention and treatment

J. A. EWING

INTRODUCTION

In the paper that I prepared for ALC. 80, 'Alcohol research in the 1980s: Implications for prevention and treatment', I restricted myself to research into the aetiology of alcoholism[1]. I demonstrated that there were four groups of factors that could supply both predisposing and protecting forces. These factors were (1) availability and price, (2) social forces, (3) psychological factors and (4) constitutional factors. Although I gave some examples of research in all of these areas I focussed mainly on the constitutional factors, since recent evidence for genetic components (in at least primary alcoholism) challenges us to understand the biological mechanisms underlying the inborn predisposition. Therefore, I discussed animal and human experimental data being accumulated with reference to such factors as willingness to drink alcohol (in the case of the experimental animal) and euphoric, and therefore presumably desirable, responses to alcohol (in the case of the human).

There already was evidence for the existence of subtypes of alcoholism − in particular a type to be called primary or familial which seems to be unassociated with any particular personality or psychiatric predisposition. Indeed, such people, once abstinent, tend to be no different from the general population. Thus, I emphasized the importance of clinical classification of patients in our therapeutic work.

Although it is less than 2 years since I prepared that paper, I am happy to say that significant new findings have been made and published in the meanwhile. Thus, even if I restrict myself to aetiologic factors in the development of alcoholism, I will have to be extremely selective in order to present an update in the space available. What I propose to do, therefore, is to comment in an explanatory way about some of the papers, hypotheses and research techniques that have excited me in the last 2 years or so.

GENETIC STUDIES

Two important papers describing the analysis of data based on Swedish adoptees have been published by the team of Bohman, Sigvardsson and Cloninger[2, 3]. These involve 862 males and 913 females who were adopted by non-relatives early in life and who were studied between the ages of 23 and 43 years (Table 45.1). This was a cross-fostering study designed to disentangle the influences provided by both genetic and environmental factors. The methods used are complex and the original papers cannot be summarized adequately in a few words. The effect of environmental factors interacting with genetic forces was demonstrated. Indeed, the authors concluded that major changes in social attitudes about drinking styles could dramatically change the prevalence of alcohol abuse, regardless of genetic predisposition. Their study demonstrated that research needs to identify subgroups of alcoholics more clearly in the future.

In the case of males they were able to demonstrate a highly hereditable type of alcoholism that passes from fathers to sons (Table 45.2). The sons born to fathers who had alcoholism early in life which called for extensive treatment and who tended to have an unskilled occupation and a serious history of criminality had nine times more alcoholism than controls. This was in spite of the fact that they were not raised by the biological father.

Table 45.1 Swedish adoption studies

Sample
862 males
913 females

Characteristics
Adopted by non-relatives
Most separated from parents in infancy
All adopted by age 3 years
Age range at follow up: 23–43 years

Table 45.2 Male alcoholism: highly hereditable type

Fathers	Mothers	Sons
Early alcoholism	No special	Nine times more
Extensive treatment	characteristics	alcoholism than
Unskilled occupation		controls
Serious criminality		

Based on Cloninger *et al.*[2]

A milder form of male alcoholism (Table 45.3) was associated with mild alcohol abuse in father or mother and this had tended to develop later in adult life. The postnatal environment provided to these sons determined the frequency and the severity of alcoholism, with the relative risk of alcoholism being twice that of controls (adoptees without alcoholic parents) when provocative factors were provided by the environment.

In the case of females, a maternal inheritance type of alcoholism was demonstrated (Table 45.4). The daughters of mothers who had mild adult onset alcoholism and minimal criminality had three times more alcoholism than controls. Also, there was an excess of alcohol abuse among the daughters of biological fathers with alcohol abuse that was mild and not associated with criminality. However, the fathers who produced sons with a severe predisposition for alcoholism (Table 45.2) had no excess of alcoholic daughters.

These exciting findings demonstrate that there are at least three types of genetic susceptibility for alcoholism and suggest that important new similar studies will be forthcoming. One of the most urgent research tasks facing us at this time is to advance our knowledge of the biological predisposition for the types of alcoholism that can be inherited.

PROSPECTIVE STUDIES

There are severe disadvantages in looking at alcoholism retrospectively. In particular, clinicians who work with alcoholics basically see only those who come for treatment. Prospective studies of alcoholism, on the other hand,

Table 45.3 Male alcoholism: milieu limited type

Fathers	or	Mothers	Sons
Mild alcoholism Minimal criminality No treatment		Mild alcoholism Minimal criminality	Two times more alcoholism than controls *with* postnatal provocation

Based on Cloninger et al.[2]

Table 45.4 Female alcoholism: maternal inheritance type

Mothers	Daughters
Mild alcoholism Minimal criminality	Three times more alcoholism than controls

Based on Bohman et al.[3]

permit one to view the natural history of alcoholism. Beginning in Boston in the 1940s some clinicians, such as the Gluecks, laid the groundwork for such prospective studies by collecting basic data on schoolboys and college students. Although the originators of this work are deceased, the archives remain available and are being used by an able custodian, Dr George Vaillant, to provide knowledge previously unavailable. Vaillant has published several articles based on these data and recently published a book on *The Natural History of Alcoholism*[4]. Vaillant and his colleagues have been able to remain in contact with the majority of the previously studied subjects. Thus, for example, in a report of 184 men, now aged 50, who were first studied as college students, Vaillant[5] was able to demonstrate that poor childhood factors, personality instability in college and adult evidence of personality disorders did *not* correlate with alcohol abuse. Instead, he concluded, the 26 problem drinkers seemed to have been depressed and unable to cope as a consequence – not a cause – of their inability to control their alcohol consumption.

Another group he has been studying were schoolboys of working class origin followed into adult life. On 400 of these, Vaillant[6] has complete drinking histories from the ages of 20 to 47. One hundred and ten showed alcohol abuse with 71 of these having evidence of dependence on alcohol. Being dependent on alcohol and having many alcohol-related problems were associated with eventual sustained abstinence. Those men who had fewer drinking problems and were not alcohol dependent were those most likely to return to controlled drinking. There was no correlation between the childhood variables that predict mental health and the eventual development of alcoholism. What, then, did predict alcoholism? There were three factors: a family history of alcoholism; a premorbid antisocial behaviour history and the absence of southern European ethnicity. In contrast, those of Irish-American background were more likely to have been very symptomatic and to achieve abstinence, when it *was* achieved, through Alcoholics Anonymous. Indeed, the self-help movement appeared more useful than clinical treatment. Vaillant found that a key to recovery seemed to be the individual's recognition that he was no longer consciously in charge of his drinking and that the use of alcohol was no longer under voluntary control. He identified non-treatment factors associated with abstinence as follows: (1) substitute dependency, (2) behaviour modification, (3) hope and (4) social rehabilitation. As he points out, AA, if regularly attended, provides all of the 'non-treatment factors' just listed.

Obviously, important conclusions come from such studies. In the first place, we see that severe alcoholism is best dealt with by seeking total abstinence. On the other hand, there probably are people who should perhaps be labelled as 'careless drinkers' who can return to asymptomatic controlled drinking. These are rarely, if ever, the severe alcoholics whom we see in clinics and hospitals. A study of this nature also points to the absurdity of a psychiatrist or other therapist saying to the patient, 'Let's try to find out why you are an alcoholic'. In my opinion this makes as much sense as saying to the diabetic, 'Let's find out why you are a diabetic'. We must recognize that the evidence points to the fact that alcoholics become anxious and depressed and lose their self-esteem because they have lost control of their use of alcohol. These appear to be cases of primary, or essential and usually familial alcoholism. They far outnumber those who have started to drink to excess because of underlying anxiety or depression[7].

THE TIQs

In my earlier paper[1] I discussed the tetrahydroisoquinolines (TIQs). Two independent groups of researchers had postulated in 1970 that these substances, which are plant alkaloids, might be elaborated within the animal body during alcohol administration. Various TIQs have indeed been demonstrated to exist within both the animal and the human during alcohol drinking[1]. There are many substances within this classification that need to be investigated. My colleague Dr Robert Myers in our animal laboratory has shown that micro-injections of several of these substances into the ventricles of the rat's brain lead to significant changes[1]. Some animals that formerly showed little interest in drinking alcohol begin to consume enough to produce a withdrawal reaction when the alcohol is no longer available. Other animals have shown a reaction very similar to that of alcohol withdrawal following the TIQ infusion itself. Researchers in Sweden have demonstrated the existence of TIQs in the cerebrospinal fluid (c.s.f.) of alcoholics during early hospitalization[1]. In a collaborative study our animal laboratory is infusing some of this c.s.f. into the ventricles of monkeys. Although some behavioural changes have been observed, it is premature to discuss the results since we have not yet broken the code to distinguish between c.s.f. from alcoholics and from non-alcoholics.

One study done with rats indicates that administering the substance naloxone can inhibit some TIQ-induced drinking in the rat[8]. Naloxone is an opiate antagonist. For example, a tiny dose of 0.4 mg will initiate a withdrawal reaction in a patient addicted to opiates. These findings suggest that there may be some common mechanism behind addiction to opiates and alcoholism. One possibility is that the endorphins (naturally occurring opiate-like substances) are mediating the response to alcohol in some way. Already there are clinical and experimental reports to suggest the existence of such a mechanism. These studies use the pharmacological properties of naloxone since it will occupy the central nervous system receptor sites that have affinity for endorphins. Thus, if naloxone antagonizes the effects of alcohol, it would suggest that the endorphins are involved in at least some of the effects of alcohol.

Studies in my human laboratory have failed to demonstrate that naloxone interferes with the mood effects of alcohol[9] or with the level of intoxication reached or a variety of physiologic measures[10]. However, at the time of my ALC. 80 paper[1] we had not yet measured performance. In a new study recently completed we evaluated this, since Jeffcoate and his colleagues[11] had shown a mild decrement in a reaction time test after subjects received alcohol. He reported that the performance was less impaired in subjects who had first received naloxone than in subjects given a placebo. In our study we used the simulated evaluation of driver impairment (SEDI) apparatus devised by my colleague Dr Kenneth C. Mills. This involves having the subject press buttons as numbers on a screen change before him and it evaluates perception, central nervous system (c.n.s.) processing and motor response. Eighty subjects who were healthy young males were divided into four groups of 20 each. On a double-blind basis they received first an injection of either naloxone or saline. Then, half of them received a gin and tonic and half of them received tonic with a fine mist of gin sprayed on top to provide at least the initial impression of a gin and tonic. Blood alcohol levels achieved were approximately 60 mg/dl and the performance of those receiving alcohol was measurably impaired on the task. However, those who received the preinjection of naloxone before receiving the alcoholic beverage were significantly less impaired[12]. Thus, it may well be that the endorphins *are* involved in some of the effects of alcohol. Much future work is called for, since alcohol has a myriad of effects on so many different parts of the body. Our work, however, primarily focusses on the effects upon the c.n.s. and particularly seeks to understand why and how alcohol produces the effects that people seek when they take a drink.

METABOLIC FACTORS

Dr Ronald G. Thurman, a pharmacologist who is associated with our research centre, has made some very exciting findings that I would like to share with you briefly. The phenomenon that he calls SIAM (Swift Increase in Alcohol Metabolism) was first demonstrated in the rat[13]. Thurman and his colleagues showed that if a rat metabolized alcohol at a certain rate, sometimes this rate would greatly increase if the rat were exposed to alcohol for some hours. This is not the increased rate of metabolism seen in human chronic alcoholics since it occurs within 2–4 hours. Thurman turned to the laboratory mouse for continued experiments since there are many genetic strains of mice available and he, along with geneticist Edward Glassman, is now studying the SIAM phenomenon in recombinant strains of mice[14]. After establishing what is the rate of metabolism of alcohol to a single dose, these mice are exposed to alcohol vapour in a chamber for several hours. Some strains show a consistent increase in metabolic rate. Other strains show no change and still others show a decreased rate. In a single preliminary study with humans, Thurman[15] has now demonstrated similar differences between humans. First, subjects were given a single dose of alcohol and their blood levels were followed down as they metabolized it. Then, they drank over several hours to maintain the blood level of alcohol before stopping drinking, at which point the rate of metabolism was again measured. Most human subjects showed no change but some showed a very great increase.

These findings are going to call for work in laboratories for several years as we try to understand the phenomenon. Meanwhile, its potential significance is tremendous. It might, for instance, explain why one subject takes a few drinks and then stops, whereas another seems to want to go on drinking. The latter may be burning the alcohol up faster and therefore drinking more in order to keep feeling the effect. The more one drinks the more one must be presumed to be at risk for tissue damage as well as for developing tolerance and dependence. As I indicated in my recently published book, *Drinking to Your Health*[16], we should never envy the person who claims to have 'a hollow leg'. Such people boast about the amount of alcohol they can consume, which simply means that they are putting themselves at increased risk for health hazards and alcoholism. Those who have a lower tolerance for alcohol and who quit drinking earlier and after drinking smaller amounts are less at risk.

CURRENT PROSPECTIVE STUDIES

The Boston prospective studies that I described called for data on a large number of young men since the prevalence rate of alcoholism is relative low. However, recent data, such as I summarized in my ALC. 80 paper[1], point strongly to the existence of a genetic component in primary alcoholism which is so often associated with a positive family history. Dr Marc Schuckit[17] has taken advantage of this to study young men who are presumably at high risk to develop alcoholism and to compare these with matched controls. Table 45.5 demonstrates the differences between family history positives (FHPs) and family history negatives (FHNs). This is a method that is being developed in other laboratories, including our own. The objective is to study any existing differences between these two groups as well as to follow them long enough to see which subjects become alcoholic. Table 45.6 shows some of the findings already published by Schuckit that demonstrate differences between the two

Table 45.5   Current prospective studies

FHPs (*family history positives*)	FHNs (*family history negatives*)

Young Males 20–25
  Not (yet) alcoholic
  No psychiatric disorder
Has one or more alcoholic
  first degree relatives
	Young Males 20–25
	  Not alcoholic
	  No psychiatric disorder
	  No alcoholic relatives

└——Matched for demography and——┘
drinking quantity and frequency

Based on Schuckit.[18]

groups[18]. The blood acetaldehyde data have been criticized as being based on inappropriate methodology and definitely must be replicated in other laboratories. However the other two items in Table 45.6 are of extreme importance. They seem to imply that the men with the positive family history feel less sense of intoxication at the same levels of blood alcohol and yet may be obtaining more tension relief than those without a family history in terms of the muscle tension measures.

Table 45.7 lists some differences reported by Schuckit in a recent presentation. Again the picture one gets is that the FHPs feel the effect of the alcohol less than the FHNs and are less affected by the alcohol. The reported differences in prolactin and cortisol levels are difficult to interpret but may be highly significant. Of certain significance is the fact that were no differences on personality tests.

I have been particularly impressed with Schuckit's method since it provides the rationale for studying much smaller numbers of subjects in much more detail. Currently available data indicate that the probability of a FHP male developing alcoholism must lie between approximately 20 and 42 %. In a recent presentation, Goodwin[19] gave the average probability figure as 27 %.

Table 45.6 Differences between FHPs and FHNs

Measure	FHPs	FHNs
Blood alcohol levels	No difference	
Alcohol metabolism	No difference	
Blood acetaldehyde levels	Higher	Lower
Feelings of intoxication	Less	More
Resting muscle-tension after alcohol	Lower	Higher

Based on Schuckit.[18]

Table 45.7 Further differences between FHPs and FHNs

Measure	FHPs	FHNs
Body sway	Less	More
Euphoria score	Lower	Higher
Performance impairment	Less	More
Reaction time	Slowed less	Slowed more
Prolactin levels	Lowered	Increased
Cortisol levels	Slower recovery	Faster recovery
Personality tests	No differences	

Based on Schuckit, M. A. Presentation at Gordon Research Conference, February 1982 (unpublished)

Based on average United States data the probability of a FHN subject developing alcoholism is $5-7\%$. Thus, the methodology involved is probably quite valid and we can anticipate exciting results from various laboratories as such studies are carried out and the prospective follow-ups are conducted.

THE PROSTAGLANDIN HYPOTHESIS

In 1980, Horrobin published[20] a very innovative hypothesis connecting alcohol drinking and the prostaglandin, PGE_1. I have attempted to present a simplified diagram of this hypothesis in Figure 45.1. Horrobin explains that alcohol enhances the conversion of dihomogamma-linolenic acid (DGLA) to PGE_1 but blocks the activity of the delta-6-desaturase which is the enzyme necessary for replenishment of DGLA stores from dietary precursors. The acute effect of ethanol is therefore an increased production of PGE_1 but chronic consumption will lead to depletion of DGLA and PGE_1. Withdrawal from alcohol will lead to a precipitous fall in PGE_1. This prostaglandin is known to have profound effects on c.n.s. and on behaviour. For example, patients with mania produce more PGE_1 than normal, while those with depression make less. Horrobin believes that alcoholics may drink to maintain

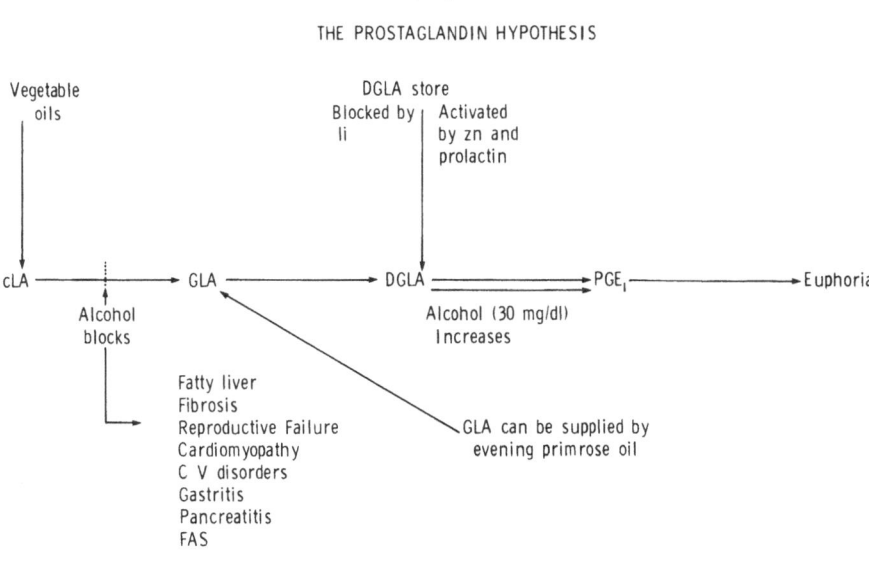

Figure 1

THE PROSTAGLANDIN HYPOTHESIS

Based on: Horrobin D. F.
          Medical Hypotheses 6:929-942, 1980

Figure 45.1   The prostaglandin hypothesis. Based on Horrobin.[20]

a normal PGE_1 level, something which will require more and more alcohol as DGLA is depleted. He reports that in both animals and humans, PGE_1, or its precursor gamma-linolenic acid (GLA) have been shown to attenuate the acute withdrawal syndrome. Injections of PGE_1, he says, prevent the development of fatty liver in alcohol-treated animals. Defective essential fatty acid (EFA) and PGE_1 metabolism are known to lead to increased fibrosis, reproductive failure, cardiomyopathy, cardiovascular disorders, gastritis and pancreatitis and could therefore be the basis for these disorders in alcoholics. A PGE_1 deficiency could also be responsible for the fetal alcohol syndrome. Three other agents are known to produce constellations of fetal defects very similar to those found in the fetal alcohol syndrome. These others are the drugs phenytoin, lithium and a deficiency of zinc. These three factors and excessive alcohol consumption all lead to PGE_1 deficiency by different mechanisms. If Horrobin's concept is correct, the key to the management of alcoholism and its medical complications lies in the provision of GLA or DGLA, fatty acids which bypass the alcohol blocked step and which are unfortunately unlikely to be present in any normal diet. Horrobin claims that unlike many concepts of alcoholism and alcohol damage, the hypothesis he provides is very readily testable and already has considerable experimental support. For example, he states that case studies in about 20 humans have shown that GLA is highly effective in preventing or abolishing hangovers and the withdrawal syndrome. One of his collaborators, Lieb, has found that the EFAs are effective in the alleviation of lithium tremor, familial tremor and alcohol withdrawal tremor.

Horrobin believes that individuals with moderately low levels of PGE_1 will feel unhappy. If they consume alcohol they will push their PGE_1 levels into the normal range or above, and will feel normal or even elated. When they stop drinking, PGE_1 levels will fall below what they were before drinking. A situation therefore will develop in which more and more alcohol must be consumed to achieve a normal PGE_1 level. Both genetic and nutritional factors might lie behind the low concentrations of PGE_1. He reports that he had the opportunity to treat an alcoholic who had failed in several attempts to stop drinking alcohol and who suffered from a disabling myopathy. Over a period of 4 months he gave the patient GLA and found that alcohol consumption dropped spontaneously and there was a dramatic restoration of muscle power and mobility.

Unfortunately, no properly controlled double-blind studies have yet been carried out and reported in the literature, as far as I know, involving GLA or the PGE_1s. A biochemist colleague in North Carolina, Dr Sam Pennington, has been studying the role of prostaglandins in the fetal alcohol syndrome[21] for some time and he tends to agree with the hypothesis of Dr Horrobin. I am happy to report that Dr Pennington is now studying the effects of acute doses of ethanol in the brain of experimental animals in terms of actual measurable levels of PGE_1. This study will either support or refute the hypothesis of Dr Horrobin.

CONCLUSIONS

It is very exciting and promising to review our knowledge in 1982 and to compare the level of our knowledge in 1980. Clearly, we now know more about the mode of action of alcohol within the animal body, in terms of both molecular and cellular mechanisms. There are more ideas for research methods and more hypotheses to be tested. I believe that we now have some promise of eventually understanding the mechanism of craving for alcoholic beverages. Although there are no new proved suggestions for us in our therapeutic work with alcoholics, the rate of progress in research should encourage us to hang in there and to keep utilizing the established methods of achieving abstinence. Subclassifying our patients is continuing to be of increasing importance, both in establishing who does best with what approach, and in increasing our awareness as to the heterogeneity of alcoholism. Finally, we should encourage more biological research in alcohol and alcoholism by showing legislators the need for increased funding. The promise for better prevention and treatment of alcoholism is almost within our grasp, but we must reach out for it.

References

1 Ewing, J. A. (1982). Alcohol research in the 1980s: Implications for prevention and treatment. In Golding, P. (ed.). *Alcoholism: A Modern Perspective*. (Lancaster: MTP)

2 Cloninger, C. R., Bohman, M. and Sigvardsson, S. (1981). Inheritance of alcohol abuse: Cross-fostering analysis of adopted men. *Arch. Gen. Psychiatry*, **38**, 861

3 Bohman, M., Sigvardsson, S. and Cloninger, C. R. (1981). Maternal inheritance of alcohol abuse: Cross-fostering analysis of adopted women. *Arch. Gen. Psychiatry*, **38**, 965

4 Vaillant, G. E. (1983). *The Natural History of Alcoholism*. (Cambridge, Mass: Harvard U.P.)

5 Vaillant, G. E. (1980). Natural history of male psychological health: VIII. Antecedents of alcoholism and "orality." *Am. J. Psychiatry*, **137**, 181

6 Vaillant, G. E. and Milofsky, E. S. (1982). Natural history of male alcoholism IV: Paths to recovery. *Arch. Gen. Psychiatry*, **39**, 127

7 Ewing, J. A. (1981). Biologic and psychotherapeutic vectors in alcoholism. In Masserman, J. H. (ed.) *Current Psychiatric Therapies*, **20**, pp. 135–144. (New York: Grune & Stratton)

8 Myers, R. A. and Critcher, E. C. (1982). Naloxone alters alcohol drinking induced in the rat by tetrahydropapaveroline (THP) infused ICV. *Pharmacol. Biochem. Behav.* **16**, 827

9 Ewing, J. A., Aderhold, R. M. and McCarty, D. (1979). Abstract: Are the endorphins implicated in human response to ethanol? *Alcoholism (NY)*, **3**, 174

10 Ewing, J. A. and McCarty, D. (1983). Are the endorphins involved in mediating the mood effects of ethanol? *Alcoholism (NY)*, **7** (In press)

11 Jeffcoate, W. J., Herbert, M., Cullen, M. H., Hastings, A. G. and Walder, C. P. (1979). Prevention of effects of alcohol intoxication by naloxone. *Lancet*, **2**, 1157

12 Ewing, J. A., Mills, K. C. and Bisgrove, E. (1982). Evidence for endorphin involvement in alcohol-impaired performance in humans. (In preparation)

13 Yuki, T. and Thurman, R. G. (1980). Mechanism of the Swift Increase in Alcohol Metabolism ('SIAM') in the rat. In Thurman, R. G. (ed.) *Alcohol and Aldehyde Metabolizing Systems-IV*, pp. 689–695. (New York: Plenum)

14 Paschal, D. L., Wallace, A. T., Bradford, B. U., Glassman, E. and Thurman, R. G. (1982). The Swift Increase in Alcohol Metabolism in inbred mice: Dose-response relations. *Alcoholism (NY)*, **6**, 285

15 Thurman, R. G., Bradford, B. U., Danis, M. and Glassman, E. (1982). The Swift Increase in Alcohol Metabolism occurs in humans: A pilot study. Presented at *Alcoholism — The Search for the Sources*, 20–22 January, Winston-Salem, NC

16 Ewing, J. A. (1981). *Drinking to Your Health*. (Reston, VA: Reston Publishing Co.)

17 Schuckit, M. A. (1980). Self-rating of alcohol intoxication by young men with and without family histories of alcoholism. *J. Stud. Alc.*, **41**, 242

18 Schuckit, M. A. (1980). Biological markers: Metabolism and acute reactions to alcohol in sons of alcoholics. *Pharmacol. Biochem. Behav.* **13** (Suppl. 1), 9

19 Goodwin, D. W. (1981). Familial alcoholism. Presented at *134th Annual Meeting, American Psychiatric Association*, 11–15 May, New Orleans

20 Horrobin, D. F. (1980). A biochemical basis for alcoholism and alcohol-induced damage including the fetal alcohol syndrome and cirrhosis: Interference with essential fatty acid and prostaglandin metabolism. *Med. Hypotheses*, **6**, 929

21 Pennington, S. N., Rumbley, R. A. and Woody, D. G. (1981). Fetal 15-hydroxy-prostaglandin dehydrogenase is altered by maternal ethanol exposure. *Biol. Neonate*, **40**, 246

46
Drinking practices and their effect on sober cognitive performance

A. GELLER

For much of this century alcohol itself has been regarded as a relatively benign substance in the human body. The damage seen in chronic alcoholics was thought to be a result of their dysfunctional habits such as poor nutrition, poor self-care and frequent trauma. Within the past 15 years it has become increasingly apparent that alcohol acts as a direct toxic agent on cells, organs and systems. The evidence has accumulated from a number of diverse studies, including those on baboon livers[1], mouse brains[2], beagle puppies[3], and rat testes[4] and is supported by clinical data from alcoholic patients.

It is not clear whether the direction of research has been influenced by a change in attitude towards the alcoholic person, from being regarded as the agent of his/her misfortune, to becoming the victim of a constitutional inability to handle alcohol or whether both research and change in attitudes have proceeded along similar paths.

Once a direct toxic action of alcohol has been shown it changes our thinking, from the comfortable assumption that tissue damage occurs only in debilitated alcoholics after prolonged extreme alcohol intake, to looking for dose response curves and thresholds for these effects. The act of undertaking dose response studies leads to a re-examination of the toxic endpoint and the search for more subtle indices of damage.

A splendid example of this is the effect of alcohol on the developing fetus. The observed toxic endpoint has been refined from the florid manifestations of the fetal alcohol syndrome to decreases in birth weight, changes in neonatal behaviour and a number of neurological 'soft signs', and the complete range of drinking practices has been surveyed to determine dose effect.

Similarly in the effects of alcohol on the adult brain, research has been liberated from contemplation of the Wernicke–Korsakoff syndrome to the less dramatic, and more pervasive, impairments seen generally in alcoholic patients. This in turn has led to the question of the threshold dose of alcohol required to produce detectable cognitive impairment.

Although alcohol abuse and alcohol dependency may be behaviourally discontinuous from non-problem drinking, the range of alcohol intake shows no such discontinuity. Heavy social drinkers may be taking in more alcohol than some alcoholics. The evidence for a direct neurotoxic effect of alcohol is overwhelming[5-9], and in animal studies appears to be dose related[10]. The most obvious, but not the only explanation for the cognitive deficits found in the vast majority of apparently non-nutritionally depleted alcoholics is that it is related to a direct neurotoxic action of alcohol. If this is so, one would expect some measure of alcohol intake to be a more important predictor of cognitive impairment than whether or not there are the behavioural manifestations of alcohol abuse and one might expect to see some effects at least at the upper end of the intake range in social drinkers.

In looking for a dose effect relationship, it is important to be aware of the magnitude of the decrements one is likely to see. Alcoholics showing deficit on neuropsychological testing are not generally on clinical examination manifesting an organic brain syndrome. In fact, one fifth[11] of the alcoholics tested may score within the normal range on the tests used. What is seen is a poorer performance of the alcoholics as a group compared with non-alcoholics as a group even when the alcoholics are performing within the normal range. With social drinkers it would be unlikely that scores in the impaired range would be found even in the heaviest drinkers. It would be predicted from a dose effect hypothesis that those scoring highest on some measure of alcohol intake would perform more poorly than those scoring lowest on that measure.

The sensitivity of the measuring instrument is of great importance when one is looking for thresholds for effect. For example, the tests which can reliably differentiate Korsakoff patients from normals[12] are not useful in detecting the less marked differences between non-Korsakoff alcoholics and normals because they are too easy to perform.

Research on the non-acute effects of alcohol intake on non-alcoholic drinkers is a new field. Only a handful of studies[13-17] have been published which examine the impact of alcohol intake on sober cognitive performance of non-alcoholics. Before interpreting these studies, it would be helpful to summarize the much more extensive literature on the cognitive performance of sober alcoholic drinkers and to point out some of the interesting questions raised by this research.

Alcoholics as a group, tested after at least 1 week of abstinence and after acute withdrawal is over, demonstrate a typical pattern of neuropsychological deficits. Verbal abilities, previously acquired knowledge and skills and overall intelligence (as measured by standard tests) are intact. Visuospatial abilities, conceptual thinking, problem solving and new learning are to varying extents impaired. On the two most widely used standard tests, the Wechsler Adult Intelligence Scale (WAIS) and the Halstead Reitan Battery (HRB), the subtests affected measure the ability to reproduce visual spatial patterns (Block Design), to solve jigsaw puzzles (Object Assembly), to decode rapidly (Digit Symbol), to form and test hypothesis about abstract geometric shapes (Category Test), to locate objects in space speedily (TPT − Time), to remember their location (TPT − Location) and to join together rapidly in sequence a series of numbered points (Trails B). Verbal learning is also impaired even though other verbal abilities are intact.

The tests on which alcoholics perform poorly are those which were selected by Reitan as particularly sensitive to the effects of brain damage and of age. Although there have been attempts to relate the particular deficits manifested by alcoholics to specific brain regions, the weight of evidence supports diffuse generalized brain damage[18].

Attempts to relate the extent of neuropsychological impairment in alcoholics to alcohol intake have met with varying success. For obvious reasons, precision on any measure of intake is unlikely to be reached. Eckhart[19], in an elegant study, examined a number of alcohol consumption variables and did find interactive relationships between recent and chronic drinking practices and some measures of cognitive performance. Of particular interest was the finding that some test scores related only to current drinking patterns whereas others related only to chronic consumption.

There are questions which have been raised in studies with alcoholics which are of particular importance both in the design and evaluation of studies of social drinkers. Normal ageing results in deficits in the same tests as those in which alcoholics do poorly. In fact, when alcoholics are divided into age groups, their performance looks very much like that of normals a decade or two older. This had led to the hypothesis that alcoholic drinking causes premature ageing or accelerates the ageing process. It seems at the present time most likely that age and alcoholic drinking result in a similar neuropsychological pattern of impairments probably by independent mechanisms[20]. It is not yet clear whether these effects are additive or interactive[21]. Age, however is a major variable which must be considered in any neuropsychological study.

Another major variable to which less specific attention has been given is the time interval between the last drink and the administration of the test. There is considerable evidence for improvement in test results with length of abstinence in alcoholics[18], though in all of the studies where controls were used, control performance was consistently better than even the most 'improved' group of alcoholics. These results have been generally taken to indicate that the cognitive deficits resulting from chronic alcohol abuse are at least partly reversible with abstinence. It is not known, however, what is being reversed. There may be a proactive effect of recent drinking upon sober performance which diminishes with time after the last drinking episode. There may be a prolonged neurophysiological perturbation from protracted withdrawal[22] interfering with test performance and abating with time. Some functions may be more disrupted by these subacute processes than they are by chronic alcohol consumption and thus show 'reversibility', whereas other functions may be mainly affected by chronic alcohol intake and show little change with the passage of abstinent time. Or, of course, there may be any combination of sensitivities.

Although retrospective alcohol intake histories are inherently unreliable, they are likely to be much more so in alcoholics. Alcoholics even after detoxification are often very fuzzy about major recent events in their lives, let alone details about how much and how frequently they have been drinking. This is probably the result of anterograde interference with memory storage during continuous drinking episodes. Social drinkers, whose drinking largely takes place during discrete periods of time are much more likely to be able to recall events, amounts and daily patterns and so in fact, would be much better subjects for establishing a dose effect curve.

All of the studies of social drinkers so far conducted have shown decrements in neuropsychological performance related to an alcohol intake measure. This finding has been consistent in different age[14], sex[15], socioeconomic status[16] samples and also with several neuropsychological measures[13].

Parker, in her studies[13, 14, 16], has shown a dose related cognitive deficit which as predicted is not within the impaired range and which resembles in magnitude the deficits associated with ageing. Neither the amount of alcohol consumed over a lifetime nor the frequency of drinking is significantly related to sober cognitive performance. The intake variable which is consistently negatively associated with sober cognitive performance is the amount of alcohol typically drunk on a drinking occasion. As a general rule, drinking patterns of seven drinks one night of the week would be expected to result in poorer cognitive performance than patterns of one drink per day for 7 days.

Parker *et al.* reported two recent studies[16]; one on men of high occupational status in California and the other a random sample of employed men in Detroit. Both samples were tested while sober and having been abstinent for 24 hours on the Shipley Institute of Living Scales. The Shipley is widely used in clinical settings but rarely in research. It is a simple pen-and-paper test with 40 multiple-choice vocabulary questions on one side and 20 verbal abstraction questions on the other side. Examples of a moderately difficult question on each side are:

Vocabulary: APPRISE = reduce   shrew   inform   delight
Abstraction: Scotland   landscape   scapegoat   —ee.

Comparison of the vocabulary score with verbal abstraction score yields a conceptual quotient which should be around 100 in a normal person. Alcoholics characteristically retain vocabulary skills but lose verbal abstraction abilities, resulting in conceptual quotients beneath 100. It is indeed extremely unusual to see even in younger alcoholics normal conceptual quotients when tested 1 week after entering treatment.

In these studies, Parker *et al.* examined the relationship between intake variables, abstraction scores, vocabulary score, age and educational level. In both groups there was a consistent effect of age, with abstraction scores decreasing one point for every 5 years of age over 30. Neither lifetime consumption of alcohol nor frequency of drinking showed a significant relationship with abstraction score. The average amount of alcohol each person reported consuming on a drinking occasion was significantly negatively correlated with abstraction score. The authors make the interesting observation that an increase in one drink in the amount of alcohol typically consumed per occasion resulted in a drop in the abstraction score equivalent to 3.7 years of ageing in the high occupation sample and 2.4 years of ageing in the random sample. (The high occupation sample had an overall abstraction score of 10 points above that of the randomly selected group.)

From these results, a 35-year-old professional drinking eight drinks on an average drinking occasion would be expected to perform much as a 65-year-old of similar background. Age and the amount of alcohol consumed on an average drinking occasion were additive in this study. An older person with a pattern of high intake on each drinking occasion would be in double jeopardy for cognitive decline. It is interesting also in this study that younger people were as vulnerable to high consumption per occasion as older people. In another study[14], 21–30-year-old students showed deficits on the Shipley Hartford also related to the amount of alcohol consumed per occasion.

Many of the neuropsychological studies with alcoholics have suggested that older alcoholics are more impaired relative to age matched controls than are younger alcoholics[23–25]. The equal vulnerability of young social drinkers would appear to conflict with this. However, there is undoubtedly more than one route to deterioration in cognitive performance. In addition to the direct neurotoxic effect of the alcohol they have consumed, older alcoholics may well have had some nutritional deficiencies, metabolic derangements, prolonged ill health and repeated minor head trauma in the course of their drinking careers.

In the study by Jones and Jones[15], women social drinkers were examined on a free recall verbal memory task both before and after drinking alcohol. All the women had been abstinent for 24 hours prior to testing. They were divided into light and moderate drinking groups on the basis of alcohol consumption over the past 1 year and were further divided into younger (below 30) and middle aged (over 37) groups.

In the baseline condition, before drinking moderate drinkers in both the younger and middle aged groups had less efficient delayed recall than did light drinkers. Age in this study was not a variable. After drinking alcohol, all subjects showed a significant decline in their recall ability. In this condition, both age and intake were variables with the older moderate drinkers showing the worst performance.

The interpretation of these results is difficult. It is not known if the observed impairments were reversible with abstinence and it is not known if there is any effect of the time interval between drinking and the testing. Cognitive decrements could be the result of minor but permanent alcohol produced central nervous system changes. They could be due to prolonged residuals of the last drinking episode. They could be the cumulative result of a low grade neurophysiologically abnormal state resulting from repeated episodes of high dosage drinking. They could be due to recent or chronic drinking practices or to a combination. Reversible or not, in practice it doesn't matter. One's drinking habits are one's drinking habits. If they do not change, they will continue to produce the same impact on one's sober cognitive performance. If these impairments are potentially reversible, this offers hope. The mere potential for reverse, however, will not lessen the impact on one's abilities.

Let us suppose that this effect is reversible and is in fact the result of a prolonged after-effect from a high dosage session. If I am a 30-year-old physician and I regularly have five or six drinks every Saturday night, I can expect to perform the next day as if I had aged 20 years. Now this is not too bad and will still be a good level of performance, but it will not represent my full capabilities. Let us suppose that over the next 6 days my performance gradually improves to near my maximal level but now it is Saturday and I am to drink my five or six drinks again. Even if the potential for recovery is there, the effect is as if the damage were permanent. Moreover, as I get older I will be adding to this 'drinking pattern' deficit the deficits resulting from my increasing age. In addition, as I get older, I can expect to be more impaired during the actual drinking session.

Decreased efficiency in any area of cognitive function is alarming to contemplate. The insidious feature of deterioration in problem solving abilities is that people are not usually aware that it has happened. Alcoholics, for example, frequently do complain of difficulties with memory as do people who are getting older. Even highly intelligent alcoholics with marked impairment of abstraction ability on the Shipley scales will not only fail to notice anything amiss with their thinking, but will vigorously assert that their thinking is as clear and sharp as ever. This is unlikely to be a purely psychological defence against impairment as the same person will readily admit to memory difficulties. Nor does it seem analogous to anosognosia. Rather it appears that built into the nature of conceptual decline is the inability to perceive that it is happening. Strategies can be devised to compensate for reduction in abilities, but only if the person is aware of it. A premature and unnoticed decline in conceptual efficiency could have a serious impact on the career of some individuals.

It is clear that more research is needed in this fascinating area. Whatever future research will bring to our understanding of alcohol dosage and neurotoxic effects, the implication of the currently available research for drinking practices is clear: it is better to spread out your drinking during the week than to concentrate it on a single evening. You are probably performing below your abilities if you are regularly consuming more than three or four drinks on a drinking occasion. The after-effects from drinking may be longer lasting than you think and you should take this into consideration when you are going to need to put out your best performance. Being young is no protection, but as you get older you are in double jeopardy from age and drinking.

References

1 Lieber, C. S., DeCarl, L. M. and Rubin, E. (1975). Sequential production of fatty liver, hepatitis and cirrhosis in subhuman primates fed ethanol with adequate diets. *Proc. Natl. Acad. Sci. USA*, **72**, 437

2 Riley, J. N. and Walker, D. W. (1978). Morphological alterations in hippocampus after long term consumption in mice. *Science*, **201**, 646

3 Ellis, F. W. and Pick J. R. (1980). An animal model for the fetal alcohol syndrome in beagles. *Alcoholism*, **4**, 123

4 Van Thiel, D. H., Gavaler, J. S., Cobb, F., Sherrins, R. and Lester, R. (1979). Alcohol induced testicular atrophy in the adult male rat. *Endocrinology*, **105**, 888

5 Freund, G. (1970). Impairment of shock avoidance learning after long term alcohol ingestion in mice. *Science*, **168**, 1599

6 Walker, D. W. and Freund, G. (1973). Impairment of timing behavior following prolonged alcohol consumption in rats. *Science*, **182**, 597

7 Bond, N. W. and DiGiuoso, E. L. (1976). Impairment of Hebb–Williams maze performance following prolonged alcohol consumption in rats. *Pharmacol. Biochem. Behav.*, **5**, 85

8 Walker, D. W. and Hunter, B. E. (1978). Short term memory impairment following chronic alcohol consumption in rats. *Neuropsychologia*, **16**, 545

9 Walker, D. W., Barners, D. E., Zornetzer, S. F., Hunter, B. E. and Kubanis, P. (1980). Neuronal loss in hippocampus induced by prolonged ethanol consumption in rats. *Science*, **209**, 711

10 Freund, G. and Walker, D. W. (1971). Impairment of avoidance learning by prolonged ethanol consumption in mice. *J. Pharmacol. Exp. Ther.*, **179**, 284

11 Goldstein, G. and Shelly, C. (1980). Neuropsychological investigation of brain lesion localization in alcoholism. In Begleiter, H. (ed.) *Biological Effects of Alcoholism* p. 731. (New York: Plenum)

12 Ryan, C., Butters, N., Montgomery, K., Adinolfi, A. and Didario, B. (1980). Memory deficits in chronic alcoholics: continuum between the 'intact' alcoholic and the alcoholic Korsakoff patient. In Begleiter, H. and Kissin, B. (eds.) *Alcohol Intoxication and Withdrawal*. (New York: Plenum)

13 Parker, E. S. and Noble, E. P. (1977). Alcohol consumption and cognitive functioning in social drinkers. *J. Stud. Alc.*, **38**, 1224

14 Parker, E. S., Birnbaum, I. M., Body, R. and Noble, E. P. (1980). Neuropsychological decrements as a function of alcohol intake in male college students. *Alcoholism*, **4**, 330

15 Jones, M. K. and Jones, B. M. (1980). The relationship of age and drinking history to the effects of alcohol on memory in women. *J. Stud. Alc.* **41**, 179

16 Parker, E. S., Parker, D. A., Brody, J. A. and Schoenberg, R. (1982). Cognitive patterns resembling premature aging in male social drinkers. *Alcoholism*, **6**, 46

17 Parker, E. S. and Noble, E. P. (1980). Alcohol and the aging process in social drinkers. *J. Stud. Alc.*, **41**, 170

18 Parsons, O. A. and Leber, W. R. (1981). The relationship between cognitive dysfunction and brain damage in alcoholics: Causal interactive or epiphenomenal? *Alcoholism*, **5**, 326

19 Eckardt, M. J., Parker, E. S., Noble, E. P., Feldman, D. J. and Gottschalk, L. A. (1978). Relationship between neuropsychological performance and alcohol consumption in alcoholics. *Biol. Psychiatry*, **13**, 551

20 Porjesz, B. and Begleiter, H. (1982). Evoked brain potential deficits in alcoholism and aging. *Alcoholism*, **6**, 53

21 Ryan, C. (1982). Alcoholism and premature aging: a neuropsychological perspective. *Alcoholism*, **6**, 22

22 Kissin, B. (1978). Biological investigations in alcohol research. *J. Stud. Alc.* (Suppl.) **8**, 168

23 Jones, B. and Parsons, O. A. (1971). Impaired abstracting ability in chronic alcoholics. *Arch. Gen. Psychiatry*, **24**, 71

24 Klisz, D. and Parsons, O. A. (1977). Hypothesis testing in younger and older alcoholics. *J. Stud. Alc.*, **38**, 1718

25 Bertera, J. H. and Parsons, O. A. (1978). Impaired visual search in alcoholics. *Alcoholism*, **2**, 9

47
Attitudes towards drinking

B. RITSON and M. DE ROUMANIE

Alcoholism as a word no longer appears in the International Classification of Diseases. The term alcoholism may have outlived its usefulness and is largely dismissed in the 1980 WHO Expert Committee report[1]. We are not concerned here with the theoretical debate about the meaning of the term or the relevance of a disease concept – see, for instance, Room[2]. We are simply concerned with recognizing that alcoholism, whatever its status as a scientific concept, is part of the label attached to many organizations concerned with alcohol related problems and is a term well implanted in the public mind along with other descriptions of drinking behaviour and problems. The study reported concerns, reported public attitudes toward drinking and alcohol related problems and we would like to use it as a jumping off point for discussion of the use of the term 'alcoholism' in describing clinical facilities.

The findings discussed here formed part of a larger study of the community response to alcohol related problems. This research was coordinated by WHO and took place simultaneously in Mexico, Zambia and Scotland[3]. Here we shall be concerned simply with the Scottish component of the project and focus on the attitudes toward drinking and alcohol problems which were reported by the population studied.

METHOD: GENERAL POPULATION SURVEY

A structured interview questionnaire was developed in collaboration with the other centres involved in the study. The main areas covered in this questionnaire were:

(1) Basic demographic and health data,

(2) Drinking Patterns

    (a) frequency, quantity, beverage type
    (b) drinking history focussing on past week

(c)   consequences of drinking and possible problems arising
(d)   attitudes towards drinking, functions of alcohol and uses of alcohol
which were construed as deviant − the subject of this paper.

The instrument was pretested and piloted. A team of experienced interviewers employed by Systems Three Scotland Ltd was trained, and the
interviewing was conducted during the period July−November 1978 and
January−February 1979. (We avoided Hogmanay and Christmas which
would clearly have proved atypical.) A total of 1007 interviews was obtained
− 608 men and 399 women − aged 17 and over and residing in Lothian; the
average interview lasted 45 minutes.

The sample was originally drawn to produce a stratified random sample of
1250 respondents (750 men and 500 women). It was planned to weight the
sample in this way because we knew men had more personal drinking
problems than women. The sample was drawn using the electoral register as a
source of households to contact. Within each of these a single respondent was
selected by the Kish Method, a system which allowed each individual in the
household an equal chance of selection. We hoped that this strategy would
enable us to interview those adults commonly not on the register (such as
17- and 18-year-olds excluded in error and those who frequently change address or are of no fixed abode).

Identifying characteristics were removed from all questionnaires and
confidentiality assured. Of the 1573 addresses attempted, 67 proved to be in
vacant premises and 81 addresses had to be removed from the sample as a
result of our method of respondent selection which specified sex of respondent
to be interviewed at each address. The sample base therefore finally numbered
1425 addresses and from these 1007 interviews were obtained. Three hundred
and three contacts refused to participate and there were 115 non-contacts.

FINDINGS

Reasons for drinking

All drinkers were asked to indicate the relative importance of a number of
reasons for drinking. Their responses are summarized in Table 47.1. By far the
most popular reasons for drinking were 'to celebrate' and 'to be sociable'.
Male drinkers attached more importance to all reasons for drinking − this was
particularly evident amongst the heaviest drinkers who, perhaps not
surprisingly, could advance most good reasons for their habit.

The differences in the importance of particular reasons between men and
women were quite wide. Younger people and particularly young women
attached somewhat greater importance to the relaxing properties of alcohol.
We found that the more socially disadvantaged gave more salience to
drinking for escapist reasons − for instance, to change mood, give confidence
and relieve tension. Social classes I and II, on the other hand, stressed more
positive pleasurable reasons for drinking. It was particularly interesting that

Table 47.1 Percentage indicating that the attached statement was an important reason for their own drinking, by age and sex

Statement	Males				Females			
	Age				Age			
	17–29	30–49	50+	All	17–29	30–49	50+	All
Drinking is a good way to celebrate	67	50	46	54	56	43	38	43
I drink because there isn't anything else to do	14	6	11	9	4	4	2	3
It is part of a good diet	3	7	19	10	4	2	5	4
I like the feeling of getting high or drunk	30	18	11	19	16	10	5	10
It is what most of my friends do	67	51	43	53	53	51	20	41
It helps me forget my worries	16	14	15	15	12	8	8	9
Gives me more confidence	34	12	17	20	33	13	6	17
I drink when I feel tense and nervous	17	14	13	15	15	12	7	11
(N)	(170)	(215)	(223)	(608)	(107)	(128)	(164)	(399)

even those who drank very little gave similar reasons for drinking to those who drank regularly. This suggests that norms surrounding drinking are firmly established and widely agreed in Lothian.

Reasons for not drinking

The relative importance attached to a number of reasons for not drinking or being careful about drinking are summarized in Table 47.2. Seventy per cent of respondents thought that the proposition 'alcohol cost too much when you need money for other things' was either 'very important' or 'somewhat important'. This was much the most significant reason for taking care about drinking. It was also widely accepted that drinking is bad for your health. Only a minority support was found for most of the reasons given. Differences of views between men and women were relatively small.

The most modest and the heaviest drinkers proved most likely to find a significant number of reasons against drinking. Personal experience may have taught the heaviest drinkers to know reasons for not drinking but it is equally probable that those who drink most are more likely to attach greater significance to any issues surrounding alcohol. The heaviest drinkers proved most concerned about developing alcoholism but in contrast they were not conspicuously concerned about losing control over their lives or damaging their health through drinking. They seemed to view alcoholism in a different light from other alcohol related problems.

Men of higher socioeconomic status were less worried about the financial implications of drinking but much more concerned that drinking might interfere with their job. Older and poorer women found many more reasons for not drinking than those who were younger and of higher socio-economic status. Better educated, younger and wealthier women seem to be the carriers of the new permissiveness amongst females in attitudes toward alcohol.

Attitudes toward drinking and drunkenness

All respondents (including on this occasion abstainers who had been excluded from the previous set of questions) were asked whether or not they agreed or disagreed with four statements about drinking and four about drunkenness. Half of these statements were phrased to emphasize the positive aspects of drinking and drunkenness and the other half to emphasize the negative. These statements and the relative agreement of respondents with them are shown in Figure 47.1.

Taking statements about drinking first, the one with the greatest amount of agreement was 'drink often brings out the worst in people'. The one showing the least amount of agreement was the statement that 'having a drink is one of the pleasures of life'. As for attitudes toward drunkenness, the one showing the greatest unanimity of agreement was 'a drunken person is a disgusting sight' and the one with the least agreement was 'it does some people good to get drunk once in a while'. Although there appeared to be a tendency for

Table 47.2 Reasons against drinking, by age and sex. Percentage agreeing that attached statement was important or very important

	Males				Females			
	Age				Age			
Reason	17–29	30–49	50+	All	17–29	30–49	50+	All
Drinking is bad for your health	66	65	62	64	71	72	58	66
It costs too much when you need money for other things	86	72	67	75	86	70	70	74
Your family and friends get upset when you drink	27	29	23	26	26	11	14	19
It may interfere with work	64	62	38	54	50	38	18	33
It goes against my religion	8	9	8	8	6	5	17	10
You are afraid of becoming alcoholic	30	20	11	20	26	23	12	19
It makes you do things you feel sorry for later	46	33	22	33	45	21	13	24
Drinking makes you feel sick	65	49	34	48	62	47	33	46
Drinking gets you into trouble with the police	54	45	34	44	41	31	19	29
Drinking leads to losing control over your life.	46	40	34	40	46	38	26	34
(N)	(170)	(215)	(223)	(608)	(107)	(128)	(164)	(399)

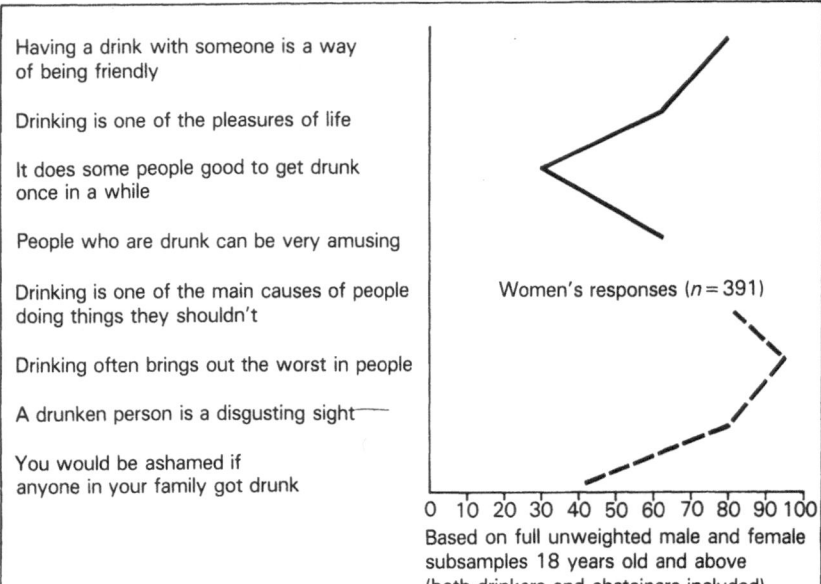

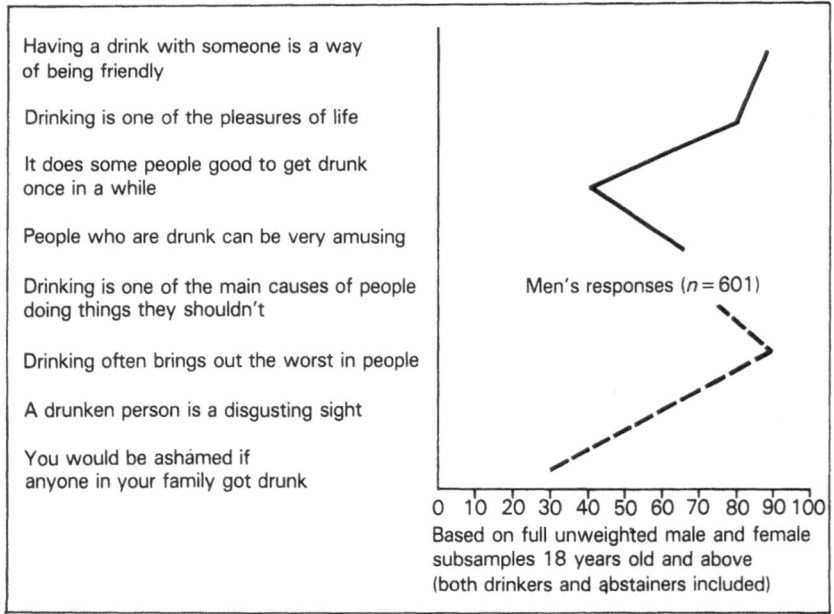

Figure 47.1 Attitudes toward drinking and drunkenness by sex (% agreeing with each statement) (in Lothian general population sample). Based on full unweighted male and female subsamples 18 years and older (both drinkers and abstainers included)

fewer people to agree with the negative statements about drunkenness as compared to drinking, this may largely be due to the fact that questions about drinking were phrased in a much less categorical way than those about drunkenness.

Women were found to display a more negative attitude than men towards all drinking and drunkenness items, particularly drunkenness ones. As women drink more they become more tolerant of drunkenness.

Age appeared to make little difference with respect to attitudes to drinking, but seemed to play more of a role with respect to attitudes towards drunkenness, with the youngest age group much less likely to express anti-drunkenness sentiments than the oldest.

With regard to socioeconomic status, it was found that there was a pattern of high status respondents having a more positive attitude toward drinking than lower status. An exception was in attitudes toward drunkenness, where there appeared to be a tendency for men who came from the lowest socioeconomic group to be most tolerant. In general, it was found that the relationship between consumption and attitudes toward drinking and drunkenness was direct, with less negative attitudes toward both as consumption levels increased. It was, however, found that there was an abrupt shift with a more critical stance in the heaviest drinking category. This may be due to the experience of this group with the negative effects and after-effects of heavy consumption.

In general the positive reasons were supported by everyone − men, women, drinkers, abstainers − suggesting a high level of acceptance that alcohol has a useful beneficial role in the community and even a drunk has his or her amusing aspect. An exception here was the belief that it did some people good to get drunk once in a while, which drew support from only a minority of drinkers. Equally, most of the negative attributes were supported − confirming the well-known Scottish ambivalence toward alcohol and the widespread support which these attitudes receive from all sections of the community.

Responses to public events

To probe respondents' attitudes towards various problems associated with drink and their opinions on various responses which might be made to them, they were presented with four descriptions of hypothetical situations or vignettes, involving alcohol-related occurrences. Two of the vignettes described relatively mundane albeit undesirable consequences of drinking, a man falling down in the street and a woman who cannot walk well because of drink. The other two described more serious outcomes, a man hitting his wife on at least two occasions and a man spending so much on drink that there is not enough food for his family. It is noteworthy that two events were public and affected only the drinker. The remaining two were more domestic and involved a victim. The exact list of these vignettes is reproduced in Table 47.3. In addition to enquiry about each event's seriousness, respondents were asked questions concerning whether or how often such things happened in their community, whether or not a bystander to the event should intervene or offer help, whether a relative should try to help the person in question, whether the Police or an outside authority should be called, whether the offending person in the vignette should be regarded as having an alcohol problem and needing treatment as well as a few questions peculiar to the specific incident.

Table 47.3 shows the proportion of men and women who thought people in the community should regard events as serious and the proportion who felt each of them happened often in their community. As can be seen, the event most often regarded as serious involved family being deprived of food. This was followed by a man hitting his wife, a woman not being able to walk well and a man falling in the street. As can be seen, there was very little difference between the sexes in the assessment of seriousness of any of these situations. As also shown in Table 47.3, the situation which was regarded as most serious, family not having enough food, was also the one which the smallest proportion of the respondents said they knew to have happened in the community. Slightly more knew of a man having hit his wife. Knowledge of a man falling down in the street and a woman who could not walk well were of intermediate frequency. Again differences between men and women were not substantial, although somewhat more women than men knew of the more serious and more domestic situations.

There was little association between age, socioeconomic status or consumption in assessment of the relative seriousness of the problems. On the other hand, a strong negative correlation was found between age and a scale measuring the relative awareness of problems, with younger people showing more awareness than older. A significant association between total consumption and awareness of problems was found among males and a rather weaker one among women. Respondents who drank more per occasion rather than those who spread their drinking out through the week seemed to show most awareness of the alcohol problems depicted in the vignettes.

Table 47.3 Seriousness evaluation of vignettes described

Vignettes	Viewed as serious (%age)		Happen often (%age yes)	
	Males	Females	Males	Females
Suppose a man drinks so much that he falls down in the road and cannot get up	56	61	23	19
Suppose a man has hit his wife when drunk	81	83	19	24
Suppose a woman in the street has drunk so much that she cannot walk well	62	64	15	15
Suppose a man spends so much time drinking that there is not enough food for the family	90	88	12	15

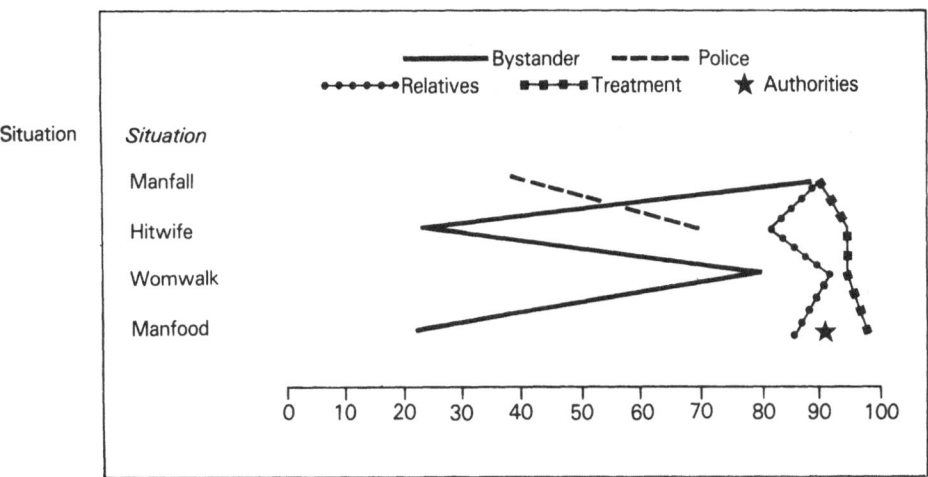

Figure 47.2 Legitimate sources of help and intervention in various hypothetical situations, as perceived by men and women in the Scottish population sample

Figure 47.2 shows the response to the question concerning the appropriateness and responsibility of a variety of different parties to provide help and intervention in each of the situations. With regard to the two more public situations, respondents were asked whether the bystanders should try to help. Although the word help was not defined and may have caused some confusion, over 80 % thought that bystanders should try to help. In contrast, in the more serious domestic situations where respondents were asked whether neighbours should intervene, only about one quarter felt that was appropriate. It was interesting that men seemed more keen on a neighbour getting involved than women. Also in the serious situations respondents saw intervention as being much more the prerogative of the police or the authorities in general, with little difference between the sexes. Substantially fewer respondents felt that authorities should be called in the less serious incidents. Respondents were more prepared to advocate the intervention of relatives in these situations. Intervention by relatives was regarded as least appropriate in the case of a man hitting his wife. Almost all respondents felt that persons described in each of these events had an alcohol problem and should be treated.

Looking at associations between these views and other variables, it was clear that those of higher socioeconomic status favoured more intervention by neighbours, bystanders and, where indicated, by the police. Younger women understandably proved more willing to assign responsibility to relatives than older ones. We also found that heavier drinkers were conspicuously unwilling to involve relatives — this may relate to personal experience!

The reasons for and against drinking *per se* are very similar to those obtained in other surveys of this kind (Cahalan *et al.*[4] and Edwards *et al.*[5]). The most relevant comparison is with Dight's Scottish population survey[6], which found that 'to be sociable' and 'to celebrate' were the most popular reasons for drinking. Dight also found, like us, that the heavier and more frequent drinkers endorsed more reasons for drinking than those who drank only rarely. It is perhaps particularly revealing that even those who abstain or drink very modestly still endorse similar reasons for drinking and not drinking, as if the responses were touching an established set of socially convenient answers which are largely agreed within the Lothian population and endorse the public image of alcohol as an aid to sociability rather than a psychotropic drug.

The relationship between attitudes and behaviour is obviously very relevant to health education. The observation that the heaviest drinkers (consuming more than 42 units of alcohol per week − more than 21 pints of beer or its equivalent − 1 unit here is 9 g alcohol) gave such strong support to reasons for not drinking or being careful about one's drinking, illustrates the unfortunate gap which exists in us all between percept and practice. They were also the group which, along with abstainers, most consistently agreed with the negative attributes of drunkenness − no need to remind the experienced drinker of the drawbacks of drinking, on this evidence he or she seems to know them already.

The vignettes of alcohol related problems represented an attempt to gain some understanding of the appreciation of such problems which already existed and the population's perception of what were considered appropriate responses. The method has many shortcomings[3], and observational studies would be a preferable means of understanding likely community reactions. It is not possible to equate a high level of reported knowledge of these incidents with prevalence, because incidents on which respondents' experience was based may be duplicated between respondents or founded on media reportage rather than personal encounter. Nonetheless the level of the alcohol related domestic violence and deprivation is disturbingly high (approximately 15−20% acknowledged such incidents). The findings are given further credibility by the specific finding that those who drank most had most knowledge of such occurrences. Most felt that bystanders would be expected to do something for the drunk in the street, but the more serious and domestic events were left partially to relatives but particularly to police or other authorities. All incidents were regarded as warranting 'treatment'. Although the nature of this 'treatment' was not spelled out, it does suggest a very high level of acceptance for medical intervention in alcohol related problems.

Respondents were also asked about their attitudes toward appropriate help for drinking problems. The findings are summarized in Table 47.4. As can be seen, there seemed to be strong popular support for the notion that some alcohol treatments are effective, combined with disagreement with the notion that excessive drinkers should be punished. These responses suggest that popular opinion has been largely won over to a medicalized notion of deviant drinking. There also was considerable agreement (almost two thirds) with the

Table 47.4 Attitudes towards seeking help with alcohol problems. Percentage agreeing with statements listed, by sex

	Males	Females
There are treatments that often succeed with people with alcohol problems	83	86
If you had a problem with your drinking you would be ashamed to tell anyone about it	44	54
If you had a problem in this community everyone would soon know about it	75	78
A man's drinking is his own business and no concern of the community	49	51
If a man drinks and does not support his wife, the community should give help	68	62
A man who is always drunk should be punished	17	18
You wouldn't want a place where people with alcohol problems get treated near where you live	37	35
Total N	(N = 393)	(N = 389)

idea that the deprived family of a deviant drinker deserves financial help from the community.

On the other hand, there seems to be substantial stigma associated with alcohol problems. About half admitted to feeling ashamed to tell anyone if they had an alcohol problem; fully three quarters indicated that people in their community would readily learn of someone with a drinking problem, an item which suggests such drinking's newsworthiness and its would-be stigma. Slightly more than a third would not want an alcohol treatment place near their home.

The belief that a man's drinking is his own business and no concern of the community was approved by half the sample. This frequency suggested that drinking behaviour may be viewed in Scotland as a territory of private life over which community institutions have little legitimate sway. The necessary warrant for overriding this barrier against intervention may well be found only in instances of particularly troublesome individuals even amongst confirmed deviant drinkers. This cultural belief may serve to keep those proffering treatment at bay.

As can be seen, the differences between men and women in response to these items were not substantial. The largest difference was in relation to the item 'if you had a problem with your drinking, you would be ashamed to tell anyone about it', with women significantly more likely than men to agree.

We examined the relationship of each of these items to consumption, socioeconomic and other variables. Belief in treatment was associated with age, with the oldest age group being least optimistic. Women, older men, abstainers and occasional drinkers were more likely to answer that they would be ashamed to tell of a drinking problem, as were those who lived outside the city. They also felt the same way about others soon knowing if they had a drinking problem – a view interestingly shared particularly by those of lower socioeconomic status.

The view that the community should help the wife and children of a man who drinks and does not support them found most agreement amongst those who were heavier drinkers (of both sexes) and higher socioeconomic groups, whereas a more punitive view was found amongst poorer women of social class V. Similar associations were found with the view that 'you wouldn't want a place where alcohol problems get treated to be near where you live'. As a sweeping generalization, it might be said that a less punitive, but more interventionist, approach was more likely to be favoured by the young, middle class and heavier drinkers.

There is a widespread belief that treatment for alcohol related problems is both necessary and useful but it needs to be offset against the stigma and shame which still surrounds owning a drinking problem.

In 1976 Dight[6] found that 51% of Scottish men and 42% of women agreed that people who become alcoholic have only themselves to blame and only 14% supported the view that 'giving treatment to alcoholics is something well worth spending public money on'. Although the concept of alcoholism is well established in the public mind in Scotland as elsewhere, and viewed by the population as a condition characterized principally by a compulsion to drink frequently and excessively[6], it is still assigned an essentially negative image which represents a barrier to seeking help.

Treatment agencies have been shown to have a pessimistic view of their capacity to help the alcoholic[7, 8]. This pessimism may have a common root in the negative stereotype assigned to the alcoholic. In view of the public readiness to support intervention for a wide range of alcohol related problems which do not themselves constitute alcoholism, coupled with the belief that early intervention at the time when problems first arise is more likely to be effective, both point to the benefits of an alcohol problem perspective amongst agencies rather than one which necessitates self-definition as alcoholic as a condition of referral.

Acknowledgement

The work upon which this publication is based was performed in whole or in part under Contract No. ADM 281-76-0028 with the US National Institute on Alcohol Abuse and Mental Health Administration; Department of Health, Education and Welfare.

Note

This collaborative project is not intended to provide data which is representative of the countries concerned but only of the communities studied. It is hoped on the basis of the several studies to develop in co-operation with the appropriate national authorities and the communities themselves a more adequate response to the problems associated with alcohol use in these communities. Whether such responses shall have relevance to other communities within the countries concerned, or to other countries, will be for others to discern.

References

1 WHO Expert Committee on Problems Related to Alcohol and Consumption (1980). Problems related to alcohol consumption. *WHO Tech. Rep. Ser.*, 650.
2 Room, R. (1981). A farewell to alcoholism? A commentary on the WHO 1980 Expert Committee response. *Br. J. Addict.*, **76,** 115
3 World Health Organization (1983). *Final Report: Community Response to Alcohol-related Problems, Phase 1.* (Geneva: WHO)
4 Cahalan, D., Cisin, J. and Crossley H. (1969). *American Drinking Practices.* (New Brunswick, NJ: Rutgers Center of Alcohol Studies)
5 Edwards, G., Hensman, C. and Peto, J. (1969). A comparison of female and male motivation for drinking. *Int. J. Addict.*, **8,** 577
6 Dight, S. (1976). *Scottish Drinking Habits.* (London: HMSO)
7 Shaw, S., Cartwright, A., Spratley, T. and Harwin, J. (1978). Responding to drinking problems. (London: Croom Helm)
8 Ritson, B. and de Roumanie, M. (1981). Agency views of alcohol problems. *Proceedings of International Conference — Alcohol and Drug Addiction*, Liverpool. (In press)

48

Chronic alcoholism in a multidisciplinary clinic in a district general hospital

– an epidemiological survey related to social, clinical, histopathological and biochemical pattern of its presentation

S. K. MAJUMDAR, G. K. SHAW, P. O'GORMAN and A. D. THOMSON

INTRODUCTION

Chronic alcoholism or the alcohol dependence syndrome (the term suggested by the World Health Organization[1]) is a serious and growing problem in Great Britain[2]. In England and Wales alone it is estimated that there are about 700 000 alcoholics (constituting 2–3 % of the population); in Scotland 10 % of the population have a drinking problem; there are two to three women to every five men in Britain who are alcoholics compared to one woman to five men 10 years ago[3, 4]. There are 15 alcoholics for an average general practitioner (of which only two may be known); 75 000 convictions for public drunkenness and 40–60 % among convicted persons have a drinking problem[5].

Though alcoholism as a social and medical 'disease' decreased in frequency during the earliest years of this century[6], the consumption of ethanol (beer, wine and spirits) in the UK has been steadily growing over the past 30 years; the average annual consumption of alcoholic beverages by adults was equivalent to 5.2 litres of absolute ethanol in 1950 and 9.7 litres in 1976 and during this period the mortality rate from cirrhosis rose from 2.3 to 3.8 per 100 000[7].

In contrast to broad-based studies of this problem in the USA and Europe, remarkably little is known about comprehensive survey of the social, clinical, pathological and biochemical patterns of presentation of chronic alcoholics in this country; the present survey was carried out to look into the above aspects in chronic alcoholic patients who attended the Area Liver, Alcohol and Nutrition Clinic, Greenwich District Hospital between June 1975 and January 1977.

DETAILS OF PATIENTS

One hundred and five chronic alcoholic patients (M = 80; F = 25; age range 19−69 years) were included in the study (Table 48.1). Most of the patients (92.3 %) were referred to the clinic by general practitioners and the rest from other sources, e.g. Salvation Army, different alcohol rehabilitation units and other hospitals. Up-to-date information on the state of health, diet, drinking habits, including preferences and duration, smoking habits, were collected from the patients themselves and/or their relatives through verbal interview at the time of presentation. Employment profile, marital status, social classification, domicile and dietary status are given in Tables 48.2−48.6 respectively.

60.9 % of our patients were heavy smokers, smoking about 20−40 cigarettes daily or the equivalent amount of tobacco ($\frac{1}{2}$ oz (14 g) = 20 cigarettes) for many years. Alcoholics, in general, seem to be chain smokers.

PROFILES OF DRINKING HISTORY

Chemical dependence characterized by morning shakes/tremors, which is relieved immediately by drinking, was present in 41 % of our patients but no

Table 48.1   Age and sex incidence of survey population

Age group	Male No. of patients	%	Female No. of patients	%
16−19	0	0	1	4
20−29	8	10	3	12
30−39	19	23.7	2	8
40−49	28	35	7	28
50−59	20	25	8	32
60+	5	6.2	4	16
Total	80		25	
Mean age	44.49		45.83	
±SD	± 10.56		± 14.49	

Table 48.2 Employment status

	Patients (%)
Employed for 3 years or more	60.0
Unemployed	15.2
Retired	7.6
Casual employment	6.6
Housewives	4.7
No information	5.7

Table 48.3 Marital status

	Patients (%)
Married	65.0
Single	12.3
Separated/divorced	10.4
No information	12.3

Table 48.4 Social classes*

Social class	Patients (%)	Total: 105 patients
I	6.6	7
II	21.9	23
III	38.09	40
IV	12.3	13
V	14.2	15
No information	6.6	7

* In accordance with *Classification of Occupations*, 1970[8] in terms of social classes by occupation

Table 48.5 Domicile profile

	Patients (%)
Living with spouse/family	68.5
Good quality lodgings	4.7
Lower class hostels	3.8
Living rough	2.8
No information	20.0

Table 48.6 Dietary status*

	Patients (%)
Fair	55.3
Poor	25.7
Excellent	2.8
No information	16.2

* Assessed subjectively by asking relevant questions and by careful clinical observations

relationship was observed between those chemically dependent and those who were chemically non-dependent but admitted they were heavy drinkers. Degree of tolerance seems to be different in different people.

Attempts were made to collect all relevant information from the patients regarding their drinking preference, type, age of starting, duration and its daily amount (Tables 48.7−48.10 respectively).

Table 48.7 Drinking preferences (first preferences only)

	Patients (%)
Beer	46.6
Whisky	27.6
Sherry	7.6
Others (vodka, spirits)	18.1

Table 48.8(a) Type of drinking

Regular	72.4%
Bout	13.4%
No information	14.2%

METHODS AND RESULTS

Clinical features of survey population

Full physical examination was carried out on each patient. Table 48.11 shows the mode of clinical presentation of the patients. Table 48.12 shows the pattern of systolic and diastolic pressures recorded at the clinic. Needle biopsy of liver was performed for tissue diagnosis in 29 patients and the findings are

Table 48.8(b) Age of starting

Age (years)	Male	Female	Total Patients
<15	6	0	6
15—20	35	5	39
21—30	3	1	4
31—40	5	1	6
41—50	—	4	4
51+	—	2	2
	49	12	61

Age range 15—50   Not recorded in 44 patients

Table 48.9(a) Formula for calculating units in terms of amount of absolute ethanol present

Beverage	Units
Sherry: 1 bottle	12
Wine: 1 bottle	6
Spirits: 1 bottle	32
Beer: 1 pint	2

Table 48.9(b) Daily amount of drinking

Units	Patients (%)	Mean + SD	Range
Up to 16	36.7		*Male*
16	50.0		5—64 units
		25 ± 14.5	
32	8.3		*Female*
32+	5.0		5—28 units

given in Table 48.13. History of past psychiatric conditions was also noted (Table 48.14).

Biochemical features of survey population

Liver function tests

Conventional biochemical liver function tests (serum bilirubin, alkaline phosphatase, aspartate transaminase, γ-glutamyl transpeptidase, serum pro-

Table 48.9(c) Drinking units in male and female patients

Units	Male	Female
0–10	3	4
10–20	16	6
20–30	17	4
30–40	11	—
40–50	4	—
50–60	1	—
60 units +	5	—
	37	14

Table 48.10 Duration of drinking

Years	Patients (%)
<5	19.1
6–10	12.3
11–20	13.3
>20	9.5
No information	45.7

Table 48.11 Clinical features of survey population ($n = 105$)

Signs	% Present	Symptoms	% Present
Hepatomegaly	60.9	Anorexia	61.9
Spider naevi	21.9	Tremors	63.8
Splenomegaly	2.8	Nausea/vomiting	57.1
Liver palm (palmar erythaema)	6.6	Malaise/fatigue	45.7
Peripheral neuropathy	10.4	Diarrhoea	21.9
Gynaecomastia	2.8	Tingling/numbness	29.5
Parotid swelling	2.8	Cramps/joint pain	15.2
Dupuytren's contracture	1.9	Amnesic episodes	12.3
Jaundice	11.4	Haematemesis/melaena	9.5
Tongue atrophy	9.5	Delirium Tremens (DTs)	4.7
Ascites/oedema legs	4.7	Abdominal pain/discomfort	28.5
Lymphadenopathy	5.7	Pruritis	8.5
Anaemia	9.5	Rash	6.6
		Heartburn	3.8
		Weight loss	3.8

Table 48.12 Systolic and diastolic pressure

Systolic (mmHg)					Diastolic (mmHg)				
100	101−130	131−150	151−180	180+	60−80	81−89	90−110	111−120	120+
Patients (%)					Patients (%)				
2.08	50.0	31.2	14.5	4.1	59.3	9.3	30.2	1.04	0.0

Table 48.13 Alcoholic liver disease: histo-
logical status

Histological status	No. of patients
Normal histology	5
Steatosis	22
Active hepatitis	3
Cirrhosis	5
Siderosis	1
Granuloma	1

Table 48.14 Past psychiatric conditions

Conditions	Patients (%)
Depression	16.1
Drug addiction	2.8
Attempted suicide	3.8
Anxiety/tension	2.8
No abnormality detected	64.5

teins and their electrophoresis) were routinely done in all patients. Serum proteins were all within normal limits. Table 48.15 shows serum bilirubin and circulating enzymes in the survey population.

Vitamin status – vitamin B₁, B₂, B₆ (pyridoxal-5-phosphate – PALP) (Table 48.16)

Vitamin status – vitamin B_1, B_2, B_6 (pyridoxal-5-phosphate – PALP) *(Table 48.16)*

4 ml of blood was collected in special vials (containing acid citrate and dextrose as preservative to prevent haemolysis) from each patient. Vitamin estimations were performed at the Department of Vitamin and Nutrition Research, F. Hoffman-La Roche and Co, Ltd, Basle, Switzerland. The following erythrocytic enzyme activation tests were used according to the methods of Heller, Salkeld and Korner[9, 10]. Erythrocyte transketolase (ETK)

Table 48.15   Clinical laboratory findings in survey population ($n = 105$)

	Mean + SD	% Present	Range for survey population	Normal range
A. Conventional liver function tests				
Total bilirubin (μ mol/l)	11.5 ± 11.76	27.4 (raised)	0.3–85	3–17
Alkaline phosphatase (ALP) iu/l	88.96 ±78.93	13.1 (raised)	40–250	20–100
Aspartate transaminase (AST) iu/l	50.5 ±10.5	36.0 (raised)	6–100	5–20
γ-glutamyl transpeptidase (GGT) iu/l	100.0 ±50.5	64.0 (raised)	10–700	4–28
B. Haematological				
Haemoglobin (g/dl)	14.27 ± 1.56	6 (low)	9.4–20 (raised in 1 patient)	12.5–18
Mean corpuscular volume (MCV), fl	92.77 ±9.12	20 (raised)	73–118 (low in 2 patients)	82–99

Table 48.16 Blood vitamin status in patients studied ($n = 25$). (Range of activity (ratio) shown in bracket)*

Vitamin status	αETK	αEGR	$P\text{-}5\text{-}PO_4(PALP)$
	Patients (%)		
Adequate	60% ($\leqslant 1.15$)	56% ($\leqslant 1.19$)	16% (10–20 ng/ml)
Marginally deficient	24%	16%	–
Inadequate (severe)	16% ($\geqslant 1.26$)	28% ($\geqslant 1.29$)	76%

* Higher the ratio, greater is the degree of deficiency of that particular vitamin

for vitamin B_1; gluthathione reductase (EGR) for B_2. Pyridoxal-5-phosphate (PALP) – the active metabolite of vitamin B_6 (pyridoxine) – was directly estimated in red blood cells by methods of Lumeng and Li[11].

α represents the activation coefficient. α ETK is a measure of vitamin B_1 (thiamine) status and is the ratio of increased erythrocyte transketolase activity (with added thiamine pyrophosphate (TPP) *in vitro*) to the original activity (without TPP). Similarly, α EGR is a parameter for vitamin B_2 (riboflavin) status and is the ratio of increased erythrocyte gluthathione reductase activity (with added flavin adenine dinucleotide (FAD) *in vitro*) to the original activity (without FAD). The higher the ratio, the greater is the degree of deficiency of the relevant vitamin. Pyridoxine is inactive as such and is converted in the body (mainly liver, etc.) to its active metabolite – pyridoxal-5-phosphate (PALP) – with the help of adenosine triphosphate (ATP) and PALP is measured directly in the erythrocytes.

DISCUSSION

The Area Liver, Alcohol and Nutrition Clinic was set up at Greenwich District Hospital in early 1975 with the following aims:

(1) To detect the chronic alcoholics at an early stage of their drinking life.

(2) To look into their medical, psychiatric, social and psychological aspects in a comprehensive way.

(3) To offer them multidisciplinary therapy with the help of physicians, psychiatrists, nursing staff (trained specially to deal with drinking problems), social workers and psychologists.

(4) Last, but not least, to make an early attempt to prevent dangerous medical and psychosocial catastrophes due to chronic alcoholism.

A χ^2 test of significance showed that there is a 99.9% probability that there is a differing age structure for males and females, but it is not possible to say that female alcoholics were in general younger or older than male alcoholics as the mean age is similar (Table 48.1). A Y-test of significance showed that difference in ages of starting drinking for male and female alcoholics had 99.9 % significance and data showed, women in general started drinking heavily later in their life (Table 48.8b).

No relationships were observed between the amount of ethanol consumed and the age of the patient or the duration of drinking. A Y χ^2 test of significance showed that the difference in amounts drunk by men and women were 99 % significant; amounts of units of ethanol taken by female alcoholics were much less than their male counterparts (Table 48.9c). No information could be obtained in 34 patients.

In this study on 105 patients, 68.5 % are living with their families (Table 48.5) and hence have a higher degree of social stability, 60 % employed for 3 years or more (Table 48.2), 65 % married, 10.4 % separated/divorced, 12.3 % single (Table 48.3) and 55.3 % have fair dietary history (Table 48.4). Regarding employment status, only 15.2 % of the patients were unemployed at the time of study (Table 48.2) while in two earlier studies − one in inpatients done by Hore and Smith in 1975[12] and in another referral study done by Edwards et al. in 1967[13] from male patients attending infor- mation centres, 30 % and 31 % were unemployed respectively at the time of study.

It is interesting to point out that in spite of reasonable degree of social stability, secure employment and fair dietary status, features of physical dependence like chemical dependence (characterized by 'morning shakes' which is relieved immediately by drinking) were present in about 41 % of our patients; clinical features presented by our patients conform to the recognized patterns suggestive of early hepatic, gastrointestinal and neurological involve- ments (Table 48.9); blood vitamin status assessed in 25 of the patients (Table 48.16) indicated deficiency of B_1 in 40 %, of B_2 in 44 % and B_6 (pyridoxal- 5-phosphate − PALP) in 76 %. Conventional biochemical liver function tests showed abnormalities in some patients (Table 48.15) and out of 29 liver biopsies carried out in our patients, five patients had histologically confirmed cirrhosis − these patients' duration of drinking seemed to be longer than others and its amounts heavier (Table 48.13). Of course, many good surveys have been carried out recently on the incidence of alcoholic cirrhosis in different parts of the United Kingdom[14-17]. Steatosis, the commonest ethanol-induced hepatic abnormality[18] was present in 75.8 % of our biopsied patients. In spite of early detection, the overall clinical and biochemical profiles of the alcohol dependence syndrome in our patients seem to warrant active attention for regular follow-up.

No significant relationships were observed between haematological para- meters and units of ethanol consumed or the duration of drinking and a variable constructed to combine the units consumed with the duration of drinking also showed no significant correlation ($r = 0.23$). It is, however, important to mention here that clinical laboratory investigations were only carried out at one point in time for each patient and the units drunk may well have varied over time for each patient.

The social classes of our patients were ascertained by occupation of the patient and in housewives by that of their husband. The social classes grossly conform with those of Hore and Smith[12] and Edwards *et al.*[13]; but in our study (Table 48.4), social class III was lower (38.09 %) compared to 50 % and 41 % respectively in those studies. It is relevant to point out that Hore and Smith's study[12] was in hospital inpatients and that by Edwards *et al.*[13] in all referrals to the Information Centre, and our study is confined to the outpatient clinic of a district general hospital.

Alcoholics are physically less healthy than non-alcoholics. Out of a total of 1020 laboratory readings in this study, one quarter were abnormal; 89 % of our patients had at least one abnormal laboratory reading, the majority between one and two abnormal readings.

Clinical implications of these findings seem to be important in the overall long term management of the patients. Chronic ethanol ingestion may lead to raised blood pressure and depression. Ethanol-induced hypercortisolaemia may be one of the mechanisms through which ethanol could cause both depression and hypertension and both conditions are alleviated on total abstinence[18]. Both systolic and diastolic blood pressures grossly conform to the pattern described by Ramsay[19] and Beevers[20]. It is fair to point out that blood pressures were recorded in our patients in the afternoon clinic as a routine procedure and that casual observation has its own limitations.

In a vast majority of our patients serum vitamin B_{12} levels are within normal limits, but 20 % of the patients showed levels higher than normal. As these patients were not given cyanocobalamin, nor had they any hepatic tumour or infection (bacterial, viral etc.), the higher levels might be due to sudden release of B_{12} stored in hepatocytes, after acute injury inflicted on them by ethanol ingestion[21]. In fact, high serum vitamin B_{12} levels have previously been reported in a number of infective conditions in which there was liver cell damage[22]. Serum folate levels were found to be lower than normal in 40 % of our patients, which could be due to its low dietary intake or its intestinal malabsorption.

Deficiency of thiamine and riboflavin in our patients might be due to their reduced intake and diminished intestinal absorption. Pyridoxine (vitamin B_6) is converted to its active metabolite — pyridoxal-5-phosphate (PALP) — in the body, mainly in the liver and erythrocytes. In our patients PALP was estimated in erythrocytes, levels of which correlated well with plasma PALP[11]. PALP is a reliable index of nutritional status. It is apparently clear that in our patients, the liver is unable to perform this metabolic activation and hence PALP levels were low in 76 % of the patients. Secondly, PALP is a co-enzyme in different enzyme systems involved in decarboxylation, trans-amination etc.[21]. Chronic alcoholism is known to induce microsomal enzymes[23]. Enzyme induction leading to increased demands for the co-factor — PALP — by enzymes thus induced might also be partially responsible for this deficiency.

Ethanol is a major cause of hepatic cirrhosis in London and also in other parts of the Western world[14, 24]. With increasing consumption of ethanol, the incidence of physical and psychosocial complications is rising and so the early diagnosis of chronic alcoholism should be given top priority in community health care. Early recognition of hepatic and other organic damage is worthwhile, because there is evidence that even when cirrhotic process has started, the prognosis can be improved by total abstinence[15] and other complications can also be prevented. Indeed, alcoholic liver disease (ALD) even in advanced cases seems to bear a fairly good prognosis (excluding, of course, early deaths from irreversible complications like ascites, gastrointestinal and variceal bleeding etc.) provided total abstinence can be achieved and indefinitely maintained[24]. Hence, regular follow-up and a multidisciplinary approach to this rising and widespread malady have become all the more important in order to prevent the dangerous sequelae of this self-inflicted syndrome which has acquired the dimension of a 'social disease'.

There is a positive relationship between *per capita* ethanol consumption and mortality from liver cirrhosis; morbidity rates among drinkers compared with non-drinkers seem even higher than mortality rates; ethanol-induced liver damage is apparently independent of the type of beverage consumed; alcoholism and excessive drinking and hence, liver disease risks, have increased in affluent areas of the world since 1945; alcoholic liver disease (ALD) among occupational groups with greater exposure to beverages (such as waiters, bartenders and brewery workers) has increased, but no comparative and objective study is available at present which indicates differences in racial or ethnic susceptibility to alcoholic liver disease including cirrhosis[25]. This is an area which needs research. The severity of alcoholic liver disease (ALD) probably depends on the duration and amount of ethanol abuse; continuous (72.4% in our study) rather than intermittent drinking are known to be more harmful to the liver (five cirrhotics in our study belong to this group).

While prognosis of non-cirrhotic alcoholic liver disease depends mainly on subsequent drinking, cirrhosis may ensue with continued drinking in 5−50% of the patients[14−17, 26]; survival rates are dependent on subsequent drinking, but when damage reaches an advanced stage of irreversible distortion of hepatocytic architecture (macronodular cirrhosis) total abstinence does not seem to prevent further worsening of the disease; 25% of these patients may develop hepatoma (primary carcinoma of the liver); this is why we have suggested regular follow-up by a multidisciplinary team including physician-hepatologist. As a note of alarm and warning, it is worthwhile to summarize the influence of alcoholism on the incidence of liver disease from an international viewpoint. A series of studies in West Germany revealed that the prevalence of alcoholic hepatic cirrhosis rose from 18% of all liver cirrhosis cases during 1946−59, to 39% during 1958−68, to 53% during 1965−75; similar studies in India revealed increases from 4.9% during 1933−62 to 16.2% during 1963−74[25]. It is really alarming.

The prognosis of alcoholism is poor, as at present its prevention is very much on a losing wicket all over the globe. Disabling intellectual impairment and brain damage may be the earliest complications of chronic alcoholism even in absence of severe hepatic damage and may arise early in the alcoholic career[27, 28]. With treatment of any sort, 20 % of alcoholics have a lasting recovery, 20 % are total failures; and 60 % have relapses and remissions[29]. Since the consequence of intellectual and physical impairment for the patient is far-reaching and the success of therapeutic measures is limited, prophylactic steps must be concentrated on the prevention of alcoholism by all possible means – medical, social, psychological, legal, commercial and religious.

In the United Kingdom, out of a population of 55 million, there are 36 million regular drinkers, 2 million heavy drinkers, 700 000 problem drinkers and 200 000 addicted drinkers; a general practitioner with a list of 1800 – 1900 adults may have about 100 heavy drinkers (of which only one in ten is known), 40 problem drinkers and ten addictive drinkers; up to one in five healthy men coming mainly from the upper social classes who attend health screening programmes is found to have some biochemical evidence of heavy ethanol consumption[30]. The problem has thus reached a stage which society can no longer ignore.

CONCLUSIONS

Our conclusions are as follows.

(1) Early detection and regular follow-up by members of a multidisciplinary team are essential pillars in the long term management of chronic alcoholics.

(2) Despite reasonable degree of social stability, secure employment and fair dietary status, about 41 % of the patients were chemically dependent; clinical, biochemical and histopathological features presented by these patients conform to the recognized pattern of hepatic, gastrointestinal and neurological involvements seen in advanced or hard alcoholics, possibly of Skid Row type.

(3) All the social classes were affected.

(4) Out of a total of 1020 laboratory readings, 25 % of the tests were abnormal; 89 % of the patients had at least one abnormal laboratory test; majority between one and two abnormal readings.

(5) Objective assessment of the various medical consequences of chronic alcoholism only offers genuine insight into the gravity of this growing self-inflicted 'social disease'.

ACKNOWLEDGEMENT

We thank the Department of Vitamin and Nutrition Research, F. Hoffman-La Roche and Co, Ltd, Basle, Switzerland, for kindly estimating the blood vitamin status (vitamin B_1, B_2, B_6) in our patients.

References

1 Edwards, G., Gross, M. M., Keller, M., Moser, J., Room, R. (eds.) (1977). *Alcohol Related Disabilities*, pp. 9–16. (WHO Offset publication, No. 32) (Geneva: World Health Organization)

2 Editorial (1977). The female alcoholic, *Lancet*, **2**, 1015

3 *The Times*, London, 20 March, 1980

4 *Guardian*, London, 9 July, 1981

5 *British Medical Journal Editorial* (1977). Drinking behaviours. *Br. Med. J.*, **2**, 914

6 Office of Health Economics (1970). *Alcohol Abuse*. (Studies in Current Health Problems, No. 34) (London: O.H.E.)

7 Royal College of Psychiatrists (1979). *Alcohol and Alcoholism*. (London: Tavistock Publications)

8 Office of Population (1970). *Classification of Occupations*. (London: HMSO)

9 Heller, S., Salkeld, R. M. and Korner, W. F. (1974). Vitamin B_1 status in pregnancy. *Am. J. Clin. Nutr.*, **27**, 1125

10 Heller, S., Salkeld, R. M. and Korner, W. F. (1974). Riboflavin status in pregnancy. *Am. J. Clin. Nutr.*, **27**, 1225

11 Lumeng, L. and Li, T. K. (1974). Vitamin B_6 metabolism in chronic alcohol abuse. Pyridoxal phosphate levels in plasma and the effects of acetaldehyde on pyridoxal phosphate synthesis and degradation in human erythrocytes. *J. Clin. Invest.*, **53**, 693.

12 Hore, B. and Smith, E. (1975). Who goes to alcoholic units? *Br. J. Addict.*, **70**, 263.

13 Edwards, G., Fisher, M., Hawker, A. and Hensman, C. (1967). Clients of alcoholic information centres. *Br. Med. J.*, **4**, 346

14 Hodgson, H. J. F. and Thompson, R. P. H. (1976). Cirrhosis in South London. *Lancet*, **2**, 118

15 Brunt, P. W., Kew, M. C., Scheuer, P. J. and Sherlock, S. (1974). Studies in alcoholic liver disease in Britain. 1. Clinical and pathological pattern related to natural history. *Gut*, **15**, 52

16 Krasner, N., Davis, M., Portmann, B. and Williams, R. (1977). Changing pattern of alcoholic liver disease in Great Britain; relation to sex and signs of autoimmunity. *Br. Med. J.*, **1**, 1497

17 Morgan, M. Y. and Sherlock, S. (1977). Sex-related differences among 100 patients with alcoholic liver disease. *Br. Med. J.*, **1**, 939

18 Majumdar, S. K., Shaw, G. K., Thomson, A. D. and Bridges, P. K. (1981). Serum cortisol concentrations and the effect of chlormethiazole on them in chronic alcoholics. *Neuropharmacology*, **20**, 1357

19 Ramsay, L. E. (1977). Liver dysfunction in hypertension. *Lancet*, **2**, 111

20 Beevers, D. G. (1977). Alcohol and hypertension. *Lancet*, **2**, 114

21 Thomson, A. D., Rae, S. A. and Majumdar, S. K. (1980). Malnutrition in the alcoholic. In Clarke, P. M. S. and Kricka, L. S. (eds.) *Medical Consequences of Alcohol Abuse*, Chap. 6, pp. 103–155. (Chichester: Ellis Horwood)

22 Neale, G., Caughey, D. E., Molin, D. L. and Booth, C. C. (1966). Effects of intra-hepatic and extra-hepatic infection on liver function. *Br. Med. J.*, **1**, 382

23 Gelehrter, T. D. (1976). Enzyme induction. *N. Engl. J. Med.*, **294**, 589

24 Basile, A. (1977). Alcoholic liver disease. *Br. Med. J.*, **2**, 319

25 Lelbach, W. K. (1976). Epidemiology of alcoholic liver disease. In Popper, H. and

Schaffner, F. (eds.) *Progress in Liver Disease.* Vol. 5, pp. 494–515. (New York: Grune & Stratton)

26 Majumdar, S. K., Shaw, G. K., Aps, E. J. and Thomson, A. D. (1981). Alcoholic liver disease among alcoholic patients in a psychiatry hospital. *Practitioner,* **225,** 1833

27 Lee, K., Moller, L., Hardt, F., Haubek, A. and Jensen, E. (1979). Alcohol-induced brain damage and liver damage in young males. *Lancet,* **2,** 759

28 Majumdar, S. K., Thomson, A. D., Shaw, G. K., O'Gorman, P., Aps, E. J., Lishman, W. A., Ron, M. and Acker, W. (1981). Brain damage and alcoholic liver disease. In Tongue, E. J. (ed.) *Proceedings of the 27th International Institute on the Prevention and Treatment of Alcoholism,* 15–20 June, Vienna, pp. 303–323. (Vienna: Findruck).

29 Edwards, G. (1968). Patients with drinking problems. *Br. Med. J.,* **4,** 435.

30 Paton, A., Potter, J. F. and Saunders, J. B. (1981). A.B.C. of alcohol – nature of the problem. *Br. Med. J.,* **283,** 1318

Part 11:
ALCOHOLISM AND EDUCATION

49
Alcohol education: does it really affect drinking problems?

M. GRANT

INTRODUCTION

There has, over the past 20 years, been a growing recognition that alcohol problems are serious enough and extensive enough to merit greater attention than is currently being paid to them. The purpose of this paper is to examine one aspect of that attention — namely, alcohol education — in order to assess what impact it has, or is likely to have, upon the severity and magnitude of the problems it is intended to alleviate. As the first stage of that examination, it is important to determine just what sort of problems are indeed caused by excessive drinking. Only then will it be possible to decide whether education, which is at best a haphazard and potentially wasteful process, is indeed an appropriate strategy upon which to be pinning scarce hopes and scarcer dollars.

ALCOHOL CONSUMPTION, ALCOHOL PROBLEMS AND PUBLIC POLICY

In most parts of the world, alcohol consumption is increasing rapidly. The United Kingdom Brewers' Society collects and publishes extremely comprehensive data on the production and consumption of beverage alcohol throughout the world. Their International Statistical Handbook[1] reveals that the vast majority of countries in the developed world have, during the same 20-year period that has seen a growing recognition of the importance of alcohol problems, experienced increases in *per capita* consumption which are, in some cases, in the order of over 100 %. Many, including the UK, show increases in consumption which, though considerable, are somewhat less steep. What is most striking about these data, however, is how very few exceptions there are to the general trend. France, for example, where *per capita* consumption of wine has actually been slowly but steadily dropping, still has the highest recorded *per capita* consumption of alcohol in the world.

Of particular concern is the situation in the developing world, where commercially produced beverages are replacing the traditional forms of drinking. Since traditional home-produced alcohol was usually relatively weak and was prepared only in sufficient quantity for immediate village and family use, and since the new commercially produced alcohol is being vigorously and successfully promoted, there can be little doubt that the *per capita* consumption in such countries, though poorly documented, is increasing particularly rapidly. Certainly, where attempts have been made to gather relevant data, as in the case of Zambia[2], the trend towards higher consumption is quite marked.

This vision of a world awash in alcohol is of concern because of an accumulation of evidence which points to the association between the overall level of consumption in a population and the incidence of various kinds of alcohol problems. The precise nature of the relationship, from a statistical and epidemiological points of view, remains the subject for complex debate[3], but it is nevertheless clear that, in general terms, as the availability of alcohol increases, so does its consumption and so do various indices of alcohol-related damage, such as prosecutions for drunkenness and deaths from liver cirrhosis.

Whilst liver cirrhosis is most frequently used as an index of all alcohol problems, it is important to remember that there is a very much longer list of disabling or fatal conditions for which excessive drinking is a potent cause. In terms of physical damage, it is not sufficient to consider specific diseases such as cancer of the oesophagus, pancreatitis, stomach ulcers, cardiomyopathy and peripheral neuropathy. It should also be remembered that in a study[4] of a general hospital ward, catering for everyday medical emergencies, approximately one fifth of the male patients were found to have some kind of alcohol-related problem. In psychiatric hospitals too, there is evidence of very widespread alcoholic morbidity. Accidents in the home, at work and on the roads, together with social problems, such as divorce, domestic violence, child abuse, and wider societal and economic concerns, such as lost productivity and absenteeism, all combine to demonstrate how very diverse and how very widespread alcohol problems are.

It has been necessary to emphasize this diversity, if only to clarify the enormity of the task which confronts those responsible for developing an integrated preventive policy and for determining the role which education might be expected to play within that policy. Recent discussion on this area[5] has concentrated upon the conflict between the principles of market justice and the principles of social justice. Thus, alcohol education, though it remains the focus of the remainder of this paper, cannot but be seen as a single plank of a much wider platform, which has its foundations in those same basic concerns for social welfare which inform other areas of public policy. The attempts of the United States National Academy of Science[6] to chart a way forward make it clear just how important it is that regulatory measures, such as taxation, and environmental measures, such as the nature of the drinking place itself, have to be developed in parallel with specific legal and educational initiatives.

ALCOHOL EDUCATION AND THE KNOWLEDGE/ ATTITUDES/BEHAVIOUR TRIAD

Educating people about drinking and about alcoholism is very different from educating them about many other topics. Although they may well lack accurate knowledge, they invariably hold opinions about drinking and alcoholism, opinions which are often as firmly held as they are erroneous. Public health education about these subjects has, therefore, to assist in a preliminary process of unlearning before useful concepts are communicated. The process of unlearning can often prove quite troublesome, particularly if cherished views are being challenged.

A pervasive problem in the whole area of health education, and one which is especially relevant to alcohol education programmes, is the assumption that there is a consecutive causal relationship between increasing knowledge, changing attitudes and changing behaviour. It is, of course, not difficult to increase people's knowledge about alcohol and alcohol problems. Indeed a review of approximately 150 alcohol education impact studies currently being undertaken by this author has failed to identify any which actually diminished or failed to increase knowledge. The central issue here, since few studies show significant behaviour change of any kind, is whether indeed attitude changes precede and predict behaviour change. At its simplest, the issue is one of consistency, and its examination as a phenomenon of social functioning begins with the classic 1934 study by La Piere[7]. In this study, La Piere reports on his cross-country travels in America with a young Chinese couple. He observed that out of 251 separate transactions for accommodation, the travellers were refused service only once. However, 6 months after each contact La Piere sent a questionnaire to the establishments they had visited asking whether members of the Chinese race were acceptable as guests there. Of those responding (128 of the 251) only one said 'yes', 7 % were uncertain and all the rest replied that Chinese guests were unacceptable.

Chastening though this fable is, the temptation must be avoided to reject totally the concept of a causative relationship in this area. The work of Ajzen and Fishbein[8] on attitude behaviour variables led them to conclude that 'a person's attitude has a consistently strong relation with his or her behaviour when it is directed at the same target and when it involves the same action'. It is this conclusion which provides the basis for sharpening very considerably the focus of alcohol education. Many educators would now suggest that if indeed it is behaviour change which is being sought, then the form, content and explicit aims of the programme, however defined, should directly confront behavioural rather than attitudinal issues.

That is why it is so important to have a clear sense of which problems it is that the education is seeking to prevent. There is sometimes, particularly amongst people who are not themselves directly involved in health education, an unrealistic expectation that really massive changes in drinking habits can be brought about as the result of the most meagre of educational interventions. In truth, the process is a much slower and more gradual one. Arguing for a recognition that alcohol education is designed to increase rationality both at an individual and at a societal level, Partanen[9] stresses the necessity to leave recipients sufficient leeway in which to consider matters for themselves. 'The success of education', he suggests, 'depends on how well the campaign really knows the behaviour which is its target and the attitudes which serve to reinforce the particular habits.'

It may be helpful at this stage to consider an example which illustrates this point. If indeed an attempt is being made to encourage particular changes in behaviour, then the desired behaviour should not only be clearly specified; the instructions for how to achieve the change should also be explicit and accessible to the target audience. There is evidence[10] that heavy drinking during pregnancy can have an adverse effect upon the health of the unborn child. A precise objective for an educational campaign might, therefore, quite properly be 'to limit or eradicate drinking during pregnancy'. For such an aim to have any chance of success, however, the educational programme would have to explain how to deal with social pressure to drink, how to develop alternative behaviours and how to adapt to an altered and possibly threatening lifestyle. It would not be sufficient simply to be aware that heavy drinking was hazardous. Knowledge, even relevant knowledge, does not carry with it instructions for its application.

This point is relevant throughout the whole health education field, and is indeed one of the striking features of the review by Gatherer et al.[11] of effectiveness of health education. Finally, in terms of aims, another message gleaned from Gatherer, the characteristics of the target group towards which the education is directed have to be consistent with the aims and the instructions. This point is of particular relevance when considering the educational needs of new and potentially indifferent target audiences, such as might be envisaged within the context of areas such as that of alcohol problems in employment. Here, the very diverse needs of sections of the workforce differentiated by job function has been analysed[12] and can serve as an object lesson for the application of the same principle in the widest range of other contexts including, for example, school programmes and mass media campaigns.

ALCOHOL EDUCATION IN THE SCHOOLS

Reference has already been made to the review of alcohol education impact studies currently being undertaken by the author. In preparing this review, all published examples of alcohol education programmes organized and evaluated in North America and Western Europe between 1960 and 1980 have been scrutinized. Of these, approximately half related to alcohol education programmes directed towards young people and located, either wholly or in part, within the school curriculum. For a variety of reasons, more than 80 % of the evaluated programmes originate from the USA. This is hardly surprising, when it emerges that by the turn of this century, virtually every State required by statutory provision that instruction about alcohol be included in the public school curriculum. Writing in the early 1940s, Roe[13, 14] reviewed the regulations governing the various curriculum requirements and also the content of textbooks in use at that time. There is ample evidence from Milgram's series of annotated bibliographies[15-18] that there has been a considerable proliferation of alcohol education resources since the time at which Roe was writing. This proliferation has been most marked during the same 20-year period that has seen the striking increases in alcohol consumption and in alcohol problems on the one hand and, on the other, in concern about how best to prevent these problems occurring.

It can be argued, therefore, that school-based alcohol education programmes have been thrust forward as one of society's main responses to the upsurge in alcohol problems. If that is so, then it is reasonable to ask whether there is any evidence that this explosion of educational activity has had any positive impact upon its recipients. The short answer is: not much.

In their report on the status of drug education in Ontario in 1977, Goodstadt and his colleagues[19] were able to demonstrate a relationship between exposure to drug education and frequency of reported drug use for tobacco education and tobacco use amongst some students, and marijuana education and marijuana use amongst rather more. They were, however, unable to find any relationship to speak of, either positive or negative, between alcohol education and frequency of drinking or between alcohol education and drunkenness. This chastening result is echoed in the analysis of the evaluated studies in the present author's review. Although no school-based alcohol education programmes were identified which either diminished or failed to increase knowledge, this represented in many cases the extent of positive reported impact. Few projects were able to claim significant alterations in terms of attitudes and even fewer could show positive impact upon any behavioural measures at all. Those which were able to point to behaviour change tended to be the programmes which had most clearly defined the objectives both of the education and of the evaluation and which had most carefully designed the content to take account of the expectations of the target audiences.

It would seem, therefore, that a great deal of effort (not to say time and money) has been expended in order to achieve comparatively little. If this situation is to be improved, then it is important to try to understand why it is that people have, for 20 years, continued to do something which has been repeatedly shown to have virtually no positive impact. Unterberger and Di Cicco[20] contend that sharp emotional disagreements concerning overall goals and plans of action have resulted in a neglect of promising instructional programmes or at best superficial coverage. It may be, however, that the problem lies at an even deeper level and has to do with whether it is, in any case, appropriate to use schools as the main arena for alcohol education.

Much confusion exists in the minds of educational theorists, in the minds of individual teachers and in the minds of parents as to the way in which schools should guide pupils and prepare them for adult life. Society charges schools with the task of bringing new generations to full citizenship. Through legislation and through the encouragement of best practices, society can have a direct influence upon the nature of that process of maturation, in a way which is much more tenuous in relation to the informal education which children receive at home. It is for this reason, presumably, that nineteenth century social reformers in the USA were so anxious to press for the statutory inclusion of alcohol education in the public school curriculum. Yet, quite apart from relaying information and establishing a code of moral values, schools do have other social tasks to perform. Today, for example, it is impossible to ignore the role of schools in alleviating youth unemployment and in streaming young people for the inequality of their future working lives. Such roles make it particularly difficult for schools to undertake the role of liberal nurturing which is implied in alcohol education.

Here, too, it is worth noting the observations of Partanen[9] when he writes: 'It is sometimes thought that the best way to alter prevalent drinking habits is to concentrate on children and young people whose behavioural patterns are as yet unformed. But one might justifiably maintain that alcohol attitudes and drinking habits are transmitted by the older to the younger, that the adult world influences its junior counterpart. Schools tend to conserve cultural values and habits, not reform them.' So it is that the possible confusion of temporal and causal sequences which Partanen describes may be at the root of the apparent lack of positive impact in school-based alcohol education. If, instead of attempting at a stroke to eliminate excessive drinking, such programmes were to concentrate upon those drinking habits and those attitudes which are actually relevant to the target audience at the time of receiving the education (rather than the habits and attitudes of the adult population responsible for the curriculum design) then, although the measures of impact might have to be redefined, at least they would be more likely, in their own terms, to achieve success.

MASS MEDIA, DRINKING AND POPULAR CULTURE

More visible, if not more pervasive, than school-based alcohol education programmes, are mass media campaigns designed to promote damage-free drinking habits. Again, referring to the analysis currently being undertaken of examples of evaluated projects, it is difficult to hold out the hope that single campaigns, no matter how many advertising awards they attract, are likely of themselves to exert a powerful influence on the population in a matter as complex as drinking behaviour. Indeed, Wallack[21] has already set out at some length what he sees as the odds stacked against finding behaviour change as a result of evaluating the impact of single campaigns using conventional experimental methodology. Where campaigns have been evaluated, as in the case of the study by Plant[22] of the Scottish Health Education Group's television spots, results are frequently bedevilled by a lack of agreement over basic objectives between those responsible for originating the programme material and those responsible for evaluating it. If, therefore, measuring individual behaviour change appears something of a blind alley for mass media evaluation, the question remains as to how alternative objective criteria may be discovered. It is possible that here the emerging concept of generativity may be of value. The media themselves produce their own measure if, instead of looking for effects upon individuals, effects upon newspapers, radio and television programmes are sought.

Areas of social concern attract comment in the media, both in relation to particular news items and in relation to issues of public policy which they imply. There is, of course, a wide range of potential areas of social concern available to newspaper editors and broadcasters. If, over a period of time, therefore, particular topics attract increasing column inches and increasing units of broadcast time, then it is reasonable to suppose that this measure of increased concern has been generated, at least in part, by those forces within society which have a particular interest in that topic. As these topics, such as alcohol problems, emerge from the woodwork to become the stuff of public debate, so the opportunities for the development of integrated preventive policies increase. It has been suggested[23] that this measure, though crude, may be of particular relevance to mass media campaigns, where the impact can more properly be seen in a societal rather than an individual context.

Such an approach, located within the context of television programmes and popular media of various kinds, has to be able to establish itself not just in terms of its relation to health education but also in relation to popular culture as a whole. What this introduces into the prevention debate is the extent to which popular culture itself can be seen to exert an influence upon people's health-related drinking behaviour. Some preliminary analysis of British and American television and feature films[24, 25] has been undertaken opening up a number of interesting avenues for further study. It is always difficult to resolve the central question of whether the media mirror society or directly influence it. Certainly, however, television programming, particularly in the areas of drama, soap opera and situation comedy, portray a great deal of drinking. Popular media do play a part in helping to define the values which people give to particular modes of behaviour and particular behavioural aspirations. If, as appears to be the case, the relative frequency with which beverage choices are made on television is (alcohol⟶ tea or coffee⟶ soft drink ⟶water) whilst in the real world it is (water⟶ soft drink ⟶ tea or coffee⟶ alcohol) then questions do have to be asked about the distorting qualities of the mirror which we are supposed to be holding up to ourselves. There is, certainly, a kind of informal educational process at work here, which it would be foolish to ignore, if an integrated preventive approach is being sought.

CONCLUSION

This paper has, of necessity, concentrated as much upon the failures and limitations of alcohol education as upon its successes and strengths. In no way is this intended to imply that the failures and limitations outweigh the successes and strengths. In reality, the opposite is the case, provided always that, in developing education programmes, due attention is paid to the salient lessons from previously evaluated attempts. It is for this reason that exercises, such as the review being undertaken by the author, are of value, in that they enable general trends to be seen over a reasonable period of time. If any single lesson emerges from the review, it is that the evidence establishes beyond doubt that, concentrating upon specific target groups and basing the education upon specific and pragmatic objectives, it is indeed possible to achieve distinct though modest success. In such an enterprise, however, a modest success is worth a great deal more than a whole cartload of repetitious failures.

Acknowledgements

Since much of this paper is based upon preliminary results of a review of alcohol education impact studies, the author wishes to acknowledge, in relation to that review, the assistance of the Alcohol Education Centre (for agreeing to the necessary sabbatical leave), the Alcohol Research Group of the School of Public Health, University of California at Berkeley (for providing research facilities) and the Social Aspects of Alcohol Committee of the Wine and Spirit Association of Great Britain (for providing financial support). Without the generosity of these three different bodies, this paper would never have been written.

References

1 UK Brewers' Society (1979). *International Statistical Handbook.* (London: The Brewers' Society)
2 Haworth, A. and Serpell, R. (1981). Community response to alcohol related problems in Zambia: a summary of the Final Report on Phase 1. Presented at the *National Conference on Community Response to Alcohol-Related Problems,* Lusaka
3 Davies, D. L. (ed.) (1977). *The Ledermann Curve.* (London: Alcohol Education Centre)
4 Quinn, M. A. (1976). Alcohol problems in acute male medical admissions. *Health Bull.,* **34,** 253
5 Beauchamp, D. E. (1980). *Beyond Alcoholism: Alcohol and Public Health Policy.* (Philadelphia: Temple University Press)
6 Moore, M. H. and Gerstein, D. R. (eds.) (1981). *Alcohol and Public Policy: Beyond the Shadow of Prohibition.* (Washington, DC: National Academy Press)
7 La Piere, R. T. (1934). Attitudes vs. Action. *Social Forces,* **13,** 230. (Reprinted (1975) in Liska, A. E. (ed.). *The Consistency Controversy.* (New York: Wiley))

8 Ajzen, I. and Fishbein, M. (1977). Attitude—behaviour relations: a theoretical analysis and review of empirical research. *Psychol. Bull.*, **84**, 888

9 Partanen, J. (1981). Teesejä valistuksesta. *Alkoholipolitiikka*, **46**, 161

10 Pratt, O. E. (1980). The fetal alcohol syndrome: transport of nutrients and transfer of alcohol and acetaldehyde from mother to fetus. In Sandler, M. (ed.) *Psychopharmacology of Alcohol*. (New York: Raven Press)

11 Gatherer, A. *et al.* (1979). *Is Health Education Effective?* (Health Education Council Monograph Series No. 2) (London: Health Education Council)

12 Grant, M. (1981). Programmes of prevention. Presented at the *International Committee on Occupational Mental Health Conference*, May 1981, Heidelberg

13 Roe, A. (1942). Legal regulations for alcohol education. *Q. J. Stud. Alc.*, **3**, 433

14 Roe, A. (1943). A survey of alcohol education in the United States. *Q. J. Stud. Alc.*, **4**, 574

15 Milgram, G. G. (1975). *Alcohol Education Materials: An Annotated Bibliography.* (Brunswick, NJ: Rutgers Center of Alcohol Studies)

16 Milgram, G. G. and Page, P. B. (1979). Alcohol educational materials, 1978—79, an annotated bibliography. *J. Alc. Drug Educ.*, **24**, 4

17 Milgram, G. G. (1980). *Alcohol Education Materials 1973—78.* (New Brunswick, NJ: Rutgers Center for Alcohol Studies)

18 Milgram, G. G. and Page, P. B. (1980). Alcohol education material, 1979—80: an annotated bibliography. *J. Alc. Drug Educ.*, **25**, 4

19 Goodstadt, M. S., Sheppard, M. A., Kijewski, K. and Chung, L. (1978). *The Status of Drug Education in Ontario, 1977.* (Toronto: Addiction Research Foundation)

20 Unterberger, J. and Di Cicco, L. (1968). Alcohol education re-evaluated. *Bull. Natl. Assoc. Secondary School Principals*, **52**, 15

21 Wallack, L. M. (1980). *Mass Media Campaigns: The Odds Against Finding Behaviour Change.* Paper F. 111, Social Research Group, University of California, Berkeley

22 Plant, M. A. *et al.* (1979). Evaluation of the Scottish Health Education Unit's 1976 Campaign on Alcoholism. *Soc. Psychiatry*, **14**, 11

23 Grant, M. (1981). Formal and informal programming decisions: the case of alcohol abuse. In Leathar, D. S., Hastings, G. B. and Davies, J. K. (eds.) *Health Education and the Media.* (Oxford: Pergamon)

24 Cook, J. and Lewington, M. (1979). *Images of Alcoholism.* (London: Alcohol Education Centre/British Film Institute)

25 Breed, W. and de Foe, J. (1979). Themes in magazine alcohol advertisements: A critique. *J. Drug Iss.*, **9**, 511

Index